编写指导委员会

丛书总主编：段 峰 王 欣

博文高等学校英语专业系列教材

医疗口译教程

Medical Interpreting

主 编◎胡敏霞
副主编◎殷明月 吉 晋 杨辉亮

四川大学出版社
SICHUAN UNIVERSITY PRESS

图书在版编目（CIP）数据

医疗口译教程 = Medical Interpreting ／ 胡敏霞主编. — 成都：四川大学出版社，2024.6
博文高等学校英语专业系列教材
ISBN 978-7-5690-5328-9

Ⅰ. ①医… Ⅱ. ①胡… Ⅲ. ①医学—英语—口译—高等学校—教材 Ⅳ. ①R

中国版本图书馆 CIP 数据核字（2022）第 019078 号

书　　名：医疗口译教程
　　　　　Yiliao Kouyi Jiaocheng
主　　编：胡敏霞
丛 书 名：博文高等学校英语专业系列教材

丛书策划：刘　畅
选题策划：余　芳　张　晶　刘　畅
责任编辑：余　芳
责任校对：周　洁
装帧设计：阿　林
责任印制：王　炜

出版发行：四川大学出版社有限责任公司
　　　　　地址：成都市一环路南一段 24 号（610065）
　　　　　电话：（028）85408311（发行部）、85400276（总编室）
　　　　　电子邮箱：scupress@vip.163.com
　　　　　网址：https://press.scu.edu.cn
印前制作：四川胜翔数码印务设计有限公司
印刷装订：成都市新都华兴印务有限公司

成品尺寸：170 mm×240 mm
印　　张：31.5
插　　页：2
字　　数：696 千字

版　　次：2024 年 6 月 第 1 版
印　　次：2024 年 6 月 第 1 次印刷
定　　价：118.00 元

扫码获取数字资源

四川大学出版社
微信公众号

总　序

　　新时代的国际形势和国家需求既对我国外国语言文学专业和学科建设提出了新挑战，也提供了发展的新契机。

　　习近平总书记在给北京外国语大学老教授的回信中指出，努力培养更多有家国情怀、有全球视野、有专业本领的复合型人才，在推动中国更好走向世界、世界更好了解中国上做出新的贡献。这是党和国家对高校外语教育工作者的殷切希望，也是时代赋予我们的重要责任。围绕新时期新要求、新文科新思考，外语人才培养需要进行全方位的改革，教材建设是其中极其重要的一环。因为教材是教育教学的基本依据和重要载体，关乎解决"培养什么人、怎样培养人、为谁培养人"这一根本问题，关乎立德树人目标的最终实现。

　　基于这样的目的，我们组织专家和一线教师编写了这套多语种的外语专业教材，教材覆盖面广，既有传统的语言技能训练、外国语言学和外国文学，也有医学口译等跨学科的主题，反映了外语学科在新文科概念的导引下所开展的尝试。我们希望以此为开端，逐渐增加教材种类，扩大教材的涉及面，为新型外语人才的培养打下坚实的基础。

　　总的说来，博文系列教材以"博雅通识，优化创新"为主要目的，具有以下特色。

　　1. 博雅教育注重培养具有扎实语言能力、深厚人文素养、宽广学术视野、强烈批判精神的高素质外语人才，对外国语言研究、外国文学研究、翻译研究、国别与区域研究、比较文学与跨文化研究有浓厚兴趣，具有一定研究潜能的高素质学术型外语人才。博文系列教材选用了中西方经典文学篇章，以人文素质教育为外语教学的根本，发掘外语语言文化的专业内涵，体现了外语教育强本固基的办学要求。

2. 博文系列教材创建 GIDE 课程体系，以"引领"（Guiding）、"浸润"（Immersion）、"深化"（Deepening）、"拓展"（Exploration）四个层次为课程目标，分阶段、分层次地将外国语言文学专业培养目标融入教材建设。引领学生形成专业意识，浸润中西方文化文明精髓，深化专业知识和人文素质，拓展思辨能力和跨文化交流能力，形成专业和学科建设的有机衔接，对培养高素质外语人才和复合型外语人才，具有重要的作用。

3. 课程思政是新时代背景下，稳步推进思想政治教育改革以形成大思政育人体系的一个重要方向。四川大学外国语学院以全课程育人大格局为理念，提升德育实效性，将育人目标贯穿于课程教育的全过程，不断升级人才培养方案，将课程思政的概念和实施，整体、科学、有序地融合进育人机制和教材建设。博文系列教材坚守中国视角、中国立场，在具备国际前沿视野的同时，将社会主义核心价值观融入教材编写，以培养精通专业领域知识，一心为公，拥有家国情怀和国际视野，具备良好的语言运用能力和深厚的人文素养的高端外语人才。

4. 教材紧扣新时代国家对高校外语人才培养的要求，参照教育部新国标，坚持课程思政建设，在上述总体思想的指导下，结合四川大学外国语学院开设的专业课程，从知识传授、技能培养、能力提升等不同层面，进行系列化设计。偏重语言技能训练的教材遵循语言地道、例证典型、解析精当的原则，同时注重选材的权威性和实效性；偏重能力提升的教材精选外国语言学、翻译学、文学与文化研究的经典原文，既传授专业基础知识，又致力培养学生的文本赏析和思辨能力。各教材均在符合学科、专业与相应课程需求的前提下，设计和安排教材的主要内容、知识体系、习题设置与考核要求等，体现了各自的鲜明特色。

四川大学外语学科源自 1896 年创办的四川中西学堂的英语和法语科目，历史悠久，传统厚重。巴金、吴虞、朱光潜、吕叔湘、钟作猷、周煦良、卞之琳、罗念生、顾绶昌、吴宓等著名学者和文化名人曾在本学科任教或就读，为本学科的发展打下了坚实的基础。博文系列教材由四川大学外国语学院教学专家与一线教师共同编写，邀请国内知名外语类专家担任顾问，编写团队既具有一线教学经验，熟悉学生需求，又具备宽广的国际视野和历史传承。当然，本系列教材的内容难免存在不足之处，编写团队恳切希望广大教师和学生提出宝贵意见。

博文系列教材编写组

前　言

编写背景

医疗卫生一直是国际交流的重要活跃领域，专业性强，影响面广。随着全球化、人口老龄化，生命科学研究、医疗技术、大健康产业等医疗卫生领域强劲增长，同时，随着新型传染病的全球性暴发和蔓延，医疗卫生领域的国际交流变得越发重要。

医疗口译作为相关语言服务，其重要性体现在三大领域或者说应用场景。

一是公共医疗服务领域（"医—患"场景）。这个领域的医疗口译属于公共服务或社区口译（public service or community interpreting）。简短的交替传译（短交传）为译员的主要工作模式。欧美国家的医疗口译体系相对成熟，外来移民较多的美国、加拿大、英国、澳大利亚等国，以及接受难民较多的瑞士和德国等欧洲大陆国家，都已制定了医疗口译的行业标准、法律法规和认证机制，为英语水平较差的病患［LEP（Limited English Proficient）patient］提供语言翻译服务。未来，随着中国经济的迅猛发展和国际地位的提升，各地举办的大型体育赛事和展会增加，来华工作、学习、旅游和生活的外籍人士增多，为解决国际人士的就医语言障碍，国家及地方势必出台相关语言服务政策。由此，中国医疗服务口译将迎来职业化的"春天"。

二是国际医学会议领域（"医—医"场景）。这个领域的医疗口译属于会议口译（conference interpreting），同声传译（同传）为译员的主要工作模式。穆雷等人（2017）发现，在全球语言服务供应商前100强发布的招聘广告中，笔译需求量最大的领域是IT行业，医疗行业次之，而口译需求量最大的领域正是医疗行业。同时，越来越多医疗领域的国际会议也使得对医学类同传译员的需求加大，而且，各种在线远程口译和语音转写技术还提高了对医学会议口译质量的要求。因此，精通医学知识、掌握同传技能的复合型人才必然是国际医疗交流中的紧缺必备人才。

三是公共卫生应急领域（"医—众"）。这个领域的医疗口译既包括社区口译也包括会议口译，译员的工作模式可以是同声传译或交替传译。SARS 疫情之后和《国际卫生条例》颁布以来，世界卫生组织（WHO）共宣布了 7 次国际公共卫生紧急事件（Public Health Emergency of International Concern，简称 PHEIC，或译"国际关注的公共卫生事件"），分别是甲型 H1N1 流感疫情、脊髓灰质炎疫情、西非埃博拉疫情、"寨卡"疫情、刚果（金）埃博拉疫情、新型冠状病毒感染疫情和猴痘疫情。面对突发疫情，病毒来源、传播防控、病例筛查、疫苗研发、疾病治疗、援助合作等相关信息需要在国际卫生和公众群体中得到及时有效的传递，译员甚至需要冒着感染风险完成高强度、高难度、紧急型、专业性的口译任务。

综上，尽管医疗口译市场需求巨大，但高水平从业人员较少，临时上场的口译员水平参差不齐。原因之一便是市场上缺乏优质医疗口译相关教材资源，教师无法给学生提供专业、系统、深入的医疗口译训练，对医疗口译感兴趣的学生，不管是医学背景还是口译背景，无法通过教材辅助完成自我训练和提升。

编写理念和篇章结构

为了让医疗口译员胜任开篇提出的"医—患""医—医""医—众"三大场景，译员首先需要具备较为全面的临床医学知识和较为扎实的口译技能，因此本教材立足科学合理的口译训练模式和全面基础的临床科室病症，以帮助学习者掌握多科室医疗口译基本功为目标，具体安排设计如下。

本书分为二十章：第一章"医疗口译简介"、第二章"突发公共卫生事件"、第三章"初级卫生保健"、第四章"门诊/急诊"、第五章"呼吸内科"、第六章"消化内科"、第七章"内分泌科"、第八章"血液科"、第九章"肿瘤科"、第十章"心学管内科/外科"、第十一章"神经内科/外科"、第十二章"骨科"、第十三章"精神科"、第十四章"眼科"、第十五章"耳鼻喉科"、第十六章"妇产科"、第十七章"儿科"、第十八章"重症科"、第十九章"中国传统医学"、第二十章"健康中国与健康世界"。

第一章"医疗口译简介"，内容包括医疗口译的定义、分类、历史、角色、功能、资质、认证、职业素养、伦理教育等，以及医疗口译的重点难点，如医学术语的词根溯源、发音特征、高低语域和文化差异等。

第二到第十九章每章都分为五个部分：导读、口译技巧、口译词汇、口译实战、口译注释与学习资源。其中核心部分为"口译技巧"和"口译实战"。"口译技巧"包括记忆技巧、笔记技巧、意义听辨、公众演讲、精力分配、双语转换、数字转换、文化调解、交际技巧、综述技巧、译前准备、应急技巧、职业伦理和口译技术。"口译实战"为3~5分钟的短篇演讲，主题是科室介绍和典型病症，包括三篇英译汉和三篇汉译英的材料（选文经过改编）。所有材料均提供参考译文。"口译词汇"安排在"口译实战"之前，是实战语篇的译前词汇准备。各个临床科室的内容与配套的医疗口译慕课的视频材料互为补充。

第二十章"健康中国与健康世界"是特别章节。为了落实习近平新时代中国特色社会主义思想进教材，我们选取了近年来习近平总书记关于全球卫生健康共同体与新型冠状病毒感染疫情防控和国际合作的重要讲话，旨在帮助学习者提升在重大国际场合讲好中国故事的能力。

适学人群和教学安排

本书适用于具有一定英语基础的医学院学生、翻译（口译）专业的本科生和研究生、医务工作者、医疗口译爱好者和自由职业者。如果将学习者背景分为"医学背景"和"口译背景"，那么《医疗口译教程》可能实现以下学习效果。

对"医学背景"学习者：
- 掌握口译技巧练习方法，并达到一定程度的技能自动化。
- 开启独特口译思维模式，"听"要"听词取意"、"说"要"言之有物"，能够自由切换双语听说。
- 理解口译员的基础角色和延伸角色，遵守口译职业伦理。

对"口译背景"学习者：
- 掌握学习、记忆医学术语和临床英语的有效方法。
- 胜任基础医疗话题的双语传译，如临床科室常见疾病的病因、症状、诊断和治疗等的双语传译。
- 了解医疗口译在知识、技能和职业素养方面的独特要求。

建议教师安排大约80个学时完成《医疗口译教程》的教学，每章4个学时。教材内容丰富多样，课堂未完成的部分可安排学生自学。但鉴于医学词汇具有特殊性，尤其是以希腊语、拉丁语为词根的派生词与一般的低语域英语单词相比记忆难度更大，需要有效的词根词缀记忆法，并结合视觉化等方法才能提高记忆效果，因此，建议任课教师根据第一章"医疗口译简介"中的技巧和方法对"口译词汇"进行译前讲解，再开始"口译实战"。另外，相关口译技巧、口译技术和口译伦理也需要教师特别关注和强调。

编写团队和团队分工

胡敏霞，博士，四川大学外国语学院副教授，硕士研究生导师，MTI 教育中心副主任，研究方向为口译认知过程，同传上千小时，获四川省第八届高等教育优秀教学成果二等奖。负责编写前言、参考文献和以下 8 章：第一章"医疗口译简介"、第六章"消化内科"、第七章"内分泌科"、第八章"血液科"、第十三章"精神科"、第十四章"眼科"、第十五章"耳鼻喉科"、第二十章"健康中国与健康世界"。

殷明月，博士，四川大学外国语学院副教授，硕士研究生导师。研究方向为口译员职业伦理、口译与国际传播、口译史。获得全国教学比赛总决赛二等奖 2 次，省级教学比赛一等奖 1 次。获得全国及省级英语演讲比赛、口译比赛优秀指导教师奖 40 余次。主持国家社科项目 1 项、省社科项目 1 项、校级项目 5 项；作为主研人员参与省教改重点项目 1 项（排名第 3）、市厅级重大项目 1 项（排名第 2）。多次为各级领导、国际组织及行业协会提供口笔译服务。负责编写以下 6 章：第五章"呼吸内科"、第九章"肿瘤科"、第十六章"妇产科"、第十七章"儿科"、第十八章"重症科"、第十九章"中国传统医学"。

吉晋，博士，四川大学外国语学院讲师，研究方向为口译和国际法。优秀共产党员，2020 年作为翻译随中国国家医疗专家组赴意大利协助开展新型冠状病毒感染疫情防控，2021 年获国家卫生健康委员会中国抗疫医疗专家组组派工作表现突出个人。负责编写以下 6 章：第二章"突出公共卫生事件"、第三章"初级卫生保健"、第四章"门诊/急诊"、第十章"心血管内科/外科"、第十一章"神经内科/外科"、第十二章"骨科"。

杨辉亮，四川大学华西临床医学院副教授，华西医院骨科主治医师。2018年四川大学医学博士毕业，2016—2017 年受中国留学基金委资助赴哈佛大学完成联合博士培养。2018—2021 年受四川大学华西医院和中国博士后科学基金会资助赴布朗大学完成博士后培养。负责全书的医学知识、科室典型病症的选择和翻译审核。

目　录

第一章

医疗口译简介

1　导读

在本章，我们将讨论医疗口译的定义、分类、历史、角色、功能、认证、伦理等基础概念和认知框架，同时也将讨论医疗口译的学习重点和练习难点，如医疗口译的术语发音、术语记忆、高低语域、语内转换和文化差异等贯穿全书的问题。

2　医疗口译的概念框架

2.1　医疗口译的定义和分类

医疗口译的英文对应表达是 medical interpreting 或 healthcare interpreting（Hsieh，2016）[1]，按工作场景可分为社区口译（"社口"）和会议口译（"会口"），按工作模式可分为交替传译（"交传"，又分为"短交传"和"长交传"）和同声传译（"同传"，又分为"有稿同传""无稿同传"或"现场同传""远程同传"等）。

社区口译，是指"在特定社会机构环境中，当公共服务提供方和使用方讲不同语言时需要的口译"（Pöchhacker，1999）[2]。社区口译也称"公共服务口译""联络口译""对话口译""陪同口译"等，口译工作方式多为"短交传"。在社区口译的框架下，医疗口译就是在医疗机构中为医患服务的口译。与医疗口译类似的社区口译还有法庭口译、教育口译、警务口译、避难口译、媒体口译等。

会议口译是指在正式、非正式或类似会议的环境中，以交传或同传方式将原语演讲翻译为译语的口译。（AIIC，1984；Pöchhacker，2013）[3-4]会议口译的具体场景主要是以"论坛""对话""圆桌""大会""研讨会"等名称命名的国际（双边或多边）会议，"但也可延伸到正式晚宴、新闻发布会、议会会议、国际法庭，甚至大学演讲厅和教堂服务"等。（Diriker，2015）[5]在会议口译的框架下，医疗口译是指各种涉及医学主题知识的会议口译。

会议口译和社区口译并非泾渭分明，职业医疗口译员完全可以既为医疗机构提供交传口译服务，也在国际会议上提供同传口译服务。作为口译专业技能，交传和同传是由多种语言、文化和思维的细分技能组成的综合技能。同传更是口译技能的顶端，在进入同传训练之前译员应该完成大量交传训练，并在完成约 1000 小时的同传技能和主题知识的训练之后再接受会议用户委托。

2.2 医疗口译的社会历史

在西方，自 20 世纪 90 年代中期以来，为了满足大量移民、难民、少数族裔和土著人群的医疗服务需求，医疗口译在法律法规、职业化、实践和研究方面都取得了巨大的发展。（Bischoff & Hudelson，2010；Bischoff，2020；Dysart-Gale，2005；Kaufert & Koolage，1984）[6-9] 例如，在人口多元化程度较高的美国，自 1990 年以来，英语能力有限的人口增加了 80%。2013 年，美国英语能力有限的人口就超过了 2550 万，约占美国总人口的 8.5%。（Zong & Batalova，2015）[10] 2014 年，美国两大医保 Medicare 和 Medicaid 中的英语能力有限的人口约 870 万，约占总医保人口的 8.4%，主要分布在东（如纽约）西（如加利福尼亚州）海岸。（Proctor，Wilson-Frederick & Haffer，2018）[11]

在中国，2010 年的全国人口普查统计显示在中国居住的外籍人员约 60 万人，2020 年的全国人口普查统计显示在中国居住的外籍人员约 85 万人，占全国 14 亿人的 0.06% 左右。各城市的外籍人口规模不一。以舒适宜人、"来了就不想走"的成都为例，公安局出入境数据显示 2018 年成都有常住外国人 17411 人，而成都常驻总人口约 2000 万，外籍人口占比约 0.1%。

在外籍人口更多的广州，詹成和严敏宾（2013）[12] 对全市 28 家医院进行了调查，他们发现只有一家三甲私立医院祈福医院（Clifford Hospital）建有"医疗口译中心"，配备了 11 名全日制医疗口译员（英语 6 名、日语 2 名、韩语 1 名和印尼语 2 名）。

我们编写《医疗口译教程》期间，也访问了四川大学华西医院的临床医生、国际合作和外事人员。初步调查发现目前该医院的外籍患者就医情况基本如下：（1）由家人、朋友或单位外事秘书陪同外籍患者往返医院；（2）双语医师负责院内的问诊治疗，或双语医师担任临时口译，协助主治医师工作；（3）家人、朋友或单位外事秘书协助院内陪同和医患语言沟通不畅时的解释。另外国际会议等大型合作项目由国际合作处牵头协调，国际患者或寻求国际会诊的国内患者也可以直接在语言服务能力较强的华西特需医疗中心就医。

Bischoff（2020）[7] 对日内瓦大学医院开展了 25 年（1992—2017）的医疗口译服务工作进行了回顾，总结了其医疗口译服务开展的五个阶段：（1）服务启动阶段，开始为难民和寻求庇护者提供简单医疗口译服务；（2）增长规范阶段，由于涌入大量讲阿尔巴尼亚语的寻求庇护者，日内瓦大学医院的所有部门开始提供阿尔巴尼亚语口译，并在医生和护士中普及口译使用；（3）质量保证阶段，关注医患沟通对医疗结果的影响，尤其是口译服务对医疗质量的提升作用；（4）制度形成阶段，明确口译资金的监管和落实以及口译员的职业角色；（5）服务公平阶段，医疗口译被纳入服务公平的总体框架。

综上，推进社区医疗口译制度性发展的最重要力量还是社会历史与人口以及宏观经济因素，因此，目前国内大部分社区医疗口译都还是零星、偶尔、随意、自然发生的非职业口译，而专门针对寻求优质医疗服务的医疗旅游者的社区口译也还在起步阶段。

医疗会议口译的情况则大不相同。医疗行业是口译服务提供商被预订订单最多的行业（穆雷，沈慧芝，邹兵，2017）[13]。同时，国际会议通常由专门机构或组织筹措会议经费、安排正式会议议程、预定会议口译服务（通过语言服务商或是直接联系译员），会议口译也有统一的资质认证和质量标准，不管是用户还是从业人员，他们的需求在医疗口译服务过程中都能得到专业保障。因此，目前在医疗行业，中国大部分口译员和口译学员的就业方向还是医疗会议口译。

2.3 医疗口译的角色功能

通过梳理前期文献，我们发现医疗口译的角色功能主要包括语言翻译、文化解释、医患协调、患者陪同、协同治疗、移民融入等。在这里"会口"和"社口"的区别也很关键。前者主要跟"信息"打交道，而后者主要跟"人"打交道，前者要确保会议期间海量信息的密集传递，后者要以语言为工具确保交流各方获得满意服务，因此两者在角色功能上有不同侧重。

（一）社区医疗口译的角色功能

Kaufert（1990）[14]认为在加拿大医疗口译的角色或功能包括：（1）语言翻译；（2）文化经纪（①向医院人员解释当地文化和语言；②向当地患者解释生物医学概念）；（3）患者赋权，维护当地患者、亲属团体或土著社群的利益。Drennan（1999）[15]认为在南非医疗口译的角色或功能包括：（1）语言专家；（2）文化专家；（3）患者赋权；（4）协同治疗。Weiss 和 Stuker（1999）[16]对瑞士医疗口译员的角色分类与此相似。

Angelelli（2004）[17]认为口译员是：（1）"侦探"，寻找破案信息；（2）"多功能桥梁"，帮助医患沟通；（3）"钻石鉴赏家"，倾听患者故事；（4）"矿工"，挖掘有用信息。Leanza（2005）[18]认为瑞士洛桑的口译员在儿童父母和儿科医生之间扮演了四种代理角色，分别是：（1）语言代理；（2）社群代理（即文化调解）；（3）融入代理，帮助移民融入主流社会；（4）制度代理，将制度性话语、规范和价值观传递给患者。Hsieh（2008）[19]认为，除担任传声筒（conduit）、赋权者（即倡导者）和协同治疗者之外，译员还是管理者，负责保护医疗资源，规范医疗伦理，优化信息交流。

Bischoff 和 Hudelson（2010）[6]对瑞士 205 名接受过医疗口译服务的医患人员进行采访后发现，受访者认为医疗口译员能够促进医患理解，帮助医生更有效地向患者传达指示和了解患者的实际情况，减少医患冲突，帮助移民了解医院情况和个人权利。Bischoff、Kurth 和 Henley（2012）对瑞士一家妇女医院的 10 名口译员和 2 名口译经理进行了调查。受访口译员和口译经理认为，他们主要扮演了四种角色：翻译、文化解释者、医患关系维护者和移民患者陪同人员。此外，他们还认为，自己在促进移民融入当地社会等方面发挥了作用。

对于译员是否应当为患者赋权或倡导患者权益，患者和医院的看法大相径庭（Drennan，1999）[15]。译员在口译实践中的赋权行为可能会超出培训范围和行业规定（Hsieh，2008）[19]。关于协同治疗，Weiss 和 Stuker（1999）[16]认为，当译员与患者、医生密切接触几个月后，译员实际上便成了协同治疗师，不过前提是专业医护人员支持其扮演这一角色。Avery（2001）[20]认为，医疗口译员的作用是促进医疗环境中讲不同语言的人们之间的理解和交流。为了确保沟通效果，译员在尊重个体和社区目标的基础上，有必要进行语言澄清、文化调解和适度赋权。Bischoff、Kurth 和 Henley（2012）发现，使用口译服务经验较少的临床医生一般会要求译员逐字翻译。如果不是逐字翻译，那么医生会担心失去对面诊的控制。

美国国家卫生保健口译委员会（National Council on Interpreting in Health Care，NCIHC）2005 年出版的实践标准（NCIHC SOP 2005）中对译员角色边界（role boundary）提出了三点要求：（1）译员在执行口译任务期间应避免与各方私下接触；（2）译员的口译专业活动应限制在会谈期间；（3）兼任其他职务的译员在口译时也要遵守所有口译实践标准。

综上，社区医疗口译员的首要角色应该是信息传译者，负责精确、完整地传译信息并对信息保密，即进行中立的语言翻译工作。在语言翻译之外，译员的其他角色需由各方协商界定。（Dysart-Gale，2007；Hsieh et al.，2010；Robb &

Greenhalgh, 2006; Rosenberg et al., 2008)[21-24] 我们建议刚刚接触客户的口译员首先完成好语言翻译的工作;其次,在口译过程中进行必要的、"透明的"文化解释;最后,当译员与客户非常熟悉之后,在客户许可的基础上,承担力所能及的额外工作,如协调医患关系、缓和医患冲突、协助治疗等。

(二)医疗会议口译的角色功能

医疗口译员的多重角色容易引发复杂的伦理决策,而伦理困境会给译员带来沉重的心理压力(Hubscher-Davidson, 2020)[25],进一步加大已经接近饱和的口译认知负荷(Gile, 2009)[26],从而给口译效果带来负面影响。在繁重议程的压力下,会议口译的工作主要集中在圆满完成信息传译上。虽然信息加工工作看似单纯,但也会涉及文化敏感信息,所以译员应先与会议组织方沟通好传译原则。如果客户希望实现完整精确的翻译,那么译员的主要角色就是在时间和认知的巨大压力下(因为大部分会议都是用同传)完成精准的信息传译。译者的主要任务如下:

(1)对于有稿的演讲,译员要在译前完成讲稿或 PPT 的预处理,尽量提前翻译好,这样才能节约精力,会议当天才能集中精力处理会议现场出现的新稿件;

(2)对于无稿或无 PPT 的演讲,根据演讲题目或对讲话人做背景梳理,整理相关要点和专业词汇,形成双语词汇表并打印出来,或是形成双语平行语料库存于电脑,便于会议期间随时搜索;

(3)快速阅读或视译会议现场获取的稿件,标出重点、难点和生僻词汇的对应译文;

(4)在完成自己负责部分的准备工作和同传工作之外,尽量辅助同传搭档查找生词的对应译文;

(5)译后配合客户完成财务手续;

(6)译后归档会议的双语信息和话题知识;

(7)重听会议原语和译语录音,找出待改进之处。

2.4 医疗口译的资质认证

美国有两个机构提供医疗口译认证:医疗口译员认证委员会(The Certification Commission for Healthcare Interpreters, CCHI)和医疗口译员认证全国委员会(The National Board for Certified Medical Interpreters, NBCMI)。

以英语/普通话的医疗口译为例,要获得 CCHI 认证或 NBCMI 认证,考生必须满足以下条件：（1）年满18岁；（2）拥有高中文凭（或通过GED考试）；（3）完成至少40小时的医疗口译培训或获得1年口译职业经历证明；（4）精通英语和普通话；（5）通过医疗口译笔试（机考）；（6）通过笔试后的口试；（7）获得CCHI认证后每两年需要完成16小时的继续教育，获得NBCMI认证后每五年需要完成30小时的继续教育。

澳大利亚国家翻译资格认证局（The National Accreditation Authority for Translators and Interpreters，NAATI）负责对澳大利亚医疗领域的专业译员进行技能和能力评估，规定持有会议口译认证的译员（certified conference interpreter）才有资格参加专业医疗口译的认证考试。

在澳大利亚，具有认证的专业医疗口译员（Certified Specialist Health Interpreters，CSHI）是经验丰富且成就卓著的口译员，是医疗领域的口译专业人士，要完成专业培训，并在专业领域持续拓展知识和技能，是能力突出的语言使用者，理解医学专业术语并拥有广泛的医学知识，对自身作为医疗团队成员的角色有着深刻理解，对文化和语言以及相关医疗伦理规范和专业标准有全面了解。

要通过CSHI认证考试，译员需要具备以下能力。（1）传译能力：能在原语和译语之间传译复杂专业的医疗信息；（2）语言能力：能使用包括术语和行话在内的原语和译语；（3）跨文化能力：能识别重要且微妙的文化信息，并能在口译任务中进行适当说明；（4）主题能力：能理解复杂专业的医疗主题，并能为专业听众进行口译；（5）伦理能力：能理解医疗口译伦理规范和临床指南，并应用于口译实践和医患互动；（6）研究能力：能使用有效工具搜索、提取和管理医疗口译所需的专业信息；（7）服务能力：能融入医疗团队，辅助医患互动，促进医疗效果的提升；（8）技术能力：能使用包括电话口译和视频口译在内的现场和远程口译技术。

2.5 医疗口译的职业素养

在医疗口译的专业协助下，"医—患""医—医""医—众"之间皆可实现跨语言和跨文化交流。我们认为医疗口译员所需的核心职业素养有以下几点。

（一）良好的语言能力

必须熟练掌握工作语言。例如，在美国医院为日本患者服务的口译人员就必须熟练掌握英语和日语。如果医学口译员掌握了多种外语，他们就能有更多的就业机会。译员必须理解患者所说的一切，并且能够准确无误地将意思翻译给医生。

（二）熟悉医学术语

鉴于医学领域的专业性，译员必须熟悉医院流程、医疗场景、医学检查、药物治疗、手术治疗和其他相关医学知识，能够快速准确地理解医生及患者的话语，准确理解患者描述的体征和症状，准确地向医生和患者传达等值信息。医学知识和医学术语的学习需要很长时间，一名优秀的口译员必须在学习这些术语时保持最佳状态。医疗口译员应该积极参加医疗健康方面的研讨会等，以扩展专业知识并在需要时使用。注意医学话语和普通话语的区别，这样才能理解医生想要说的话，并用普通人的语言传达给患者。只有通过严格培训和累积实践经验，才能满足以上要求。

（三）耐心和文化同理心

专业译员需要成为交流双方的良好倾听者，并耐心地与客户打交道，即使他们已经是经验丰富的译员。同时，译员还必须具有文化敏感性，以关怀心和同理心来对待患者。了解医患文化差异，译员就能更顺畅地与患者沟通并向医生解释医患文化间的细微差别。

（四）诊（译）前交流

在与患者见面之前，如果临床医生和译员能够进行简短沟通，双方就有机会相互认识，了解患者基本情况和可能的病症、病因、检查和治疗术语以及本次交流的目的。在医患对话前，医生给患者自我介绍时也要顺带介绍译员。译员在对话开始前可以向病人强调"您说的每一句话我都会完整地翻译给医生，而医生的话我也都会准确翻译给您"。这个声明将避免病人跟译员说了一些重要信息之后又不让翻译给医生听的情况，那将使译员陷入两难境地。这些"仪式性"的交流有助于医生、患者和译员更好地交谈。

（五）获得认证

尽早获得医疗口译相关认证和资质。拥有认证可以让译员迅速获得用户认可，并获得薪水更高的、更好的工作机会。医疗保健的提供方也越来越认识到与有资质、有认证的译员合作的好处。在国外，已经有一些地方和机构强制要求医疗口译员获得认证。在中国，目前还没有针对医疗口译的专门认证，但有志于在医疗领域工作的译员可以先获得交传或同传口译认证，再辅以医学教育或医疗口译经验说明自己的资质。

（六）让患者放松，能够讨论敏感问题和自我心理调适

患者在医院需要应对的情况很多，包括应对陌生环境中的焦虑感以及对自己健康状况的担忧等。所以，医疗口译员要尽量让患者放松，并向患者保证将提供

专业透明的语言服务。医生与患者讨论敏感问题时，译员必须保持镇静。即使在手术过程中进行口译，译员也不能因胆怯而影响自己的工作。即使不是在医院现场，有些医学会议的 PPT 也可能引起心理不适，所以译员需要调整和克服。

（七）节省医院时间

凭借在工作语言之间准确完整翻译关键医疗信息的能力、强大的人际交往能力、灵活的客户服务能力、对医疗信息和记录保密的能力、强大的抗压能力，以及在电话上或远程视频中与人互动交流的能力，医疗口译员能够弥合跨文化交流的沟通缺口，规范医疗流程，也能节省医院的宝贵时间。

（八）口译通用技能

除了上述医疗口译的特定技能和职责，医疗口译员还必须掌握众多的通用口译技能，包括良好的听力和分析能力、公众演讲能力、记忆能力、笔记能力、精力分配能力、多任务协调能力、语言转换能力、数字转换能力、概述能力、临场反应能力、译前准备能力、文化调解能力、遵守职业准则和伦理规范的能力、口译技术和设备的操控能力等。将这些技能整合在一起，才能顺利完成交传和同传两种口译服务。以上都还只是入行的口译基本技能，以认知能力和语言能力为主，入行之后，商务能力、人际交往能力、客户教育能力、议价交付能力等也是成功译员必备的。

2.6　医疗口译的伦理教育

在上一节，我们已经了解到医学口译人才既要是通才（generalist），也要是专才（specialist）。医学口译领域有大量的伦理规范和要求。经过系统培训的职业译员必须严格遵守医疗和口译伦理准则。首先，我们来看看职业译员和非职业译员在进行医疗口译时的角色差异，以及非职业译员工作期间可能出现的不符合伦理要求的行为。

职业译员会将重要的医疗信息在医生和语言能力有限的患者之间进行准确的口头传译。根据具体要求，医疗口译员可能还需要协助病人填写表格或帮助医院翻译医疗文献。在这个过程中，职业译员必须坚持提供优质服务，并与医护人员、患者及家属积极互动。职业译员在必要时还要协助患者随访，联系和提醒预约患者。职业译员会严格按照医院政策为患者保密。职业译员还要参加持续的医疗口译实训，以保持技能水平和熟练程度。职业译员可能还需履行医院分配的相关职责。

因此，按照职业伦理要求，职业译员至少需要：（1）接受过系统的技能培训，训练有素，具有岗位胜任力；（2）完整、透明和中立地传译所有重要的医疗信息；（3）确保医学术语的准确性，减少医疗误判和事故；（4）遵守保密原则，避免利益冲突。

非职业译员又称临时译员。目前，由于大部分医院都没有受过专业培训的职业译员，而临时雇用译员也费时耗力，所以在很多情况下只能依靠诸如患者家属（包括儿童或未成年人）、朋友、志愿者或懂英语的医生、护士、护工等非职业口译员临时承担医疗口译任务。这种情况在西方国家医院也相当常见。还有研究显示，移民患者对非职业口译员的信任超过了职业译员。（Zendedel et al.，2016）[27]

使用非职业译员的不利之处以及可能会出现的问题如下：未经培训的口译员在传译时容易出现遗漏、增补、替换、加入自己意见或自己替代回答提问等情况。有研究发现，在患者的陪同者充当医疗口译员的情况下，口译准确率和完整率会大幅降低，而且会出现剥夺患者话轮、损害患者自主决定权等问题。（Cox et al.，2019）[28]医生和患者可能会因为不能完整了解医疗信息而承担不良的医疗后果，例如误诊或治疗失误。比如，家人或朋友觉得没有必要翻译患者所说的每一句话，从而总结、概述或省略病人所述信息。他们也可能在口译时插入自己的意见、强加自己的判断或替病人做出选择（虽然大多时候是出于好意）。再如，担任口译的家人和朋友可能发现自己的英语能力有限，尤其是碰到完全不熟悉的医学术语时。在自己也没有听懂的情况下，有的家人和朋友会如实相告，有的则直接省略或胡乱猜测。此外，许多患者可能不便向家人和朋友透露敏感或私人信息。例如，一名受虐待的妇女被施虐者带到医院，然后由施虐者为她翻译，那么受虐待的妇女就不太可能完整说明自己受伤的原因和程度。如果担任口译的是儿童或未成年人，那更可能造成医疗信息的歪曲和丢失，更重要的是可能会使儿童或未成年人承受有害的心理和认知负担。

现在让我们谈谈由医院员工担任口译的不利之处。即使医院的医生、护士、护工或志愿者精通英语，由他们担任译员还是会有诸多不利之处。（1）他们不可能精通所有科室的专业术语，他们还有自己的本职工作，因此不能像职业译员那样全身心投入译前准备，专注地完成某个口译任务，任何未知的医学术语或是口译流程上的不合规都可能使对话交流陷入困难，增加医疗成本，甚至危及患者健康。（2）因为也懂专业，所以他们更有可能在对话中添加或省略信息，更可能会去解读意思而不是忠实地口译，还可能会插入个人意见和判断。（3）他们没有受过口译技巧培训，也没有跨文化交流的经验，一些中国文化中习以为常的说法或表达或许会引起具有外语文化背景的人的反感或不适。（4）他们可能已经与患者存在某种职业关系，这将干扰其作为译员的公正和中立立场。

综上，我们应该根据具体的医疗情境与工作任务性质来判断是否应当使用非职业口译。（Pines et al., 2019）[29] 在不得不使用非职业译员的情况下，最好在译前对非职业译员进行培训，让他们了解基本的口译伦理准则，如立场中立、信息保密、交流透明、传译忠实等。

3 医疗口译的重点难点

3.1 医疗口译的术语发音

很多学习者放弃学习医疗口译的原因之一就是医学词汇太长，发音太难。译员自己发音不熟练，理解讲话者的发音就会受到影响。译员说不清、听不明，口译时自然就开不了口。具有医学背景的学生虽然医学英语词汇量大，但也存在一定程度的英语发音障碍，这将会直接影响国际交流效果。在本书各个临床专科的专业术语中，也有部分难发音的专业术语，而在真正的国际会议上，生僻词汇更是俯拾皆是。为此，我们推荐几个医学术语发音突破策略。

（一）找准重音

首先通过词典获取音标，然后确认重音。重音对了，发音就对了一半。重读音节的发音最为清晰，是表述和识别单词的关键；非重读音节会因连读、略读等发音习惯而听上去比较模糊。同时，由于医学英语的单词很长，多由词根、前缀及后缀组合而成，因此很多单词都可能有双重音或亚重音，应注意所有重读音节都需要较为清晰的发音。例如：

消化科：食管 esophagus/iːˈsɔfəgəs/，食管癌 esophageal/iːˌsɔfəˈdʒiːəl/cancer，肝肿大 hepatomegaly/ˌhepətəʊˈmegəli/，脾肿大 splenomegaly/ˌspliːnəʊˈmegəlɪ/，便血 hematochezia/hiˌmætəʊˈkiːziə/，黑便 melena/məˈliːnə/，呕血 hematemesis/ˌhiːməˈtemisis/。

内分泌科：糖原 glycogen/ˈglaɪkədʒ(ə)n/，下丘脑 hypothalamus/ˌhaɪpə(ʊ)ˈθæləməs/，脑垂体 pituitary/pɪˈtjuːɪt(ə)rɪ/，骨质疏松症 osteoporosis/ˌɒstɪəʊpəˈrəʊsɪs/，雌激素 estrogen/ˈestrədʒən/，睾丸素 testosterone/teˈstɒstərəʊn/。

在以生物抗衰或肿瘤治疗为主题的国际医学会议中，以下生僻词汇可能会出现，请同学们试试能不能根据音标念出单词：

白藜芦醇 resveratrol/rɪsˈverəˌtrɒl/，类黄酮 flavonoid/ˈflevənɔɪd/，番茄红素 lycopene/ˈlaikəpiːn/，虾青素 astaxanthɪn/ˌæstəˈzænθɪn/，花青素 anthocyanin /ˌænθə(ʊ)ˈsaɪənɪn/。

（二）重音移动

随着词性的变化或词义的丰富，单词的重音可能会后移。例如：

消化内科：内镜 endoscope/ˈendəskəʊp/，内镜检查 endoscopy/enˈdɒskəpi/，腹腔镜 laparoscope/ˈlæpərəuskəʊp/，腹腔镜检查 laparoscopy/ˌlæpəˈrɒskəpi/，结肠镜 colonoscope/kəʊˈlɒnəˌskəʊp/，结肠镜检查 colonoscopy/ˌkəʊləˈnɒskəpi/。

耳鼻喉科：咽 pharynx/ˈfærɪŋks/，咽炎 pharyngitis/ˌfærɪnˈdʒaɪtɪs/，喉 larynx /ˈlærɪŋks/，喉炎 laryngitis/ˌfærɪnˈdʒaɪtɪs/，耳科 otology/əʊˈtɒlədʒɪ/，耳炎 otitis /ə(ʊ)ˈtaɪtɪs/，耳鼻喉科 otolaryngology/ˌəʊtə(ʊ)lærɪnˈgɒlədʒɪ/。

内分泌科：胰岛素 insulin/ˈɪnsjʊlɪn/，胰岛素瘤 insulinoma/ˌɪnsjuliˈnəʊmə/，尿酮 ketone/ˈkiːtəʊn/，酮症酸中毒 ketoacidosis/ˌkiːtəʊæsiˈdəʊsis/。

抗衰老：胡萝卜 carrot/ˈkærət/，类胡萝卜素 carotenoid/kəˈrɒtənɔɪd/。

（三）识别不发音的字母

"h"，在含 rh-或 rrh-的词中，h 都是不发音的，rr 只发一个 r。如昼夜节律 circadian rhythm/ˈrɪð(ə)m/，肝硬化 cirrhosis/siˈrəʊsis/，腹泻 diarrhea /ˌdaiəˈriːə/。

"n"，在以 cn-、gn-或 mn-开头的词中，"n"前的字母"c""g""m"不发音。如刺细胞 cnidoblast/ˈnaidəʊblaːst/，手指粗糙 gnarled/nɑːld/ fingers，记忆术 mnemonics/nɪˈmɒnɪks/。但如果在单词中间，"c""g""m"也可与前面元音组成音节发声，如失忆症 amnesia/æmˈniːzɪə/。

"p"，在以 psy-、pt-或 pn-开头的词中，"p"不发音。如精神科 psychiatry /saɪˈkaɪətri/，精神分析 psychoanalysis/ˌsaɪkəʊəˈnælɪsɪs/，（眼科）翼状胬肉 pterygium/təˈrɪdʒiːəm/，肺炎 pneumonia/njuːˈməʊnɪə/。

（四）两个字母一起发音

ph 发音为/f/，如恐惧症 phobia/ˈfəʊbɪə/，脑病 encephalopathy /enˌsefəˈlɔpəθi/，（分隔胸腔和腹腔的）膈膜 diaphragm/ˈdaɪəfræm/。

sc 的发音为/s/，如腹水 ascites/əˈsaitiːz/。

ch 发音为/k/，如胆道镜 choledochoscopy/kəˌledəˈkɔskəpi/。

eu 发音为/juː/，如呼吸正常 eupnea/juːpˈnɪə/。

（五）特别发音

"c"在"a""o""u"之前发/k/，如卡路里 calorie/ˈkæləri/，软骨 cartilage

/ˈkɑːt(ɪ)lɪdʒ/，有疗效的 curative/ˈkjʊərətɪv/，康复期血浆 convalescent /kɒnvəˈles(ə)nt/ plasma。

"c" 在 "i" "e" 之前发/s/，如脐带瘢 umbilical cicatrice /ˈsɪkətrɪs/，大脑 cerebrum/ˈserɪbrəm/。

"dys" 的发音为/dɪs/，如吞咽困难 dysphagia/dɪsˈfeɪdʒɪə/，言语困难 dysphasia/dɪsˈfeɪzɪə/。

（六）其他策略

（1）按照音标或示范发音进行朗读或跟读练习，重复朗读多次就能流畅地发音。在突破单个生词后，在句子、段落或篇章中进行朗读。"影子练习"（即滞后跟读）是改善发音的有效方法，因为对全篇演讲的音频或视频进行"影子跟读"，能够强迫学生在语音干扰下完成单词发音。

（2）在真实多样的语境中进一步熟悉单词。上面的音标都是英式音标，而美式发音可能有所不同。英语是当前的世界语言，我们可以尽量获取世界各地的音频或视频材料，听辨口音不同的讲话者对同一话题中同一单词的发音，通过反复练习实现自动灵活的表达和识别。

3.2 医疗口译的术语记忆

很多学习者放弃医疗口译的另一个原因就是医学单词太多、太难记了。通过学习本书，学习者可打下一定的医学英语词汇基础。但在现实会议中，任何一个 15～30 分钟的演讲都有 2000～5000 个字词，里面肯定有大量生词和陌生术语需要译者做额外的译前准备。但是，我们希望大家能够通过本书的学习，掌握医学术语的快速记忆方法，提升未来译前准备的效率。

现在我们给大家推荐以下几种医学词汇的记忆方法。前三种方法与词根（root）、前缀（prefix）、后缀（suffix）及其组合有关。词根是词的基本部分，词缀包括前缀和后缀。前缀是出现在单词开头的一组字母，后缀是出现在单词末尾的一组字母。

以下举例说明如何通过希腊语或拉丁语词根来记忆医学术语。

（一）词根记忆法（The Root Method）

（1）消化内科：

gastro-表示 "胃"：胃炎 gastritis/gæˈstraɪtɪs/，胃肠科 gastroenterology /ˌgæstrəʊentəˈrɒlədʒi/，胃癌 gastric/ˈgæstrɪk/cancer，胃功能 gastric function 等。

entero 表示 "肠"：（小）肠炎 enteritis/ˌentəˈraɪtɪs/，痢疾（腹泻）dysentery

/ˈdɪsəntɛri/。

colic 表示"结肠（或大肠）"：结肠 colon/ˈkəʊlən/，结肠炎 colitis/kəˈlaɪtɪs/，大肠埃希菌（大肠杆菌）E. coli/ˈkəʊlai/。

hepatic 表示"肝的"：肝炎 hepatitis/ˌhepəˈtaɪtɪs/，肝病科 hepatology /hepəˈtɒlədʒi/，肝素 heparin/ˈhepərɪn/。

（2）血液科：

hemat- 表示"血"：血液科（血液病学）hematology /ˌheməˈtɒlədʒi/，血液病学家 hematologist/hiːməˈtɒlədʒɪst/，血液病的 hematological/hiːmətəˈlɒdʒɪkl/，呕血 hematemesis/hiːməˈteməsɪs/，便血 hematochezia/hemətəˈkiːzɪə/等。

该词根还有变体 hemo-：血友病 hemophilia/ˌhiːməˈfɪlɪə/，血红蛋白 hemoglobin/ˌhiːməʊˈgləʊbɪn/，血液透析 hemodialysis/ˌhiːmədaɪˈælɪsɪs/，血细胞 hemocyte/ˈhiːməsaɪt/。

（3）学生可以使用以下常用词根进一步整理相关主题或科室词汇：

Cardi/o：Related to the heart 与心脏相关

Derm/a/o，dermat/o：Pertaining to the skin 与皮肤相关

Encephal/o：Related to the brain 与大脑相关

My/o：Related to muscle 与肌肉相关

Oste/o：Related to bone 与骨相关

Pulmon/o：Refers to the lungs 与肺相关

Rhin/o：Related to the nose 与鼻相关

Sclerosis：Hard or hardening 硬化

Stasis：Slowing or stopping the flow of a bodily fluid 瘀滞

Therm/o：Indicates heat 与"热"相关

（二）词缀记忆法（The Suffix Method）

（1）前缀：

anti-（抗）：抗凝 anticoagulation/ˈæntɪkəʊˌægjʊˈleɪʃən/。

cryo-（冷）：冷沉淀 cryoprecipitate/ˌkraɪəʊprɪˈsɪpɪtət/。

hyper-（过高，过多）：分泌过多 hypersecretion，高血糖 hyperglycemia /ˌhaɪpəglaɪˈsiːmɪə/，甲状腺功能亢进（甲亢）hyperthyroidism/ˌhaɪpəˈθaɪrɒɪdɪz（ə）m/。

hypo-（过低，过少，下部）：分泌过少 hyposecretion，低血糖 hypoglycemia /ˌhaɪpəʊglaɪˈsiːmɪə/，甲状腺功能减退（甲减）hypothyroidism /ˌhaɪpəʊˈθaɪrɒɪdɪz(ə)m/，下丘脑 hypothalamus/ˌhaɪpə(ʊ)ˈθæləməs/。

para-（副，旁）：甲状旁腺 parathyroid/ˌpærəˈθaɪrɔɪd/，宫外孕 paracyesis /ˌpærəsaiˈiːsɪs/。

peri-（包、膜）：心包 pericardium/ˌperɪˈkɑːdɪəm/，心包炎 pericarditis /ˌperɪkɑːˈdaɪtɪs/，软骨膜 perichondrium/ˌperɪˈkɒndrɪəm/，软骨膜炎 perichondritis /ˌperɪkɒnˈdraɪtɪs/。

（2）后缀：

-itis 表示"炎症"（inflammation）：结肠炎 colitis/kəˈlaɪtɪs/，小肠炎 enteritis /entəˈraɪtəs/，胃炎 gastritis/gæˈstraɪtɪs/，肝炎 hepatitis/hepəˈtaɪtɪs/，甲状腺炎 thyroiditis/ˌθaɪrɔɪˈdaɪtɪs/（thyroid-itis），胰腺炎 pancreatitis/ˌpæŋkrɪəˈtaɪtɪs/ （pancreat-itis）。

-scope 表示"镜"，-scopy 表示"镜检查"：内镜 endoscope，内镜检查 endoscopy；腹腔镜 laparoscope/læpərəˌskəʊp/，腹腔镜检查 laparoscopy /ˌlæpəˈrɒskəpi/。

-emia 表示"血或血液中存在的某种物质"：贫血 anemia（lack of blood），白血病 leukemia/luːkiːˌmɪə/（血液中异常或不成熟的白细胞增多，increased numbers of immature or abnormal leukocytes），血容量过高 hypervolemia/haɪpəːvəˈliːmɪə/ （too high a volume of blood）。

-oma 表示"肿"或"瘤"：血肿 hematoma/ˌhiːməˈtəʊmə/，水肿 edema /ɪˈdiːmə/，淋巴瘤 lymphoma/lɪmˈfəʊmə/，骨髓瘤 myeloma/ˌmaɪəˈləʊmə/，癌或肿瘤 carcinoma/ˌkɑːsɪˈnəʊmə/，黑色素瘤 melanoma/ˌmeləˈnəʊmə/。

-osis（疾病）：硬化（症）sclerosis/sklɪəˈrəʊsɪs/，（细胞）凋亡 apoptosis /ˌæpəˈtəʊsɪs/，神经（官能）症 neurosis/njʊəˈrəʊsɪs/，精神病（失常）psychosis /saɪˈkəʊsɪs/，酮症酸中毒 ketoacidosis/ˌkiːtəʊæsiˈdəʊsɪs/（keto-acid-osis），骨质疏松症 osteoporosis/ɒstɪəʊpəˈrəʊsɪs/（osteo-por-osis）。

-in（e），-en，-on（e）（激素）：肾上腺素 adrenaline/əˈdrenəlin/，胰岛素 insulin，血清素 serotonin/ˌserəˈtəʊnɪn/，雌激素 estrogen/ˈestrədʒən/，胰增血糖素 glucagon/ˈgluːkəg（ə）n/，睾丸素 testosterone/teˈstɒstərəʊn/，激素 hormone。

-opia（视力障碍）：近视 myopia/maɪˈəʊpɪə/，老视（老花）presbyopia /ˌprezbɪˈəʊpɪə/，弱视 amblyopia/ˌæmblɪˈəʊpɪə/。

（三）组合记忆法（The Combination Method）

更多词根（root）和词缀（affix）组合举例：

光老化 photoaging（光 photo + 老化 aging）。

致癌 carcinogenesis/ˌkɑːsinəʊˈdʒenəsɪs/（癌 carcino + 生成 genesis）。

光致癌 photocarcinogenesis/ˈfəʊtəʊˌkɑːsinəʊˈdʒenəsɪs/（光 photo + 癌 carcino + 生成 genesis）。

直肠癌 colorectal/ˌkəʊləˈrektəl/cancer（结肠 colon + 直肠 rectum + 癌症 cancer）。

气胸 pneumothorax/ˌnjuːmə(ʊ)ˈθɔːræks/（pneumo-气 + thorax 胸）。

间充质干细胞 mesenchymal/ˈmezənˌkɪməl/stem cells（MSCs）（间充质 mesenchyme/mezənkaɪm/来自希腊语词根 mesos "middle" 中间 + enkhuma "infusion" 充注）。

巨噬细胞 macrophage/ˈmækrə(ʊ)feɪdʒ/（巨 macro + 噬 phage = eater）。

吞噬细胞 phagocyte/ˈfægə(ʊ)saɪt/（吞噬 phago + 细胞 cyte）。

（清除衰老细胞的）抗衰药物 senolytics/ˌsɪnɒˈlitiks/［衰老 senescence/sɪnesns/，senolytics 由 seno + 摧毁 lytic 组合而成，直译 "摧毁衰老"，是选择性清除衰老细胞（senescent cells，SCs）的药物］。

（清除衰老细胞的）抗衰疗法 senotherapeutics（seno + therapeutics）。

（细）胞外囊泡 extracellular vesicle/ˈvesɪk(ə)l/（外 extra + 细胞 cellular + 囊泡 vesicle）。

外泌体 exosome/ˈeksəzəʊm/（exo + some，胞外囊泡的一种，益于组织再生）。

染色体 chromosome/ˈkrəʊməsəʊm/（色或色素 chromo + some）。

蛋白组 proteome/ˈprəʊtɪəʊm/（prote + ome），分泌组 secretome/ˈsiːkritəʊm/（secret + ome），转录组 transcriptome/transˈkriptəʊm/（transcript + ome）。

线粒体 mitochondrion/ˌmaɪtəˈkɑndrɪən/（丝线 mitos "thread" + 颗粒 chondrios "granule"，复数 mitochondria）。

端粒 telomere/ˈteləmə/（尾巴 telo + 部分 mere，即染色体的尾端）。

端粒酶 telomerase/teˈlɔməreɪs/（telomer 端粒 + ase 酶 - enzyme）。

肝源性低血糖 hepatogenic hypoglycemia/haɪpəʊglaɪˈsiːmɪə/（肝 hepato + 源头 genic + 低 hypo + 血糖 glycemia）。

血红蛋白病 hemoglobinopathy/hiːməʊgləʊbɪˈnɒpəθi/（血红蛋白 hemoglobin + 病 opathy）。

血友病 hemophilia（血 hemo + 友好/亲和 phil + 病 ia）。

血色素沉着症 hemochromatosis/ˈhiːməˌkrəʊməˈtəʊsɪs/（血 hemo + 色或色素 chromat + 病症 osis）。

血栓症 thrombosis/θrɒmˈbəʊsɪs/（血栓 thrombus + 症 osis）。

栓塞 embolism/ˈembəlɪz(ə)m/（栓塞 embolismos "insert"），肺栓塞 pulmonary /pʌlmənəri/embolism，脑栓塞 cerebral/serəbrəl/embolism，气泡栓塞 air embolism。

抵抗 resistance，胰岛素抵抗 insulin/ɪnsjəlɪn/resistance，甲状腺激素抵抗 thyroid/θaɪrɔɪd/hormone resistance。

紊乱/障碍/病症 disorder：甲状腺紊乱 thyroid disorder，钙稳态紊乱 calcium homeostasis/həʊmɪəsteɪsɪs/disorder，葡萄糖稳态紊乱 glucose/gluːkəʊz/ homeostasis disorder。

（四）缩略词记忆法（The Abbreviation Method）

由于部分医学词汇过长，所以医生或医学研究者也会用缩略词来表示。学习者可按主题或科室分类，在下面例子（见表1-1至表1-5）的基础上自行整理更多的常用缩写，既方便脑记也方便笔记。

表 1-1　问诊（Medical Interview）

原语（中文）	译语（英文）	缩写
主诉	chief complaint	CC
既往史	past medical history	PMH
现病史	history of present illness	HPI
社会史/病人基本资料	social history/patient profile	SH/PP
家族史	family history	FH
系统回顾	review of systems	ROS

表 1-2　消化内科（Gastroenterology Department）

原语（中文）	译语（英文）	缩写
消化科医生/胃肠病学家	gastroenterologist	GI
胃溃疡	gastric ulcer	GU
炎症性肠病	inflammatory bowel disease	IBD
肠易激综合征	irritable bowel syndrome	IBS
溃疡性结肠炎	ulcerative colitis	UC

续表

原语（中文）	译语（英文）	缩写
消化道出血	gastrointestinal bleed	GIB
消化道	gastrointestinal tract	GIT
胃食管反流病	gastroesophageal reflux disease	GERD
弥漫性血管内凝血	disseminated intravascular coagulation	DIC
经内镜逆行性胰胆管造影术	endoscopic retrograde cholangiopancreatography	ERCP
内镜黏膜切除术	endoscopic mucosal resection	EMD
内镜黏膜下剥离术	endoscopic submucosal dissection	ESD

表1-3　血液科/肿瘤科（Hematology/Oncology Department）

原语（中文）	译语（英文）	缩写
白细胞	white blood cell	WBC
红细胞	red blood cell	RBC
血小板活化因子	platelet activating factor	PAF
促进细胞生产素	erythropoietin/ɪˌrɪθrə(ʊ)pɒiˈetɪn/	EPO
血液肿瘤学	hematology oncology	HO
急性髓性白血病	acute myelogenous leukemia	AML
急性髓细胞白血病	acute myeloid leukemia	AML
急性淋巴细胞白血病	acute lymphoblastic leukemia	ALL
慢性髓性白血病	chronic myelogenous leukemia	CML
慢性淋巴细胞白血病	chronic lymphoblastic leukemia	CLL
移植物抗宿主病	graft versus host disease	GvHD
移植物抗肿瘤	graft-versus-tumor	GVT

表1-4　内分泌科（Endocrinology Department）

原语（中文）	译语（英文）	缩写
1型糖尿病	type 1 diabetes	T1D
2型糖尿病	type 2 diabetes	T2D
生长激素	growth hormone	GH

续表

原语（中文）	译语（英文）	缩写
人类生长激素	human growth hormone	HGH
胰岛素样生长因子	insulin-like growth factor	IGF
甲状腺激素	thyroid hormone	TH
甲状腺素	thyroxine	T4
三碘甲状腺原氨酸	triiodothyronine	T3
促甲状腺激素	thyroid-stimulating hormone	TSH
促甲状腺素释放激素	thyrotropin-releasing hormone	TRH

表 1-5 急救科（Emergency Department）

原语（中文）	译语（英文）	缩写
高级生命支持	advanced life support	ALS
验血	blood work	Bl wk
体重指数	body mass index	BMI
血压	blood pressure	BP
心率	heart rate	HR
心肺复苏	cardiopulmonary resuscitation	CPR
颈椎	cervical spine	C-spine
请勿复苏	do not resuscitate	DNR
急诊科/室	emergency department/emergency room	ED/ER
心电图	electrocardiogram	EKG
手术室	operating room	OR
术前	preoperative	Pre-op

（五）视觉记忆法（The Visualization Method）

建议在学习人体系统器官时，利用 Free Medical Education 和 Osmosis 等医学教育资源平台以及 Google Images、Bing Images、百度图片等中英文搜索工具中的图像和视频辅助理解和记忆，然后再自己总结和整理。例如：

内分泌系统（endocrine system）：人体的内分泌腺（endocrine glands）或内分泌器官（endocrine organs），有三个位于大脑，七个分布于身体其他部位。位于大脑的三个内分泌器官分别是下丘脑（hypothalamus/ˌhaɪpə(ʊ)ˈθæləməs/），垂体（也称脑下垂体、脑垂体、下垂体，pituitary/pɪˈtjuːɪt(ə)rɪ/），以及松果体（pineal/pɪˈnɪəl/gland）。往下是颈部的甲状腺（thyroid/ˈθaɪrɔɪd/）和甲状旁腺（parathyroid/pærəˈθaɪrɔɪd/glands），胸部的胸腺（thymus/ˈθaɪməs/），位于两个肾上方的肾上腺（adrenal/əˈdriːn(ə)l/gland）、附近的胰腺（pancreas/ˈpæŋkrɪəs/），以及负责生殖功能的男性的睾丸（testes/ˈtestiːz/，单数 testis）和女性的卵巢（ovaries/ˈəʊv(ə)rɪz/，单数 ovary）。

呼吸系统（respiratory system）：呼吸系统由参与氧气和二氧化碳交换（the exchange of oxygen and carbon dioxide）的器官组成。这些器官包括鼻（nose）、口（mouth）、会厌（epiglottis/ˌɛpɪˈglɒtɪs/）、咽（pharynx）、喉（larynx）、气管（trachea/ˈtreɪkiːə/）、支气管（bronchus/ˈbrɒŋkəs/，复数 bronchi/ˈbrɒŋkaɪ/）、细支气管（bronchiole/ˈbrɒŋkɪəʊl/，复数 bronchioles）和肺（lungs）。

上呼吸道（upper respiratory tract）：由鼻、鼻腔（nasal cavity）、鼻窦（sinus/ˈsaɪnəs/，复数 sinuses）、喉（larynx）、气管（trachea）组成。

下呼吸道（lower respiratory tract）：由肺（lungs）、支气管（bronchi）、细支气管（bronchioles）、气囊（air sacs）、肺泡（alveolus/ælˈvɪələs/，复数 alveoli/ælˈvɪəlai/）组成。

3.3　医疗口译的高低语域

语言的基本语域从高到低可能分为非常正式、正式、中性、非正式和粗俗（high formal, formal, neutral, informal, and vulgar）。我们日常感觉比较舒适的语域是在中间（neutral）附近，但作为医疗口译员，我们使用的语域应该尽量靠近讲话者的语域。医疗话语的典型特征之一就是高低语域的共存与转换。

普通患者的表达会比较口语化。在医—患对话时，为了便于交流，医生会尽量使用低语域（正式程度较低）的表达，所以译员在口译时也应该使用低语域表达。例如，在医—医对话中，"吞咽困难"可以说 dysphagia/dɪsˈfeɪdʒɪə/，但在医—患对话中，患者可能无法理解，所以"吞咽困难"需要表述为 difficulty in swallowing。同样，医生可能会把消化不良（dyspepsia/dɪsˈpepsɪə/）表述成日常英语中的 indigestion 或 difficulty in digesting food。或者对"胃轻瘫"（gastroparesis/ˌgæstrəʊpəˈriːsɪs/）进行基本解释：a condition that affects the stomach muscles and prevents proper stomach emptying（一种影响胃部肌肉并阻止胃部正常排空的病症）。

下面是一些高低语域转换的练习范例（见表1-6）。

表 1-6 高低语域转换练习范例

原语（中文）	医—患/众（英文）	医—医（英文）
胃灼热（烧心）	a burning sensation in your chest	heartburn
喉炎	inflammation of the throat	laryngitis
血栓症	blood clot that gets stuck in the vascular system and reduces the flow of blood	thrombosis
胎儿	unborn baby	fetus
羊水	a clear, slightly yellowish liquid that surrounds the unborn baby during pregnancy	amniotic/ˌæmniˈɔnik/ fluid
黑便	dark or black stool	melena
便血	blood in the stool	hematochezia
呕血	vomiting blood	hematemesis
黄疸	a condition in which the skin, whites of the eyes and mucous membranes turn yellow	jaundice
胆红素	a yellow-orange bile pigment that causes jaundice	bilirubin/ˌbɪlɪˈruːbɪn/
凝血	clotting	coagulation
血友病	an inherited bleeding disorder in which the blood does not clot properly	hemophilia

在国际会议上，专业听众则比较适应中高语域的表达。一位医生上台做报告，需要在有限时间内分享自己的最新研究成果，这时的听众可能是从事基础或临床研究的同行或者对会议主题感兴趣的业界人士，这位医生可能会使用中高语域（正式、学术、精炼）的表达，那么译员也应使用相应的语域。同时，医生的学术报告过程可能会分为引入、研究方法阐释、结果及讨论、研究意义或应用前景、总结等环节，重要专业术语甚至会中英文混用外加解释，以便于准确交流，毕竟在研究中也存在"隔行如隔山"的现象。

因此，会议发言人在演讲过程中会进行语域的转换。以下是 2021 年 10 月 24 日我们在现场同传时对一位北京大学肿瘤医院教授发言的录音转写片段。他的演讲的题目是"你的健康谁做主——氢分子与活性氧"。这个题目中学生们也许不能马上翻译出来的部分"氢分子与活性氧"就是高语域，而"你的健康谁做主"就是中低语域。

这位讲话者的现场交流效果较好，我们觉得这与讲话者高低语域结合的策略有关。接下来看看他在演讲中语域的使用和转换。学习者可将下面转写材料中高语域的部分画出来，这些一般也是会出现传译困难的语段。

00：00：00-00：03：00

"各位朋友，各位同道，下午好！今天利用这个时间跟大家分享一点'你的健康谁做主'，因为这个（会议）是跟医美和抗衰老有关的，所以呢，我想，长寿先要健康，健康才能长寿。另外，就是想跟大家分享在生命过程中如何科学利用古今中外的医学智慧防止过早衰老。衰老是不可抗拒的，但过早衰老是有点问题的。这个里面呢，我们可以看到，人呢，衰老的过程是渐进性的，但是应该有三个节点，它是比较关键的。一个就是36岁，34~36岁，我把它总结成这样，60岁，80岁。这三个点对人一生来说是非常重要的。中间大概隔了两个12，现在叫7×12，你可以算一下，我们人，我们一个人的健康状况基本上12年一个周期，就是你的变化基本上是在这个范围之内。所以在这个过程中呢，我们会知道医药科学的发展，特别是近现代医学，过去200年来，我们从防控瘟疫，解除痛苦，延长寿命，到今天，需要健康管理。我们今天看到的这些问题，就是说，一个缺血缺氧，到内科系统去看病的，实际上很多病都是跟衰老相关的；另外一个就是恶性肿瘤。大家都知道，我们知道，到45岁以后，癌症，恶性肿瘤的发生率是呈指数级增长的。那么这个过程我们就会提示要抗癌症，我自己一直是做癌症（研究与治疗）的，为什么来跟大家谈衰老的问题呢？就是说癌症防控，实际上癌症防控很多年前人们就提出了，首先要抗衰老。这个过程我们要知道，人类发展的过程中，我们学会用火，然后寿命就从20岁活到40岁，特别是工业革命解放体力，有青霉素的发现，抗生素的应用，人就比较容易地从40岁活到60岁，这个是很稳定的，加上饮用水、公共卫生、冲水马桶、现代医学，还有现在生活水平的改变，所以现代人很容易活到80岁。这个过程里面呢，会产生很多问题，待会儿我们会讲到。"

00：08：00-00：11：01

"比如说，绿茶和大蒜都有很好的抗氧化作用，抗ROS的作用。我今天待会儿跟大家分享一下大蒜素的作用。这个工作是这样，是我们在30年前，这个红的就是……我们国家胃癌高发，差不多一半的胃癌呢发生在中国。然后，这里呢，我们在山东这里有一个地方呢，就是胃癌高、低发区，这两个地方就差300公里，但是它们胃癌的发生率却差10倍。找了几十年的因素，发现有一个因素，就是消耗大蒜的量跟胃癌的发生率有非常密切的关系。高发区每天每个人只吃两颗大蒜，低发区平均每天每人要吃 20 颗新鲜大蒜，就是在山东苍山那个地方。而且这个里面，我们可以看到一个非常重要的癌前病变。在常化以前，两个县一样的；从常化以后，他们就差别开了。癌症的发生率很高，这个就非常有关系。那这里面我们知道，大蒜有一个很好的作用，它有蒜氨酸，在蒜氨酸酶的作用下转化成大蒜素。当然，大蒜素遇到空气氧化以后呢就形成了……有非常强的抗菌作用，不论是革兰氏阴性、阳性细菌，真菌，病毒，都有很好的作用，所以你出差的话，带上点大蒜到一个地方是最安全的。另外一个就是它参与细胞的基本代谢。后面我的研究主要是研究它的基本的代谢过程。在这里面，我们发现一个很重要的基因叫 Metallothionine IIA，叫金属硫蛋白 2A，是个 6kD 的应激蛋白，就是说我们人体每天都会碰到各种各样的应激反应。这个蛋白经过大蒜素处理之后呢，它会在细胞里表达上调。上调联系到胃是这样：因为大家知道，胃是这样，大家都会有胃的毛病。胃会有一个很重要的功能，就是黏膜屏障和分泌功能，因为你把乱七八糟的东西稀里晃荡全部吃进去，吃到你胃里，好不好就看你的屏障功能。分泌功能就是要分泌各种东西，其中要分泌盐酸，然后用来消化这些食物。当然我们现在的癌症研究都在很靠后的功能。那么这个黏膜屏障功能、分泌功能，受的第一打击就是 stress，就是应激。应激以后就引起了一系列的代谢过程。这是一个很重要的蛋白，有非常清楚的作用，ROS 的作用跟这个的关系非常密切。所以我们可以看到，在细胞癌变、老化的过程中，它是逐渐减少的，到癌的时候它就没有了。大家可以看到这个过程，这里有一系列的变化，大家可以看到，在临床上，凡是有 M2A 高表达的患者，手术以后的预后就好。"

00：18：40－00：19：35

"这里面我们讲的葡萄糖分子变成 ATP，就是三磷酸腺苷，有一系列的转换过程，最后进入 TCA，就是三羧酸循环，产生能量。但是对于肿瘤患者，它产生的能量是非常少的，消耗一个葡萄糖分子只能产生两个 ATP。在这个过程里面呢有一个很重要的通路。就是这些糖如果多了，怎么办呢？就有一个糖异生的通路。结果代谢下来以后，它会产生很多的丙酮酸。这些东西，丙酮酸、乳酸，可以回去产生糖原，储存在肝脏。所以这个过程是很重的，现在人们可能对……糖异生的价值被低估了，就是我们在日常生活中，所以我的研究呢，正好是聚焦这个方面，发现果糖-1,6-二磷酸酶，叫激酶，叫 FBP2，它是糖异生的限速酶。如果你这些东西多了，回不去了，堆积在体内就是一个问题。"

00：20：35 - 00：21：14

"喝氢水也好，呼吸氢气也好，都有助于清除活性氧，清除 AGE 受体。另外呢，可以提供电子，增加 ATP，有了 ATP，那你不就有力了吗？就不乏力了，对不对？所以吸氢有一个很好的作用，首先解决的是乏力。另外有很好的营养价值，因为这个分子很小，跟很多的物质有非常好的相容性。增加各种营养物质吸收，所以国家也通过了氢作为食品添加剂的国家标准。所以这个产业会有很好的发展，将来大家如果做化妆品的话，加在里面也应该是好的。"

00：25：35 - 00：26：05

"如果你要抗衰老，那你就要完整记录生命过程的信息，系统采集健康窗口期的数据。我们每一个人，6 年也好，甚至对指甲那些，半年要换一遍。我们身上的细胞，大概六七年要换一遍。12 年，你整个身体的状态就会改变一遍。所以，大家可以关注自己的动态变化。一句话，原则上人这个最大的遗传度是要保护的，所以生命要省着点用！谢谢大家。"

3.4　医疗口译的语内转换

不管是在中文还是在英文里，即使抛开语域的问题不谈，也还有一些相同的医学概念似乎有好几种不同的表达，这给医疗口译员的学习带来了不少困难。其中，有些是源于希腊语词根与拉丁语词根的区别，也有些是源于英美拼写体系的不同，还有些是源于使用习惯的差异。以下分别进行解析。

（一）希腊语、拉丁语、日耳曼语词根的区别

以"肺"这个词为例，英语 lung 是日耳曼语词根，是日常英语，而希腊语词根是 pneumonos，拉丁语词根则是 pulmo。由此引申而来的与"肺"相关的概念是不是每个都会有希腊语、拉丁语、日耳曼语三个并行词呢？也不一定。因为语言是一种社会契约，所以某种表达用的人多了就会成为主要表达。比如"肺癌"一般是 lung caner（日耳曼语词根），"肺炎"是 pneumonia（希腊语词根），而"慢性阻塞性肺疾病"，即"慢阻肺"是 chronic obstructive pulmonary disease（拉丁语词根）。另外，如"肺气肿"，既可以是 pulmonary/ˈpʌlmən(ə)rɪ/（拉丁

语词根), emphysema /ˌemfɪˈsiːmə/ (拉丁语词根), 又可以是 pneumonectasis/njuːˌməʊnekˈteisis/ (希腊语词根), 也可以是 distention of the lungs with air (拉丁语词根 + 日耳曼语词根)。

（二）美式英语和英式英语的拼写差异

例如，在血液科，表示"血"（blood）的希腊语词根在美式英语和英式英语中会有拼写差异。在表示"血"（blood）的词缀或词根中，"e"为美式拼写，"ae"为英式拼写，如 hem-, haem-; hemo-, haemo-; hema-, haema-; hemato-, haemato-; hemat-, haemat-; -hemia, -haemia; -hemic, -haemic; -emia, -aemia。

具体单词拼写对比举例：血液学 hematology（美），haematology（英）；血液学家 hematologist（美），haematologist（英）；贫血 anemia（美），anaemia（英）；白血病 leukemia（美），leukaemia（英）；血友病 hemophilia（美），haemophilia（英）等。

（三）一词多义/译

（1）disorder, condition, disease：disorder 可以译为障碍或失常（如精神科）、紊乱、问题、疾病，condition 可以译为疾病、病变、障碍、紊乱等。因此，disorder 和 condition 都与 disease 相关，译员可根据病症严重程度选择合适译语。

（2）procedure：在英语中，procedure 是包括医学检查、诊断、治疗、手术、麻醉等在内的医学操作。所以，在翻译为中文时，需要根据上下文或语境确定恰当的译语。

（3）symptom, sign：这两个词经常在一起出现，但事实上有细微差别，症状（symptom）是病人的主观感受，而体征（sign）则是医疗人员的客观检查结果。

（四）表达习惯差异

中文中的很多医学术语是由英语翻译而来。由于不同的归化（偏译语习惯）和异化（偏原语习惯）策略，所以会看到一些能指（表达）有差异，但所指（意义）相同的表达。

比如"胃肠科""消化科""消化内科"对应的英语都是 Gastroenterology 或 GI，属于内科，也会涉及各种内镜检查。"肠胃炎""胃肠炎"对应的英语都是 gastroenteritis（简称 gastro），即胃肠道的炎症 inflammation of the gastrointestinal tract，医生对病人解释时可能说 stomach flu（肠胃感冒/胃肠型感冒）。

又如，"睾丸素"和"睾酮"的英文是同一个词 testosterone/teˈstɒstərəʊn/;

"孕酮""孕激素"和"黄体酮"的英文也是同一个词 progesterone /prəˈdʒestərəʊn/，而与之相似的 progestin/prəʊˈdʒestin/则是人工孕激素，是一种药物；另外，"花色苷""花青苷""花色素苷""花青素"的英文都是 anthocyanin /ˌænθə(ʊ)ˈsaɪənɪn/。

还有就是细微差异被省略而造成的多种表达。例如，英语中有许多词都可能被译为"肠炎"，包括 enteritis，enterocolitis，IBD，IBS 等。那么具体有什么不同呢？精确地说，enteritis 是小肠炎，即 inflammation of the small intestine；enterocolitis 是肠炎/小肠结肠炎，即 inflammation of the small intestine and the colon；IBD 是指炎症性肠病，即 inflammatory bowel disease，是回肠（ileum）、直肠（rectum）、结肠（colon）的慢性炎症，包括溃疡性结肠炎（ulcerative colitis，UC）和克罗恩病（Crohn's disease，CD）；而 IBS（irritable bowel syndrome）是肠易激综合征，不涉及炎症，只是大肠运动过快或过缓引起的功能/动力失调（functional/motility disorder）。

3.5 医疗口译的文化差异

医疗口译中的语际转换需要注意文化差异。接下来我们以中美医疗文化差异为例，举例分析两国在医学教育、医科职称、医疗职业以及医院/医疗级别上的差异。

（一）医学教育

在医学教育方面，美国的医科教育之前有 4 年的本科教育，在本科毕业之后，学生必须通过"医学院入学考试"（medical college admission test，MCAT）才能进入医学院学习，医学院毕业之后再要进行 3~7 年的住院医师培训（residency training）以及 1~3 年的（亚）专科培训（fellowship）。在毕业后（post-graduate，PG）的培训中，门诊训练（clinical training）是很重要的环节，其中就包括"持续门诊训练"（continuity clinic）。第一年的住院医师（resident），也称实习医生（intern，post-graduate-year 1，PGY-1），需要在专科导师（主任/主治医师 attending physician/doctor）的指导下，每周进行 1~2 个半天（一般是下午）的门诊训练；第二年的住院医师（PGY-2），可能需要有每周 2~3 个半天的门诊实习；第三年的住院医师（PGY-3），则可能需要有每周 3~4 个半天的门诊实习。持续性门诊实习有助于住院医师提升医疗水平，与病人和导师建立稳定关系，也便于长期观察病人和病情发展。中美医学教育对比详见表 1-7。

表 1-7　中美医学教育对比

阶段	中国	美国
本科阶段	通过高考，考入医学院就读（一般为 5 年），获取医学学士学位。	本科没有医学专业。学生通过大学入学考试进入非医学院就读（4 年），完成医学预科（pre-medical, pre-med）课程，获取学士学位。
研究生阶段	通过参加研究生入学考试，在医学院就读，获取学术性/专业性医学研究生学位（3 年）。	通过医学院入学考试（MCAT），申请进入医学院就读（4 年）。 1～2 年：完成基础医学课程。 2 年末：参加美国医师执照考试（USMLE）STEP 1 考试。
博士阶段	通过申请各医院的博士，在医学院就读，获取学术性/专业性博士研究生学位（3~4 年）。	3～4 年：完成临床医学课程及见习。 4 年末：参加美国医师执照考试（USMLE）STEP 2 考试。 完成医学院培训后获得医学博士学位（Doctor of Medicine, MD）。
规范化培训	通过参加各个培训基地的考试，获取名额，进入住院医师规范化培训（3 年）。	通过全美统一的住院医师遴选系统（National Resident Matching Program, NRMP）进行匹配（match），进入住院医师培训（residency training）（3~7 年）。 第 1 年为实习（internship），在第 1 年末通过 Step 3 考试，获得住院医师许可（residency permit），再经过 1～2 年培训获得普通许可（regular license），获得独立处理病人的权限。 部分住院医师在培训后期可以做住院总医师（chief resident），成为能基本胜任临床工作，独立开展基础手术的医生。
专科培训	自愿参加（2~4 年）	专科医生培训（fellowship training）（2~5 年），在主治医师（attending physician）的监督下，独立治疗绝大多数病人，主刀完成大部分的手术。完成培训，申请 Board 认证后获得专业医生资质。
就业	可在任意阶段参加工作，之后再完成毕业后培训。获取主治医师职称后，还有副主任医师、主任医师职称。	完成住院医师培训后即可获取行医资格，无论工作单位大小，都成为主治医生（attending physician），对医疗决策有最高决定权，可以独立行医。家庭科、内科、儿科、妇产科的医生可以直接去当初级治疗医生（primary care physician, PCP），即全科/家庭医生，也可以进一步完成专科医生培训后获得专科医生（specialists）认证，获得在更好医院就业的竞争力。

（二）医科职称

虽然国内一般将 attending physician 译为"主治医师"，但两者级别实际上并不相同。在美国，一般需要经过 4 年本科、4 年医学院、3～7 年的住院医师培训（residency）以及 1～3 年的（亚）专科培训（fellowship）后才能成为 attending physician（12～18 年）。在中国，医师级别大致分为医士、住院医师、主治医师、副主任医师、主任医师。中专或大专刚毕业职称是医士，考得医师证自动晋升为医师。医士和住院医师都是初级职称。本科毕业从事临床工作 4 年、硕士毕业从事临床工作 2 年、专科毕业从事临床工作 6 年可以考主治医师，考试合格自动晋升为主治医师（中级职称，至少需要 8～9 年）。本科或硕士毕业获得中级职称后 5 年或博士毕业获得中级职称后 3 年且符合各项条件，可以评副主任医师（副高，至少需要 13～14 年）。本科或硕士毕业获得副高职称后 5 年或博士毕业获得副高职称后 3 年且符合各项条件，可以评主任医师（正高，至少需要 18～19 年）。因此，从职称所需年限来看，美国的 attending physician 实际上对应中国的"副主任医师或主任医师"，在 attending physician 之上还有 consulting physician（与主任医师年资相似），而中国的"主治医师"与美国的专科培训的年资更为接近。中美医科职称用语情况详见表 1-8。

表 1-8　中美医科职称用语对比

职称	中国大陆用语（卫健委科教司）	中国香港用语（医管局）	美国用语
初级	临床住院医师（第一年住院医师规范化培训阶段）	Intern	Intern
初级	临床住院医师（住院医师规范化培训阶段）	Resident	Resident
初级	专科住院医师［专科医师规范化培训阶段（非强制要求）］	Resident Specialist	Fellow
中级	主治医师	Specialist	Attending
副高级	副主任医师	Associate Consultant（副顾问医生）	/
高级	主任医师	Consultant（顾问医生）	Consulting physician

（三）医疗职业

（1）急救。

美国救护车上的"急救员"叫 paramedic，但应注意美国 911 救护车的车上人员不同于中国 120 救护车上的医生和护士（doctors and nurses），他们是 paramedics，是独立于医师和护士之外的职业，而国内则是轮班的医生、护士或急诊科的医生、护士。

（2）医学技术。

之前，一位同事问："'医学技术学科'中的'医学技术'怎么翻译？"我们脱口而出："Medical Technology，或简称 Medtech。"同事微微一笑，说"再想想"。下面是我们"再想想"之后的结果：

"医学技术学科"对应的英文是"allied health professions"或"allied health"。《美国联邦法典》（Title 42，Chapter 6A，Subchapter V，Part F，Sec. 295）规定，allied health professional 是指未获得医学、牙科学、整骨学、脊椎医学、兽医学、视光学、足病医学、药学或临床心理学博士学位或同等学位，以及公共卫生、卫生管理、社工、咨询硕士或同等学位的其他所有医学专业人员（注册护士或医师助理除外）。可见，医学技术学科种类繁多，而各国的定义又稍有不同，可理解为临床、护理、牙科、药学之外，未获得博士学位的医学专业人员。

在国内，2011 年国务院学位委员会批准通过四川大学华西医院/华西临床医学院提出的《新设"医学技术"一级学科调整建议书》，将医学技术由临床医学下的二级学科调整为医学类一级学科。医学技术主要包括医学检验、医学影像、呼吸治疗、眼视光学、听力学、临床营养、康复治疗（含物理治疗、作业治疗及假肢矫形技术）、电生理技术等。

总之，这又是一例由英文翻译成中文，再回译为英文之后，回译的英文与最初的译文发生偏移的现象，我们可称之为"回译偏移"。

（四）医院/医疗级别

在国内，按照《医院分级管理标准》，医院经过全国统一评审，确定为三级，每级再划分为甲、乙、丙三等。划分标准包括医院规模、科研力量、人才技术、医疗硬件等。

世界卫生组织按照其专业程度将医疗服务分为初级保健（primary care，相当于国内的一级医院）、二级保健（secondary care，相当于国内的二级医院）、三级保健（tertiary care，相当于国内的三级医院）以及四级保健（quaternary care，相当于目前国内还不存在的三特医院）。

以上只是大致对应。学习者可能碰到过将"三甲医院"翻译为 First-class Hospital at Grade 3，Grade 3 A Hospital 的情况。只能说这些只是精确表达了语言层面的意思，但却未做到文化沟通。按文化翻译策略，我们可以将"三甲医院"翻译为 a tertiary hospital 或 one of the best tertiary hospitals，英语听众一下就能明白这个医院的"江湖地位"。

综上，我们在本章讨论了社区医疗口译和会议医疗口译的定义、分类、历史、角色、功能、认证、伦理等基础概念和认知框架，同时也讨论了医疗口译的学习重点和练习难点，如医疗口译的术语发音、术语记忆、高低语域、语内转换和文化差异等贯穿全书的问题。

参考文献

[1] Hsieh, E. （2016）. *Bilingual health communication working with interpreters in cross-cultural care.* London/New York：Routledge, Taylor & Francis Group.

[2] Pöchhacker, F. (1999)."Getting organized"：The evolution of community interpreting. *Interpreting*, 4 (1), 125 - 140.

[3] AIIC (1984). Random selection from reports and notes on the Brussels seminar. *AIIC Bulletin* 12 (1), 21.

[4] Pöchhacker, F. (2013). Conference interpreting. In K. Malmkjaer & K. Windle (eds). *The Oxford handbook of translation studies.* Oxford：Oxford University Press, 307 - 325.

[5] Diriker, E. (2015). Conference interpreting. In F. Pöchhacker (ed.), *Routledge encyclopaedia of interpreting studies.* London/New York：Routledge, 78 - 82.

[6] Bischoff, A. & Hudelson, P. (2010). Access to healthcare interpreter services：Where are we and where do we need to go? *International Journal of Environmental Research and Public Health*, 7 (7), 2838 - 2844.

[7] Bischoff, A. (2020). The evolution of a healthcare interpreting service mapped against the bilingual health communication model：A historical qualitative case study. *Public Health Reviews*, 41 (1). https：//doi. org/10. 1186/s40985 - 020 - 00123 - 8.

[8] Dysart-Gale, D. (2005). Communication models, professionalization, and the work of medical interpreters. *Health Communication*, 17 (1), 91 - 103.

[9] Kaufert, J. M. & Koolage, W. W. (1984). Role conflict among "culture brokers"：The experience of native Canadian medical interpreters. *Social Science & Medicine*, 18 (3),

283 - 286.

[10] Zong J., Batalova J. (2015). *The limited English proficient population in the United States.* Washington, DC: Migration Policy Institute.

[11] Proctor K., Wilson-Frederick S. M., Haffer S. C. (2018). The limited English proficient population: Describing Medicare, Medicaid, and dual beneficiaries. *Health Equity*, 2 (1), 82 - 89.

[12] 詹成，严敏宾. 国内医疗口译的现状、问题及发展——一项针对广州地区医疗口译活动的实证研究 [J]. 广东外语外贸大学学报, 2013 (3): 47 - 50.

[13] 穆雷，沈慧芝，邹兵. 面向国际语言服务业的翻译人才能力特征研究——基于全球语言服务供应商 100 强的调研分析 [J]. 上海翻译, 2017 (1): 8 - 16.

[14] Kaufert J. M. (1990). Sociological and anthropological perspectives on the impact of interpreters on clinician/client communication. *Santé Culture Health*, (7), 209 - 35.

[15] Drennan, G. (1999). Psychiatry, post-apartheid integration and the neglected role of language in South African institutional contexts. *Transcultural Psychiatry*, 36 (1), 5 - 22.

[16] Weiss, R. & Stuker, R. (1999). Wenn PatientInnen und Behandelnde nicht dieselbe Sprache sprechen — Konzepte zur Übersetzungspraxis (When patients and doctors don't speak the same language — concepts of interpretation practice). *Sozial- und Präventivmedizin*, 44 (6), 257 - 263.

[17] Angelelli, C. V. (2004). Medical interpreting and cross-cultural communication. Cambridge: CUP.

[18] Leanza, Y. (2005). Roles of community interpreters in pediatrics as seen by interpreters, physicians and researchers. *Interpreting*, 7 (2), 167 - 192.

[19] Hsieh, E. (2008). "I am not a robot!" Interpreters' views of their roles in health care settings. *Qualitative Health Research*, 18 (10), 1367 - 1383.

[20] Beltran Avery, M. P. (2001). The role of the health care interpreter — an evolving dialogue. Chicago: National Council on Interpreting in Health Care (NCIHC). http://www. ncihc. org/mc/page. do (accessed 24 February 2009).

[21] Dysart-Gale, D. (2007). Clinicians and medical interpreters: Negotiating culturally appropriate care for patients with limited English ability. *Family & Community Health*, 30 (3), 237 - 246.

[22] Hsieh, E., Ju, H. & Kong, H. (2010). Dimensions of trust: The tensions and challenges in provider-interpreter trust. *Qualitative Health Research*, 20 (2), 170 - 181.

[23] Robb, N. & Greenhalgh, T. (2006). "You have to cover up the words of the doctor": The mediation of trust in interpreted consultations in primary care. *Journal of Health Organization and Management*, 20 (5), 434 - 455.

[24] Rosenberg, E. , Seller, R. & Leanza, Y. (2008). Through interpreters' eyes: Comparing roles of professional and family interpreters. *Patient Education and Counseling*, 70 (1), 87 – 93.

[25] Hubscher-Davidson, S. (2020). Ethical stress in the translation and interpreting professions. In: K. Koskinen & N. Pokorn (eds.), *The Routledge handbook of translation and ethics*. London/New York: Routledge, 415 – 430.

[26] Gile, D. (2009). *Basic concepts and models for interpreter and translator training*. Rev. ed. Amsterdam: John Benjamins.

[27] Zendedel, R. , Schouten, B. C. , van Weert, J. C. , & van den Putte, B. (2016). Informal interpreting in general practice: The migrant patient's voice. *Ethnicity & Health*, 23 (2), 158 – 173.

[28] Cox, A. , Rosenberg, E. , Thommeret-Carrière, A. , Huyghens, L. , Humblé, P. , & Leanza, Y. (2019). Using patient companions as interpreters in the emergency department: An interdisciplinary quantitative and qualitative assessment. *Patient Education and Counseling*, 102 (8), 1439 – 1445.

[29] Pines, R. L. , Jones, L. , & Sheeran, N. (2019). Using family members as medical interpreters: An explanation of healthcare practitioners' normative practices in pediatric and neonatal departments in Australia. *Health Communication*, 35 (7), 902 – 909.

第二章

突发公共卫生事件

1　导读

本章重点为口译技巧之记忆技巧和突发公共卫生事件的 6 篇"口译实战"练习。口译实战练习中英译汉、汉译英各 3 篇，内容涵盖突发公共卫生事件介绍、2019 冠状病毒病流行、严重急性呼吸综合征冠状病毒 2、埃博拉病毒病、中东呼吸综合征和疫苗与免疫接种。请结合本章口译技巧练习 6 篇口译实战文本。

2　口译技巧——记忆技巧

口译记忆，特别是在交替传译场景下，分为长时记忆（long-term memory）和短时记忆（short-term memory）。

长时记忆是指平时对该学科、该主题的背景知识和词汇的积累和记忆。在医学、法学、科技、金融等专业性较强的领域中，长时记忆对译员能否胜任口译工作起着决定性作用。正因如此，我们可以观察到一种新兴的现象，即没有接受过任何口译技巧训练的医生，可以担任其特定领域的交替传译甚至同声传译工作。因为在口译过程中，医生调动的是该领域丰富的长时记忆。反观之，如果译员希望做好医学领域口译，那么译员也需要长期系统性输入医学背景知识和词汇。

短时记忆是指在口译过程中，通过一定的技巧，结合口译笔记，对信息进行分析和重组的记忆能力。"三分在记，七分在听"，这句话笼统地概括了口译笔记和短时记忆的比例关系。但是在不同的场景和不同的译员身上，该比例是浮动的。如在医学口译中，如果译员的长时记忆（背景知识）储备足够，则可选择将更多精力放在听、理解和输出上。如果该部分内容数字密集，则译员可选择将更多的精力放在记笔记上。

短时记忆是可训练、可塑造的。短时记忆提升的关键在于"逻辑"（logic），即通过信息组织（organization）和信息组块化（chunking）的方式梳理原文逻辑、重建原文结构，数字、人名等内容可以通过大脑重复（mental repetition/rehearsal）等方式记忆，译员也可自由使用信息视觉化（visualization）和信息联想（association）等方式记忆信息。

信息组织是指梳理原文的逻辑结构，边听边把原文分为有意义的意群。信息组块化是指将片段化的信息通过有意义的方式进行重组。信息视觉化是指将信息以思维导图、画面、图示等方式呈现。

　　接下来我们通过本章中口译实战的篇章节选演示以上记忆技巧的应用。如接下来这一段：

　　　　当感染者咳嗽、打喷嚏、说话、唱歌或呼吸时，病毒可以从感染者的嘴或鼻子中以小液体颗粒形式传播出来。这些颗粒从较大的呼吸道飞沫到较小的气溶胶不等。练习呼吸礼仪很重要，例如咳嗽时弯曲肘部遮挡口鼻，如果感觉不适，请留在家中自我隔离，直到康复。

　　该段中有意义的意群有三个：（1）病毒以颗粒形式传播；（2）颗粒的范围；（3）呼吸礼仪。

　　划分意群后，我们怎样才能记住意群中的细节呢？这就需要调动其他的记忆技巧了。我们可以将咳嗽、打喷嚏、说话、唱歌或呼吸这一系列的动作视觉化，想象自己先咳嗽，继而打了个喷嚏，然后想唱唱歌，再缓口气儿等，通过有趣的视觉化和联想，记忆第一个意群的细节。最后一个意群的信息同样可以通过视觉化和联想的方式记忆，可以想象自己弯曲肘部打了个喷嚏，仍然感觉不适，决定居家隔离，最终痊愈。

　　正如上文所说，短时记忆可训练、可塑造，但是过程确实是比较漫长和艰难的。口译初学者一旦接触了口译笔记，就很容易将过多精力放在记笔记上，以为这样就能记住更多的信息。但是口译过程中，笔记过多非但不利于口译实践，反而会影响对原文的整体性理解和对译文的输出。这也是为什么现在口译教学和训练通常把记忆技巧安排在口译笔记之前。

　　训练短时记忆的方法如下：

　　（1）选取较有逻辑的原文（中文和英文皆需要训练）。切忌一开始训练短时记忆就选用没有逻辑、语速太快和难度太大的文本。

　　（2）听第一遍，进行原语复述。

　　（3）听第二遍，进行译语复述，只需记住意群。

　　（4）听第三遍，进行译语复述，要求记住意群中的细节信息。

　　（5）根据需要，重复以上步骤，直至较为完整地复述出篇章内容。

3　口译词汇

3.1　英译汉

（一）Public Health Emergency 突发公共卫生事件

occupational poisoning 职业中毒

Public Health Emergency of International Concern（PHEIC）国际关注的突发公共卫生事件

International Health Regulation（IHR）《国际卫生条例》

National Emergency Plan for Public Health Emergencies《国家突发公共卫生事件应急预案》

pneumonic plague 肺鼠疫

pulmonary anthrax 肺炭疽

atypical pneumonia 非典型肺炎

pathogenic avian influenza 高致病性禽流感

virulent strain 烈性病菌株

pathogenic factor 致病因子

（二）COVID-19 Pandemic 2019 冠状病毒病流行

mild to moderate respiratory illness 轻度至中度呼吸道疾病

underlying medical condition 基础疾病

cardiovascular disease 心血管疾病

diabetes 糖尿病

chronic respiratory disease 慢性呼吸道疾病

respiratory droplet 呼吸道飞沫

aerosol 气溶胶

flexed elbow 弯曲肘部

self-isolate 自我隔离

social distancing 社交距离

well-ventilated 通风良好

sore throat 咽痛

diarrhea 腹泻

rash 皮疹

discolouration 变色

shortness of breath 呼吸急促

（三）SARS-CoV-2 严重急性呼吸综合征冠状病毒 2

International Committee on Taxonomy of Viruses（ICTV）国际病毒分类委员会

severe acute respiratory syndrome coronavirus 2（SARS-CoV-2）严重急性呼吸综合征冠状病毒 2

Severe Acute Respiratory Syndrome（SARS）严重急性呼吸综合征（通称非典型肺炎）

Rhinolophus 菊头蝠属

genome sequence 基因组序列

human cell receptor 人类细胞受体

spillover 溢出

genetic mutation 基因突变

lineage 谱系

variant 变体

the Delta variant 德尔塔变体

contagious 传染的

unvaccinated people 未接种疫苗的人群

viral genetic material 病毒遗传物质

3.2 汉译英

（一）埃博拉病毒病 Ebola Virus Disease

埃博拉出血热 Ebola haemorrhagic fever（EHF）

人畜共患 zoonotic

灵长类动物 primate

排泄物 excretion

病原体 causative agent

丝状病毒科 Filoviridae family

埃博拉病毒属 the genus Ebolavirus

宿主 host

果蝠 fruit bats（Rousettus leschenaulti）

几内亚 Guinea

塞拉利昂 Sierra Leone

利比里亚 Liberia

刚果民主共和国 Democratic Republic of the Congo

乌干达 Uganda

流行病学关联 epidemiological link

几乎没有任何风险 negligible to no risk

（二）中东呼吸综合征 Middle East Respiratory Syndrome

输入性 imported

中东呼吸综合征冠状病毒 Middle East Respiratory Syndrome Coronavirus
（MERS-CoV）

沙特阿拉伯 Saudi Arabia

阿联酋 United Arab Emirates（UAE）

约旦 Jordan

科威特 Kuwait

阿曼 Oman

卡塔尔 Qatar

也门 Yemen

埃及 Egypt

突尼斯 Tunisia

呼吸衰竭 respiratory failure

机械通气 mechanical ventilation

支持治疗 supportive treatment

肾衰竭 renal failure

感染性休克 septic shock

单峰骆驼 dromedary camel

免疫力低下 weakened immunity

（三）疫苗与免疫接种 Vaccine and Vaccination

白喉 diphtheria

破伤风 tetanus

百日咳 pertussis

流感 influenza

麻疹 measles

抗体 antibodies

病菌 germ

宫颈癌 cervical cancer

霍乱 cholera

乙型肝炎 hepatitis B

流行性感冒 influenza

日本脑炎 Japanese encephalitis

脑膜炎 meningitis

腮腺炎 mumps

肺炎 pneumonia

脊髓灰质炎 polio

狂犬病 rabies

轮状病毒 rotavirus

风疹 rubella

伤寒 typhoid

水痘 varicella

黄热病 yellow fever

口服小儿麻痹糖丸 oral Poliomyelitis vaccine

脊髓灰质炎病毒 polio virus

4 口译实战

4.1 英译汉

（一）Public Health Emergency 突发公共卫生事件[1-2]

Public health emergencies refer to major infectious disease outbreaks, mass diseases of unknown causes, major food and occupational poisonings, and other events that seriously affect public health that occur suddenly and cause or may

突发公共卫生事件，是指突然发生，造成或者可能造成公众健康严重损害的重大传染病疫情、群体性不明原因疾病、重大食物和职业中毒以及其他严重影响公众健康的事件。

cause serious damage to public health.

A Public Health Emergency of International Concern (PHEIC) is defined in the International Health Regulation (IHR 2005) as, " an extraordinary event which is determined to constitute a public health risk to other States through the international spread of disease and to potentially require a coordinated international response". This definition implies a situation that is: serious, sudden, unusual or unexpected; carries implications for public health beyond the affected State's national border; and may require immediate international action.

According to the classification of China's " National Emergency Plan for Public Health Emergencies ", based on the nature, severity, and scope of public health emergencies, public health emergencies are classified into the following four levels including especially serious emergency (Level I), serious emergency (Level II), large emergency (Level III) and ordinary emergency (Level IV).

Among them, especially serious

《国际卫生条例》（2005）将国际关注的突发公共卫生事件定义为"通过疾病的国际传播构成对其他国家的公共卫生风险，以及可能需要采取协调一致的国际应对措施的不同寻常事件"。该定义意味着：情况严重、突然、不寻常或意外；公共卫生影响超出了受影响国家的边界；可能需要立即采取国际行动。

根据中国《国家突发公共卫生事件应急预案》的分级，基于突发公共卫生事件性质、危害程度、涉及范围，突发公共卫生事件划分为特别重大（I级）、重大（II级）、较大（III级）和一般（IV级）四级。

其中，特别重大突发公共卫生事

public health emergencies （Level Ⅰ） mainly include：（1）The occurrence of pneumonic plague and pulmonary anthrax in large and medium-sized cities with a tendency to spread, or pneumonic plague and pulmonary anthrax that have spread to more than two provinces and have a tendency to spread further.

（2）Cases of infectious atypical pneumonia and human infection of highly pathogenic avian influenza, with a tendency to spread. （3）Massive diseases of unknown origin involving multiple provinces, with a tendency to spread. （4）The occurrence of a new infectious disease or the occurrence or introduction of an infectious disease that has not yet been discovered in China, with a tendency to spread, or it is discovered that an infectious disease that has been eliminated in China has returned to epidemic.

（5）Loss of virulent strains, virus strains, and pathogenic factors. （6） Incidents of severe infectious disease outbreaks and imported cases in the surrounding areas and countries and regions that are in transit with China, seriously endangering my country's public

件（Ⅰ级）主要包括：（1）肺鼠疫、肺炭疽在大、中城市发生并有扩散趋势，或肺鼠疫、肺炭疽疫情波及2个以上的省份，并有进一步扩散趋势。

（2）出现传染性非典型肺炎、人感染高致病性禽流感病例，并有扩散趋势。（3）涉及多个省份的群体性不明原因疾病，并有扩散趋势。（4）发生新传染病或中国尚未发现的传染病发生或传入，并有扩散趋势，或发现中国已消灭的传染病重新流行。

（5）发生烈性病菌株、毒株、致病因子等丢失事件。（6）周边以及与我国通航的国家和地区发生特大传染病疫情，并出现输入性病例，严重危及我国公共卫生安全的事件。（7）国务院卫生行政部门认定的其他特别重大突发公共卫生事件。

health safety. （7） Other particularly major public health emergencies recognized by the health administration department of the State Council.

（二）COVID-19 Pandemic 2019 冠状病毒病流行[3]

Coronavirus disease 2019 （COVID-19） is an infectious disease caused by the SARS-CoV-2 virus. Most people infected with the virus will experience mild to moderate respiratory illness and recover without requiring special treatment. However, some will become seriously ill and require medical attention. Older people and those with underlying medical conditions like cardiovascular disease, diabetes, chronic respiratory disease, or cancer are more likely to develop serious illness. Anyone can get sick with COVID-19 and become seriously ill or die at any age.

The best way to prevent and slow down transmission is to be well informed about the disease and how the virus spreads. Protect yourself and others from infection by staying at least 1 metre apart from others, wearing a properly fitted mask, and washing your hands or using an alcohol-based rub frequently.

2019 冠状病毒病（新冠肺炎）是一种由严重急性呼吸综合征冠状病毒2引起的传染病。大多数感染该病毒的人会出现轻度至中度呼吸道疾病，无须特殊治疗即可康复。然而，有些人会病得很重，需要就医。老年人和患有心血管疾病、糖尿病、慢性呼吸道疾病或癌症等基础疾病的人更有可能发展为重症。任何人在任何年龄都可能感染该病，转为重症甚至死亡。

预防和减缓传播的最佳方法是充分了解疾病以及病毒的传播方式。通过与他人保持至少1米的距离、佩戴合适的口罩、勤洗手或经常使用含酒精的免洗洗手液来保护自己和他人免受感染。

The virus can spread from an infected person's mouth or nose in small liquid particles when he or she cough, sneeze, speak, sing or breathe. These particles range from larger respiratory droplets to smaller aerosols. It is important to practice respiratory etiquette, for example by coughing into a flexed elbow, and to stay home and self-isolate until you recover if you feel unwell.

To prevent infection and to slow transmission of COVID-19, do the following: Get vaccinated when a vaccine is available to you. Stay at least 1 metre apart from others, even if they don't appear to be sick. Wear a properly fitted mask when social distancing is not possible or when in poorly ventilated settings. Choose open, well-ventilated spaces over closed ones. Open a window if indoors.

Wash your hands regularly with soap and water or clean them with alcohol-based hand rub. Cover your mouth and nose when coughing or sneezing. If you feel unwell, stay home and self-isolate until you recover. COVID-19 affects different people in different ways. Most infected

当感染者咳嗽、打喷嚏、说话、唱歌或呼吸时，病毒可以从感染者的嘴或鼻子中以小液体颗粒形式传播出来。这些颗粒从较大的呼吸道飞沫到较小的气溶胶不等。练习呼吸礼仪很重要，例如咳嗽时弯曲肘部遮挡口鼻，如果感觉不适，请留在家中自我隔离，直到康复。

为预防感染和减缓该病的传播，请采取以下措施：当有疫苗可用时接种疫苗。与他人保持至少 1 米的距离，即使他们看起来没有生病。当无法保持社交距离或处于通风不良的环境中时，请佩戴合适的口罩。选择开放、通风良好的空间而不是封闭的空间。如果在室内，请打开窗户。

定期用肥皂和水洗手，或用含酒精的免洗洗手液清洁双手。咳嗽或打喷嚏时捂住口鼻。如果您感到不适，请待在家里并自我隔离，直到您康复为止。该病以不同的方式影响不同的人。大多数感染者会出现轻度到中度呼吸道疾病，无须住院即可康复。

people will develop mild to moderate illness and recover without hospitalization.

最常见的症状包括发烧、干咳、疲倦以及失去味觉或嗅觉。不太常见的症状包括咽痛、头痛、腹泻、皮疹、手指或脚趾变色、眼睛发红或发炎。严重症状包括呼吸困难或呼吸急促、失去言语或行动能力、意识模糊和胸痛。

Most common symptoms include fever, cough, tiredness and loss of taste or smell. Less common symptoms include sore throat, headache, diarrhea, a rash on skin, discoloration of fingers or toes, and red or irritated eyes. Serious symptoms include difficulty in breathing or shortness of breath, loss of speech or mobility, confusion and chest pain.

Seek immediate medical attention if you have serious symptoms. Always call before visiting your doctor or health facility. People with mild symptoms who are otherwise healthy should manage their symptoms at home. On average it takes 5−6 days from when someone is infected with the virus for symptoms to show, however it can take up to 14 days.

如果出现严重症状，请立即就医。在去看医生或去医疗机构之前一定要打电话预约。症状轻微但其他方面健康的人应该居家恢复。从感染病毒到症状显现平均需要 5~6 天，但也可能需要 14 天。

（三）SARS-CoV-2 严重急性呼吸综合征冠状病毒 2 [4-7]

International Committee on Taxonomy of Viruses（ICTV）announced "severe acute respiratory syndrome coronavirus 2（SARS-CoV-2）" as the name of the new virus on 11 February 2020. This name was chosen because the virus is genetically related to the coronavirus

2020 年 2 月 11 日，国际病毒分类委员会宣布将此新病毒命名为"严重急性呼吸综合征冠状病毒 2（SARS-CoV-2）"。选择这一名称是因为该病毒与导致 2003 年严重急性呼吸综合征（SARS）疫情的冠状病毒在基因上相互关联。这两个病毒虽然相关，

responsible for the Severe Acute Respiratory Syndrome（SARS）outbreak of 2003. While related, the two viruses are different.

All SARS-CoV-2 isolated from humans to date are closely related genetically to coronaviruses isolated from bat populations, specifically, bats from the genus Rhinolophus. SARS-CoV, the cause of the SARS outbreak in 2003, is also closely related to coronaviruses isolated from bats.

These close genetic relations suggest that they all have their ecological origin in bat populations. Bats in the Rhinolophus genus are found across Asia, Africa, the Middle East, and Europe. SARS-CoV-2 is not genetically related to other known coronaviruses found in farmed or domestic animals. The analysis of the virus genome sequences also indicates that SARS-CoV-2 is very well adapted to human cell receptors, which enables it to invade human cells and easily infect people.

All the published genetic sequences of SARS-CoV-2 isolated from human cases are very similar. The analyses of

但却有不同。

迄今为止，从人类身上分离的所有该病毒在基因上都与从蝙蝠种群中分离出的冠状病毒密切相关，特别是从菊头蝠属蝙蝠中分离出来的冠状病毒。SARS 冠状病毒导致 2003 年非典型肺炎暴发，它也与从蝙蝠身上分离出的冠状病毒密切相关。

这些密切的遗传关系表明它们都起源于蝙蝠种群。菊头蝠属蝙蝠遍布亚洲、非洲、中东和欧洲。该病毒与在养殖或家养动物中发现的其他已知冠状病毒在基因上没有关系。对病毒基因组序列的分析也表明，该病毒高度适应人类细胞受体，使其能够侵入人体细胞并轻松感染人类。

从人类病例中分离出的所有已发表的该病毒基因序列都非常相似。对已发表的基因序列的分析则进一步表

the published genetic sequences further suggest that the spillover from an animal source to humans happened during the last quarter of 2019.

Viruses like SARS-CoV-2 continuously evolve as mistakes（genetic mutations）occur during replication of the genome. A lineage is a genetically closely related group of virus variants derived from a common ancestor. A variant has one or more mutations that differentiate it from other variants of the SARS-CoV-2 viruses.

The Delta variant is more contagious：The Delta variant is highly contagious, more than twice as contagious as previous variants. Some data suggest the Delta variant might cause more severe illness than previous variants in unvaccinated people.

People infected with the Delta variant, including fully vaccinated people with symptomatic breakthrough infections, can transmit the virus to others. For people infected with the Delta variant, similar amounts of viral genetic material have been found among both unvaccinated and fully vaccinated people.

明，病毒从动物到人类的传播发生在2019年最后一个季度。

严重急性呼吸综合征冠状病毒2这样的病毒会随着基因组复制过程中发生的错误（基因突变）而不断进化。谱系是来自共同祖先的、基因密切相关的一组病毒变体。变体具有一个或多个突变，突变将新冠病毒的一个变体与其他变体区分开来。

Delta变体更具传染性：Delta变体具有高度传染性，其传染性是之前变体的2倍以上。一些数据表明，在未接种疫苗的人群中，与以前的变体相比，Delta变体引起的疾病可能更严重。

感染了Delta变体的人，包括完成疫苗接种的有症状的突破性感染者，可以将病毒传播给他人。对于感染了Delta变体的人，在未接种疫苗和完成疫苗接种的人群中都发现了相似数量的病毒遗传物质。

4.2 汉译英

（一）埃博拉病毒病 Ebola Virus Disease [8-10]

埃博拉病毒病（EVD）也被称为埃博拉出血热，被认为是一种新出现的人畜共患疾病。它是一种影响人类和非人类灵长类动物的严重传染病，可以通过直接接触受感染的人类或动物的组织、血液、其他体液和排泄物传播给人类。

Ebola virus disease （EVD） is also known as Ebola haemorrhagic fever and is considered to be an emerging zoonotic disease. It is a severe contagious disease affecting humans and non-human primates. It can be transmitted to humans through direct contact with tissue, blood, other body fluids, and excretions from an infected human or animal.

其病原体归入丝状病毒科的埃博拉病毒属。在人类埃博拉病毒病暴发期间，人与人之间的传播是通过接触感染者的体液或排泄物而发生的。埃博拉病毒的天然宿主尚未得到证实，但果蝠可能是埃博拉病毒的天然宿主，目前被认为是主要的动物宿主。

The causative agent is classified in the genus Ebolavirus of the Filoviridae family. During Ebola outbreaks in humans, human to human transmission occurs through contact with body fluids or excretions of an infected person. The natural host of Ebola has not yet been confirmed, but fruit bats （Rousettus leschenaulti） may be natural hosts and are currently thought to be the principal animal host.

1976 年，首次埃博拉病毒病暴发发生在中非偏远村庄的人类身上。此后，它在几内亚、塞拉利昂和利比里亚等国家之间蔓延。在刚果民主共和国目前暴发的埃博拉病毒病和乌干达的埃博拉事件中的传播机制都是人与人之间的病毒转移。迄今，没有在此次疫情暴发中发现人类病例与接触动

The first Ebola outbreaks occurred in humans in remote villages in Central Africa in 1976. It has since spread between countries from Guinea to Sierra Leone and Liberia. The mechanism of spread of Ebola in the current outbreak in the Democratic Republic of the Congo and the Ebola event in Uganda is human-

物或动物产品之间的流行病学关联。

蝙蝠被认为是埃博拉病毒的主要动物宿主。除蝙蝠外，捕杀、屠宰、处理和食用健康的野生动物时如果保持良好的卫生习惯、正确保护自己并采用适当的烹饪方法，对人类几乎没有任何风险。

食用经过妥善料理和烹饪的健康家畜的肉是安全的。不要处理、出售、料理或消费因不明原因生病或死亡的野生动物或家畜的肉。不要食用野生动物生肉或用野生动物血液制作的未煮熟的菜肴。这么做会使人有较高的感染风险。

联合国粮食及农业组织（FAO）通过启动组织内部的埃博拉事件协调小组，充分参与国家、区域和国际各级的多部门协调。世界卫生组织

to-human transfer of the virus. To date, there is no epidemiological link between human cases in this outbreak and exposure in this outbreak to animals or animal products.

Bats are believed to be the principal animal hosts of Ebola viruses. With the exception of bats, healthy, wild animals hunted, slaughtered, handled and consumed as wild meat present negligible to no risk to humans if good hygiene, proper protection and appropriate cooking practices are followed.

Meat from healthy livestock that is safely prepared and cooked remains safe to eat. People should not handle, sell, prepare or consume meat that originates from wild animals or livestock that are sick or that have died from unknown causes. Raw wild meat or uncooked dishes based on the blood of wild animals should not be consumed. These practices place people at high risk of contracting any number of infections.

Food and Agriculture Organization of the United Nations （FAO） is fully engaged in the multisectoral coordination at the national, regional and international

（WHO）是有关疫情的人类健康方面的权威和主要信息来源。

levels through the activation of an internal FAO Ebola Incident Coordination Group. The World Health Organization （WHO） is the authority and primary source of information regarding the human health aspects of this outbreak.

（二）中东呼吸综合征 Middle East Respiratory Syndrome[11-12]

2015 年 5 月 29 日，中国首例输入性中东呼吸综合征（Middle East Respiratory Syndrome，MERS）患者在广东惠州确诊。中东呼吸综合征是一种由称为中东呼吸综合征冠状病毒（MERS-CoV）的病毒（更具体地说是冠状病毒）引起的疾病。

On May 29, 2015, the first imported Middle East Respiratory Syndrome （MERS） patient in China was diagnosed in Huizhou, Guangdong Province. MERS is an illness caused by a virus （more specifically, a coronavirus） called Middle East Respiratory Syndrome Coronavirus （MERS-CoV）.

中东呼吸综合征冠状病毒于 2012 年 9 月在沙特阿拉伯首次被发现，它与曾经在中国流行的 SARS 病毒同属冠状病毒，但分属不同的分支。中东呼吸综合征主要流行于中东地区，如沙特阿拉伯、阿联酋、约旦、科威特、阿曼、卡塔尔和也门，以及非洲的埃及和突尼斯等国；中东以外地区报告的所有病例最初均在中东被感染，然后输入中东以外地区。

MERS-CoV was first discovered in Saudi Arabia in September 2012. It belongs to the same coronavirus as the SARS virus that once circulated in China, but belongs to different branches. MERS is mainly prevalent in the Middle East, such as Saudi Arabia, UAE, Jordan, Kuwait, Oman, Qatar and Yemen, and Egypt and Tunisia in Africa; all cases reported outside the Middle East were initially infected in the Middle East and then imported outside the Middle East area.

中东呼吸综合征患者一般在感染后2～14天发病，典型病例常出现发热、咳嗽、气促等症状，在检查中经常发现肺炎表现。重症病例可能出现呼吸衰竭，需要在重症监护室内机械通气和支持治疗。部分病例可出现器官衰竭，尤其是肾衰竭和感染性休克。病死率为40%左右。

目前的研究表明，单峰骆驼是人类最可能的感染源，蝙蝠可能是宿主之一，但整个感染源尚不完全清楚。传染途径也尚未得到充分确认，目前主要认为通过密切接触和飞沫传播。患有糖尿病、慢性肺病、肾衰竭或免疫力低下的人群被认为是中东呼吸综合征冠状病毒感染的高危人群。因此，这些人应避免与骆驼接触、饮用生骆驼奶、接触骆驼尿液或食用未煮熟的肉。

MERS patients generally develop symptoms 2 - 14 days after infection. Typical cases often present symptoms such as fever, cough, and shortness of breath. Pneumonia is often found during the examination. Severe cases can experience respiratory failure, requiring mechanical ventilation and supportive treatment in the intensive care unit. Organ failure may occur in some cases, especially renal failure and septic shock. The case fatality rate is about 40%.

Current research shows that dromedary camels are the most likely source of human infection, and bats may be one of the hosts, but the entire source of infection is not fully understood. The route of transmission has not yet been fully confirmed. At present, it is mainly thought to be spread through close contact and droplets. People with diabetes, chronic lung disease, kidney failure, or weakened immunity are considered to be at high risk of MERS-CoV infection. Therefore, these people should avoid contact with camels, drinking raw camel milk, contact with camel urine or eating uncooked meat.

（三）疫苗与免疫接种 Vaccine and Vaccination [13-15]

免疫接种是全球健康和发展的成功典范，它每年拯救几百万人的生命。疫苗通过与身体的天然防御系统协同作用来建立保护网，从而降低感染疾病的风险。当接种疫苗时，人体的免疫系统会做出反应。

Immunization is a successful example of global health and development, saving millions of lives every year. Vaccines reduce risks of diseases by working with your body's natural defences to build protection. When you are vaccinated, your immune system responds accordingly.

我们现在拥有的疫苗可以预防20多种危及生命的疾病。目前，免疫接种每年防止200万至300万人死于白喉、破伤风、百日咳、流感和麻疹。

We now have vaccines to prevent more than 20 life-threatening diseases. Immunization currently prevents 2-3 million deaths every year from diseases like diphtheria, tetanus, pertussis, influenza and measles.

疫苗能训练人体的免疫系统产生抗体，就像人体暴露在疾病下一样。然而，因为疫苗只含有已灭活或减毒的病毒或细菌，它们不会让人生病，也不会使身体出现并发症。

Vaccines train your immune system to create antibodies, just as it does when it's exposed to a disease. However, because vaccines contain only killed or weakened viruses or bacteria, they do not cause the disease or put you at risk of its complications.

疫苗可以预防许多不同的疾病，包括宫颈癌、霍乱、白喉、乙型肝炎、流行性感冒、日本脑炎、麻疹、脑膜炎、腮腺炎、百日咳、肺炎、脊髓灰质炎、狂犬病、轮状病毒、风疹、破伤风、伤寒、水痘、黄热病等。

Vaccines protect against many different diseases, including cervical cancer, cholera, diphtheria, hepatitis B, influenza, Japanese encephalitis, measles, meningitis, mumps, pertussis, pneumonia, polio, rabies, rotavirus, rubella, tetanus, typhoid, varicella, yellow fever, etc.

通过口服脊髓灰质炎疫苗，自1995年后，中国即阻断了本土脊髓灰质炎病毒的传播，使成千上万名儿童避免了肢体残疾。普及新生儿乙肝疫苗接种后，中国5岁以下儿童乙肝病毒携带率已从1992年的9.7%降至2014年的0.3%。普及儿童计划免疫前，白喉每年可导致数以十万计儿童发病，2006年后，中国已无白喉病例报告。国家免疫规划的实施有效地保护了广大儿童的健康和生命安全。不断提高免疫服务质量，维持高水平接种率是全社会的责任。

Through oral Poliomyelitis vaccine, China has blocked the spread of local polio virus since 1995, and has prevented thousands of children from physical disabilities. After the popularization of neonatal hepatitis B vaccination, children under 5 years of age in China have been vaccinated against hepatitis B. The virus carrying rate dropped from 9.7% in 1992 to 0.3% in 2014. Before universal childhood immunization, diphtheria affected hundreds of thousands of children every year. Since 2006, there have been no reports of diphtheria cases in China. The implementation of the national immunization program has effectively protected the health and life safety of children. It is the responsibility of the whole society to continuously improve the quality of immunization services and maintain a high level of vaccination rate.

5　口译注释与学习资源

5.1　口译注释

（一）科/属

科/属是本章中涉及的比较专业且容易混淆的概念之一。现代生物分类采用界（Kingdom）、门（Phylum）、纲（Class）、目（Order）、科（Family）、属（Genus）、种（Species）7个必要的阶元。从界到种，均可设"亚级"（Sub），如亚门（Subphylum）、亚目（Suborder）、亚科（Subfamily）等。在目和科上，有时可加上"总级"（Super），如总目（Superorder）、总科（Superfamily）。亚科和属之间，有时加"族级"（Tribe）。

（二）贮主/宿主

与科/属一样，贮主/宿主也是本章中涉及的比较专业且容易混淆的概念。先来看一下下面这段文字。

2020年5月第73届世界卫生大会要求，世界卫生组织总干事与合作伙伴一道查明引发Covid-19疫情的新型冠状病毒的人畜共患来源及其传播给人的途径，包括中间宿主可能发挥的作用。溯源的目的是预防动物和人类被该病毒再次感染，避免形成新的人畜共患的贮主，以及降低人畜共患疾病出现和传播的更大的风险。

以上这段文字摘抄自中国—世界卫生组织新型冠状病毒溯源研究联合专家组新闻发布会，同时出现了"贮主"和"宿主"两个表达。在实际应用中，出现较多混用和错用的情况。从病毒学角度来说，"贮主"和"宿主"是两个不同的概念。

（1）贮主 reservoir。

贮主是指传染因子能在其中正常存活、繁殖并传给易感宿主的任何人、兽、节肢动物、植物、土壤或物质（或以上的联合）。It refers to any person, animal, arthropod, plant, soil or substance (or combination of these) in which an infectious agent normally lives and multiplies, on which it depends primarily for survival, and where it reproduces itself in such manner that it can be transmitted to a susceptible host.

（2）宿主 host。

宿主也称为寄主，是指为寄生生物包括寄生虫、病毒等提供生存环境的生物。寄生生物通过寄居在宿主的体内或体表获得营养，寄生生物往往损害宿主，使其生病甚至死亡。It refers to the organisms that provide a living environment for parasites including parasites and viruses. Parasites obtain nutrition by inhabiting the host's body or surface. Parasites often damage the host, causing its illness or even death.

5.2 学习资源

登陆中国大学MOOC（慕课），学习"医疗口译"课程中"突发公共卫生事件"的口译实战示范视频。此外，还可登录世界卫生组织、中国疾病预防控制中心等组织机构官网，学习相关知识。

参考文献

[1] 中国疾病预防控制中心. 突发公共卫生事件 [EB/OL]. [2021 - 08 - 15]. https://www. chinacdc. cn/jkzt/tfggwssj/.

[2] Chinese center for disease control and prevention. (n. d.). *Health emergency*. Retrieved May 14, 2021, from https://www. chinacdc. cn/en/.

[3] World Health Organization. (n. d.). *Coronavirus*. Retrieved November 14, 2021, from https://www. who. int/health-topics/coronavirus#tab = tab_ 1.

[4] Centers for Disease Control and Prevention. (n. d.). *Delta variant: What we know about the science*. Retrieved November 14, 2021, from https://www. cdc. gov/coronavirus/2019 - ncov/variants/delta-variant. html.

[5] World Health Organization. (n. d.). *COVID-19 FAQ virus origin 2020. 1*. Retrieved November 14, 2021, from https://apps. who. int/iris/bitstream/handle/10665/332197/WHO - 2019 - nCoV-FAQ-Virus_ origin - 2020. 1 - eng. pdf.

[6] 世界卫生组织. 2019 冠状病毒病（COVID-19）及其病毒的命名 [EB/OL]. [2021 - 08 - 11]. https://www. who. int/zh/emergencies/diseases/novel-coronavirus - 2019/technical-guidance/naming-the-coronavirus-disease - （covid-2019） - and-the-virus-that-causes-it.

[7] Centers for Disease Control and Prevention. (n. d.). *SARS-COV-2 variant classifications and definitions*. Retrieved November 14, 2021, from https://www. cdc. gov/coronavirus/2019 - ncov/variants/variant-info. html.

[8] 联合国粮食及农业组织. 埃博拉病毒常见问题 [EB/OL]. [2021 - 08 - 22]. https://www. fao. org/3/mm092c/mm092c. pdf.

[9] World Organisation for Animal Health. OIE. (2021, October 20). *Ebola virus disease*. Retrieved November 14, 2021, from https://www. oie. int/en/disease/ebola-virus-disease/.

[10] Food and Agriculture Organization of the United Nations. (n. d.). *Ebola*. Retrieved November 14, 2021, from http://www. fao. org/ebola/en/.

[11] 中国疾病预防控制中心. 中东呼吸综合征释疑 [EB/OL]. [2021 - 08 - 20]. http://www. chinaivdc. cn/mers/mersfangkongzhishi/201506/P020150605381855442340. pdf.

[12] Centers for Disease Control and Prevention. (n. d.). *About Middle East respiratory syndrome (MERS)*. Retrieved November 14, 2021, from https://www. cdc. gov/coronavirus/mers/

about/index. html.

[13] 中国疾病预防控制中心. 免疫规划 [EB/OL]. [2021 - 08 - 20]. https://www. chinacdc. cn/jkzt/ymyjz/.

[14] World Health Organization. (n. d.). *Vaccines and immunization*. Retrieved November 14, 2021, from https://www. who. int/health-topics/vaccines-and-immunization? adgroupsurvey = % 7Badgroupsurvey% 7D&gclid = CjwKCAjwhuCKBhADEiwA1HegOXF0hJ-BTMfV-W804sB1tJQPoewFhdhtVYaGx2p9Z85dmwLzMr9D4hoCjEoQAvD_ BwE#tab = tab_ 1.

[15] 世界卫生组织. 疫苗和免疫接种 [EB/OL]. [2021 - 08 - 24]. https://www. who. int/zh/ health-topics/vaccines-and-immunization? adgroupsurvey = % 7Badgroupsurvey% 7D&gclid = CjwKCAjwhuCKBhADEiwA1HegOeMdeairWMsxDEuKCN8IFGMchVpciiZV0zRbVmQDWk GNhlpNXsH78xoC1hwQAvD_ BwE#tab = tab_ 2.

第三章

初级卫生保健

1 导读

本章重点为口译技巧之口译笔记（1）和初级卫生保健的6篇"口译实战"练习。口译实战练习中英译汉、汉译英各3篇，内容涵盖初级卫生保健/全科医生介绍、社区康复、社区慢性病管理、分级诊疗及社区首诊制度、重性精神疾病管理和传染病管理。请结合本章口译技巧练习6篇口译实战文本。

2 口译技巧——口译笔记（1）

上一章我们讲口译技巧时提到了"三分在记，七分在听"。译员在掌握短时记忆技巧后，接下来需要掌握口译技巧中的另外一项重要技巧——口译笔记。

与普通的课堂会议记录和速写不同，口译笔记有其独特的结构和特点，甚至自成一套"符码"系统。口译笔记通常呈现以下特点：

（1）个人化。译员在记笔记过程中，出于个人习惯，大多数时候采用适合自己的自创的"符码"系统，选择"原语"或"译语"或两者混杂记录。由于精力分配的差别，笔记所体现出的篇章信息也存在差异。这就是为什么译员相互之间很难解读对方的笔记。

（2）瞬时性。译员在口译过程中，调动短时记忆，辅以口译笔记进行信息的转码和解码。记录下的信息仅与当时的口译内容强关联，且与相应的短时记忆相配合才能组成有意义的信息群。这也是过一段时间，口译员即使看着自己的笔记也很难回想起当时的口译内容的原因。

（3）结构化。资深译员的笔记结构会特别清晰，重点突出，而初学译员的笔记结构则较为混乱，记下的大都不是关键词语或符号。译员的笔记架构应反映语言架构和信息架构。如果在笔记环节能完成结构梳理，译员就能分配更多的精力在提升语言质量上。

（4）逻辑性。口译笔记的重要性不仅仅体现在辅助记忆上，更关键的作用在于理清信息逻辑。译员在记笔记的同时应分析和整理原文的逻辑重心和信息模块，深入理解原文，并完成译文的初次加工。

口译笔记的格式主要有缩进式和纵写式。

如图 3-1 所示，通常一行代表一个小意群的关键词，接下来的小意群关键词提行往下写。同一个大意群内容每提一行，往右缩进，直至下一个大意群出现再顶格。图中右下方的三条平行线代表列举内容，显示其并列关系。

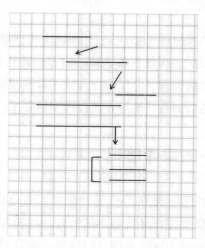

图 3-1 口译笔记格式示例

接下来我们通过本章口译实战的篇章节选演示缩进式和纵写式笔记（见图 3-2 和图 3-3）。

示例 1：PHC entails three inter-related and synergistic components, including comprehensive integrated health services that embrace primary care as well as public health goods and functions as central pieces, multi-sectoral policies and actions to address the upstream and wider determinants of health, and engaging and empowering individuals, families and communities for increased social participation and enhanced self-care and self-reliance in health.

示例 2：截至 2009 年，中国疾病预防控制中心精神卫生中心数据显示，中国各类精神疾病患者人数在 1 亿人以上，重性精神疾病患者人数已超过 1600 万。精神疾病在中国疾病总负担中排名首位，约占疾病总负担的 20%，预计到 2020 年这个比率将上升至 25%。

关
PHC　3
协
基
全&综
公共　品&功
策&动
上&大+
人
参&能
家
区
参与&自

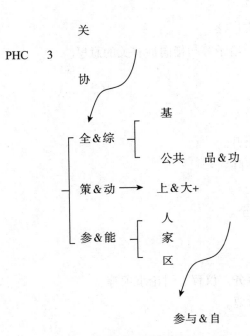

图3-2　示例1的口译笔记

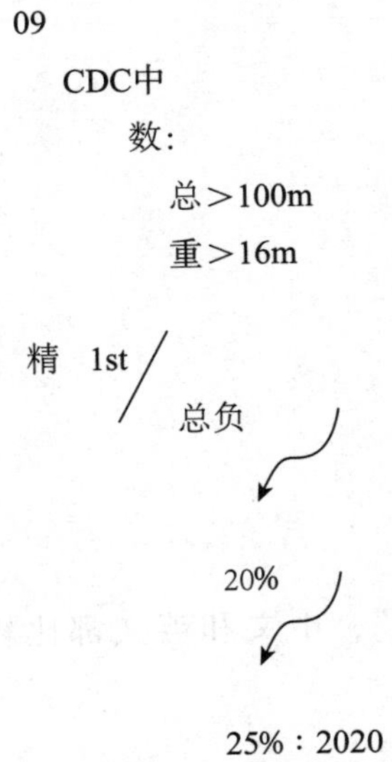

09
CDC中
数:
总>100m
重>16m
精　1st
总负
20%
25%：2020

图3-3　示例2的口译笔记

口译笔记的“符码”包括线条、基本形状（方形、圆形等）、数学符号、中文拼音、标点符号等。

（1）线条：如图3-1、图3-2和图3-3所示，线条，包括箭头符号，在口译笔记中应用非常广泛。

→：表示导致、给予等与指向性有关的意思。

←：表示倒退。

↑：表示上升。

↓：表示下降。

↗：表示缓慢上升。

↘：表示缓慢下降。

↗]：表示上升至。

↘]：表示下降至。

（2）基本形状。

□：表示国家。

≡：表示重要事务、议程、讨论事项等。

☆：表示非常重要。

（3）数学符号。

＋：表示和，加。

≠：表示不等于。

×：表示错误，不选择。

℃：表示温度。

&：表示和。

#：表示影响力。

≈：表示约等于。

☑：表示正确，选择。

@：表示对某人说。

¥：表示金额。

（4）中文拼音。如"繁"，中文和英文都比较复杂，可以用拼音"fan"代替。

（5）标点符号。

!：表示感叹，如非常荣幸"－h!"，非常欢迎"－欢!"。

?：表示提出问题。

::：表示讲话，说，指出。

（）：表示包括。

在接下来的"门诊/急诊"一章中，我们将通过更多的段落示例展示口译中记笔记的方法。

3 口译词汇

3.1 英译汉

（一）初级卫生保健/全科医生 Primary Health Care/General Practitioner

rehabilitation 康复

palliative care 姑息照护

synergistic 协同的

determinant 影响因素

self-care 自我护理

self-reliance 自立

maternal and child health care 母婴保健

endemic disease 地方病

general practitioner（GP）全科医生

family doctor 家庭医生

refer 转诊

（二）Community-based Rehabilitation 社区康复

person with disabilities（PWD）残疾人

Declaration of Alma-Ata《阿拉木图宣言》

functional limitation 功能限制

rehabilitation therapy 康复治疗

eye care 眼保健

hearing 听力

physiotherapy 理疗

occupational therapy 职业治疗

orientation and mobility training 定向和移动训练

speech therapy 言语治疗

psychological counselling 心理辅导

orthotics 矫形器

prosthetics 假肢

intervention 干预

regular schooling 正规教育

special school 特殊学校

sign language 手语

Braille training 盲文培训

（三）Community-based Chronic Disease Management 社区慢性病管理

morbidity 发病率

mortality 死亡率

social ecological perspective 社会生态学观点

patient-physician relationship 医患关系

heart disease 心脏病

community health worker（CHW）社区卫生工作者

cardiovascular disease 心血管疾病

comorbidity 多种合并疾病

mental health 精神健康

3.2 汉译英

（一）分级诊疗及社区首诊制度 Stratified Medical System and Community-based First-contact Healthcare Services

"十三五"规划 The 13th Five Year Plan

分级诊疗制度 stratified medical system

转诊机制 referral system

医疗保险制度 medical insurance system

社区首诊制 community-based first-contact system

新农合的门诊统筹制度 New Rural Cooperative Outpatient Coordination System

（二）重性精神疾病管理 Severe Mental Illness Management

精神分裂症 schizophrenia

双向障碍 bipolar disorder

偏执性精神病 paranoid psychosis

分裂情感障碍 schizoaffective disorder

自知力 insight

中国疾病预防控制中心 Chinese Center for Disease Control and Prevention

疾病总负担 total burden of disease

三级防治网络 three-tier mental illness prevention and treatment network

康复站 rehabilitation station

（三）传染病管理 Infectious Disease Management

《中华人民共和国传染病防治法》Law of the People's Republic of China on Prevention and Treatment of Infectious Diseases

甲类传染病 infectious diseases under Class A

鼠疫 plague

霍乱 cholera

乙类传染病 infectious diseases under Class B

传染性非典型肺炎 infectious SARS

获得性免疫缺陷综合征（艾滋病）acquired immune deficiency syndrome（AIDS）

病毒性肝炎 viral hepatitis

脊髓灰质炎 poliomyelitis

人感染高致病性禽流感 highly pathogenic avian influenza

麻疹 measles

流行性出血热 epidemic hemorrhagic fever

狂犬病 rabies

流行性乙型脑炎 epidemic encephalitis B

登革热 dengue fever

炭疽 anthrax

细菌性和阿米巴性痢疾 bacillary and amebic dysentery

肺结核 pulmonary tuberculosis

伤寒和副伤寒 typhoid and paratyphoid

流行性脑脊髓膜炎 epidemic cerebrospinal meningitis

百日咳 pertussis

白喉 diphtheria

新生儿破伤风 tetanus infantum

猩红热 scarlet fever

布鲁氏菌病 brucellosis

淋病 gonorrhoea

梅毒 syphilis

钩端螺旋体病 leptospirosis

血吸虫病 schistosomiasis

疟疾 malaria

丙类传染病 infectious diseases under Class C

流行性感冒 influenza

流行性腮腺炎 epidemic parotitis

风疹 rubella

急性出血性结膜炎 acute hemorrhagic conjunctivitis

麻风病 leprosy

流行性和地方性斑疹伤寒 epidemic and endemic typhus

黑热病 kala-azar

棘球蚴病 echinococcosis

丝虫病 filariasis

感染性腹泻 infectious diarrhea

病原携带者 pathogen carrier

隔离 isolation

疑似病人 suspected patient

传染病疫情 epidemic situation of infectious disease

流行病学调查 epidemiological investigation

卫生行政部门 health administration department

划定疫点 delimitation of epidemic spot

卫生处理 sanitary treatment

密切接触者 person in close contact

医学观察 medical observation

暴发 break out

流行 prevail

4　口译实战

4.1　英译汉

（一）初级卫生保健/全科医生 Primary Health Care/General Practitioner [1-3]

Primary Health Care（PHC）is a whole-of-society approach to health that aims at ensuring the highest possible level of health and well-being and their equitable distribution by focusing on people's needs and as early as possible along the continuum from health promotion and disease prevention to treatment, rehabilitation and palliative care, and as close as feasible, to people's everyday environment.

初级卫生保健是一种全社会参与卫生事业的方法，旨在确保实现最高可能水平的健康和福祉及其公平分配。从健康促进、疾病预防到治疗、康复和姑息治疗的全过程中，初级卫生保健尽可能在早期介入，满足大众日常生活中的医疗需求。

PHC entails three inter-related and synergistic components, including comprehensive integrated health services that embrace primary care as well as public health goods and functions as central pieces, multi-sectoral policies and actions to address the upstream and wider determinants of health, and engaging and empowering individuals, families, and communities for increased social participation and enhanced self-care and self-reliance in health.

初级卫生保健由以下三个相互关联和协同的部分组成：全面的综合卫生服务，其核心为初级卫生保健、公共卫生产品和功能；跨部门政策和行动，从上游和更广范围关注影响健康的因素；个人、家庭和社区的调动和赋能，社会参与度的提高，卫生方面自我护理和自立能力的增强。

Everyone in the community should

社区中的每个人都应享受初级卫

have access to it and everyone should be involved in it. Related sectors in addition to the health sector should also be involved. At the very least, it should include education for the community on the prevalent health problems and on methods to prevent health problems from arising or to control them. The healthy diet and adequate nutrition should be promoted, with sufficient safe water and basic sanitation, and maternal and child health care, including family planning. The prevention and control of local endemic diseases should be strengthened, with immunization against the main infectious diseases, appropriate treatment of common diseases and the provision of essential drugs.

General Practitioner (GP) is general doctor, or family doctor, who is the first point of contact with the health services for all non-emergency cases. GPs treat all common medical conditions and refer patients to hospitals and other medical services for urgent and specialist treatment. They focus on the health of the whole person, combining physical, psychological and social aspects of care.

生保健，并且参与其中。除卫生部门外，相关部门也应参与。这些部门应至少为大众提供健康教育，普及常见健康问题以及预防和控制该问题的方法，宣传健康的饮食和充足的营养，提供充足的安全用水和基本卫生设施，提供母婴保健，包括计划生育，加强地方病防治，开展主要传染病的免疫接种和常见疾病的正确治疗，并提供基础性药物。

全科医生也称家庭医生，是指非紧急情况下提供医疗服务的第一联系人。全科医生治疗所有常见疾病，并将患者转介到医院和其他医疗服务机构进行紧急和专科治疗。他们注重患者整体健康，结合身体、心理和社会方面的治疗。

（二）Community-based Rehabilitation 社区康复[4-5]

Community-based Rehabilitation (CBR) is a community development strategy that aims at enhancing the lives of persons with disabilities (PWD) within their community. CBR was initiated by WHO following the Declaration of Alma-Ata in 1978 in an effort to enhance the quality of life for people with disabilities and their families, meet their basic needs, and ensure their inclusion and participation.

The components of a CBR programme should include creating a positive attitude towards people with disabilities, which is essential to ensuring equalization of opportunities for people with disabilities within their own community. Positive attitudes among community members can be created by involving them in the process of programme design and implementation, and by transferring knowledge about disability issues to community members.

Often PWDs require assistance to overcome or minimize the effects of their functional limitations (disabilities). In communities where professional services are not accessible or available, CBR workers

社区康复是一项社区发展战略，旨在改善社区内残疾人的生活。社区康复是世界卫生组织在1978年《阿拉木图宣言》之后发起的，旨在提高残疾人及其家人的生活质量，满足他们的基本需求，并确保他们的融入和参与。

社区康复计划的组成部分应包括建立对残疾人的积极态度，这一组成部分对于确保残疾人在其社区内获得平等机会至关重要。通过让社区成员参与计划设计和实施过程，以及将有关残疾问题的知识传授给社区成员，可以在社区成员中建立积极的态度。

残疾人通常需要他人帮助以克服或尽量减少其功能限制（残疾）造成的影响。在无法获取专业服务的社区，社区康复工作者应接受培训，为其提供初级康复治疗和服务，包括眼保健

should be trained to provide primary rehabilitation therapies, including eye care services, hearing services, physiotherapy, occupational therapy, orientation and mobility training, speech therapy, and psychological counselling, and provide devices such as orthotics and prosthetics.

服务、听力服务、理疗、职业治疗、定向和移动训练、言语治疗、心理辅导，并提供矫形器、假肢等设备。

PWDs have equal access to educational opportunities and to training that will enable them to make the best use of the opportunities that occur in their lives. In communities where professional services are not accessible or available, CBR workers should be trained to provide basic services in the following areas: early childhood intervention and referral, especially to medical rehabilitation services, education in regular schools, non-formal education where regular schooling is not available, special education in regular or special schools, sign language training, Braille training, and training in daily living skills.

残疾人应获得平等教育和培训，使他们能够尽量抓住生活中的机会。在无法获得专业服务的社区，社区康复工作者应接受培训以为其提供以下领域的基本服务：幼儿干预和转诊，尤其是转诊至医疗康复机构，普通学校教育，无法接受正规教育时的非正规教育，普通或特殊学校的特殊教育，手语培训，盲文培训和日常生活技能训练。

（三）Community-based Chronic Disease Management 社区慢性病管理[6-7]

With the growing burden of chronic disease, the medical and public health communities are reexamining their roles and opportunities for more effective prevention and clinical interventions. The

随着慢性病负担的增加，医疗和公共卫生界正在重新审视他们的角色和机会，以实现更有效的预防和临床干预。可以通过以下方式有效预防慢性病，显著降低慢性病的发病率和死

potential to significantly improve chronic disease prevention and impact morbidity and mortality from chronic conditions is enhanced by adopting strategies that incorporate a social ecological perspective, realigning the patient-physician relationship, integrating population health perspectives into the chronic care model, and effectively engaging communities using established principles of community engagement.

Chronic diseases such as heart disease, cancer, hypertension, stroke, and diabetes now account for 80% of deaths in the United States (US) and 75% of health care costs. In 2005, 44% of all Americans had at least one chronic condition and 13% had 3 or more. By 2020, an estimated 157 million US residents will have one chronic condition or more. With this growing burden of chronic disease, the medical and public health communities are reexamining their roles and envisioning innovative partnership opportunities for more effective interventions for chronic disease prevention and management at a population level.

Community health workers (CHWs) are locally based health care workers who

亡率：采用社会生态学战略，调整医患关系，开展慢性病护理时纳入人口健康因素，通过现有的社区介入方式充分调动社区。

因心脏病、癌症、高血压、中风和糖尿病等慢性病死亡的人口现在占美国死亡人数的80%，花费的医疗保健费用占总费用的75%。2005年，44%的美国人至少患有一种慢性病，13%患有三种甚至更多。到2020年，估计有1.57亿美国居民患有一种或多种慢性病。随着慢性病负担日益加重，医疗和公共卫生界正在重新审视自己的作用，并希望创新合作方式，在人口层面对慢性病预防和管理进行更有效的干预。

社区卫生工作者是当地的保健工作者。他们的作用非常特殊，他们与

are uniquely situated to provide ongoing behavioral support to a cohort of patients in conjunction with the broader health care team. CHWs have shown to improve health in a wide range of chronic conditions, such as cancer, diabetes, cardiovascular disease, multiple medical comorbidities, and mental problems. The root of their effectiveness relies on their close connection to the community, ability to influence patient behaviors, and effective interaction with the larger health care team. CHWs are powerful drivers of decreased costs, especially among patients with high starting health care costs and among underserved and minority populations.

基础医疗团队合作，共同为患者提供持续的行为支持。社区卫生工作者可以改善许多慢性病患者的健康状况，例如癌症、糖尿病、心血管疾病、多种合并疾病和精神疾病患者。社区卫生工作者高效工作的原因在于其与社区的密切联系，他们有能力影响患者行为，可与规模更大的医疗团队开展有效沟通。社区卫生工作可有效降低医疗成本，尤其是对起步医疗花销特别高的人群和弱势及少数族裔人群来说。

4.2 汉译英

（一）分级诊疗及社区首诊制度 Stratified Medical System and Community-based First-contact Healthcare Services[8-9]

"十三五"规划（2016—2020）深化医疗卫生体制改革，旨在到2020年基本建立符合中国国情的分级诊疗制度。该规划寻求建立各级医疗机构根据患者病情轻重、急迫程度收治患者的分级诊疗制度。大多数常见的健康问题应该在基层医疗机构进行治疗，医疗机构之间也应该有患者转诊机制。

The 13th Five Year Plan（2016 – 2020）for deepening medical and health system reform aims to basically establish a stratified medical treatment system in accordance with China's actual conditions by 2020. It seeks to establish a stratified medical treatment system in which medical institutions at various levels treat patients according to severity and urgency of their disease. Most common health issues should be treated at primary medical institutions, with a proper referral system in between institutions.

分级诊疗制度被认为是解决许多地区存在的医疗资源不足和不平衡问题的关键。专家预计，分级诊疗制度将使各医疗机构各司其职，让患者得到更好的服务。为实现这一目标，专家建议进一步完善医疗保险制度和基层医疗设施。目前中国的基层医疗服务还有很多不足之处，这在一定程度上使得哪怕只是最常见的健康问题患者也要去大医院。

The stratified medical treatment system is regarded as the key to solving the problem of insufficient and unbalanced medical resources in many areas. Experts expect that the stratified medical treatment system will enable medical institutions at various levels to perform better and provide better services to patients. To achieve that goal, experts suggest the medical insurance system as well as primary healthcare facilities be further improved. China's current primary healthcare services awaits to be improved, giving patients no other options than to visit large hospitals for even the most common health issues.

社区首诊制是指当居民患病需要就诊时（除急诊外），必须先到社区卫生机构接受全科医生诊疗的一种制度。早在 2006 年中国就首次提出探索开展社区首诊制试点。此后，深圳、北京、青岛、上海、武汉、重庆六市先后颁布相应的政策法规积极响应。

The community-based first-contact system requires residents to visit the general practitioner except for emergencies in the community healthcare institutions as their first stop of medical services. China proposed the test run of community-based first-contact system as early as 2006. After that, Shenzhen, Beijing, Qingdao, Shanghai, Wuhan and Chongqing promulgated policies and regulations as a positive response.

根据服务对象的类型，可将社区首诊制开展方式分为两类：第一类以深圳、北京和青岛为代表，以特定人群为突破口，借助医疗保险或医疗保障制度，引导这些目标人群在社区首诊，逐步推广至所有城乡居民。第二类以上海、武汉和重庆为代表，以农村居民为切入点，通过新农合的门诊统筹制度，吸引农村居民在基层首诊，后推广到全体居民。

The community-based first-contact system, based on the type of patients, is practiced in two ways. First, in Shenzhen, Beijing and Qingdao, a certain target group of community residents is encouraged to visit the community healthcare institution as their first stop facilitated by the medical insurance and care system. With initial success, such service then covers the whole population within the community. Second, in Shanghai, Wuhan and Chongqing, rural residents as the target group are firstly encouraged to visit the primary healthcare institutions facilitated by the New Rural Cooperative Outpatient Coordination System. With initial success, such service then covers the whole population within the community.

（二）重性精神疾病管理 Severe Mental Illness Management [10-11]

重性精神疾病主要包括精神分裂症、双向障碍、偏执性精神病、分裂情感障碍等。发病时，患者丧失对疾病的自知力或者对行为的控制力，并可能导致危害公共安全行为，长期患病者可以造成社会功能严重损害。

Severe mental illnesses mainly include schizophrenia, bipolar disorder, paranoid psychosis, schizoaffective disorder, etc. With the onset of the illness, patients lose insight of the disease or behavioral control, and may develop behaviors harmful to public safety. Patients with enduring severe mental illness are subjective to substantial damage of their social functions.

截至2009年，中国疾病预防控制中心精神卫生中心数据显示，中国各类精神疾病患者人数在1亿以上，重性精神疾病患者人数已超过1600万，精神疾病在中国疾病总负担中排名首位，约占疾病总负担的20%，预计到2020年这个比率将上升至25%。全国至少有5600万各类精神障碍患者尚未接受过任何医疗服务。仅有1/4重性精神疾病患者接受过正规的精神科医疗服务。

As of 2009, data from the Mental Health Center of the Chinese Center for Disease Control and Prevention showed that there were more than 100 million people with various types of mental illness in China, and more than 16 million people had severe mental illness. Mental illness ranked first in the total burden of disease in China, accounting for about 20% of the total disease burden. This figure was expected to rise up to 25% in 2020. There were at least 56 million people with various mental illnesses in China who had not received health services of any kind. Only a quarter of patients with severe mental illness received formal psychiatric medical services.

2004年"686"项目的实施推动了中国精神疾病三级防治网络的建设，启动了如社区精神疾病患者康复站、家庭病床等多种形式的社区精神康复服务。从2009年开始，中国将重性精神疾病患者的社区管理纳入基本公共卫生服务项目，重性精神疾病患者的社区管理在全国得以普遍开展，但由于此项服务不仅涉及精神卫生专科服

The implementation of the "686" project in 2004 helped develop a three-tier mental illness prevention and treatment network in China. Various forms of community-based mental rehabilitation services including community mental illness rehabilitation stations and family beds are launched. Since 2009, China has incorporated community management

务，还涉及政府和社会服务，各地服务质量差异较大，重性精神疾病患者所带来的社会问题依然严峻。

of patients with severe mental illness into the basic public health service projects. Community management of patients with severe mental illness has been provided throughout China. However, as such management involves not only psychiatric specialty treatment, but also government and social services, which might differ from place to place in quality, we still face grave challenges against social problems caused by patients with severe mental illness.

（三）传染病管理 Infectious Disease Management [12]

《中华人民共和国传染病防治法》规定的传染病分为甲类、乙类和丙类。甲类传染病是指鼠疫、霍乱。乙类传染病是指传染性非典型肺炎、艾滋病、病毒性肝炎、脊髓灰质炎、人感染高致病性禽流感、麻疹、流行性出血热、狂犬病、流行性乙型脑炎、登革热、炭疽、细菌性和阿米巴性痢疾、肺结核、伤寒和副伤寒、流行性脑脊髓膜炎、百日咳、白喉、新生儿破伤风、猩红热、布鲁氏菌病、淋病、梅毒、钩端螺旋体病、血吸虫病、疟疾。①

The infectious diseases governed by the Law of the People's Republic of China on Prevention and Treatment of Infectious Diseases are divided into Classes A, B and C. Infectious diseases under Class A are plague and cholera. Infectious diseases under Class B are infectious SARS, AIDS, viral hepatitis, poliomyelitis, highly pathogenic avian influenza, measles, epidemic hemorrhagic fever, rabies, epidemic encephalitis B, dengue fever, anthrax, bacillary and amebic dysentery, pulmonary tuberculosis, typhoid and paratyphoid, epidemic cerebrospinal meningitis, pertussis, diphtheria, tetanus

---

① 2023 年 10 月十四届全国人大常委会第六次会议对《中华人民共和国传染病防治法（修订草案）》进行了审议，该修订草案对乙类传染病进行了调整，参见中国人大网（www.npc.gov.cn）。

infantum, scarlet fever, brucellosis, gonorrhoea, syphilis, leptospirosis, schistosomiasis and malaria.

丙类传染病是指流行性感冒、流行性腮腺炎、风疹、急性出血性结膜炎、麻风病、流行性和地方性斑疹伤寒、黑热病、棘球蚴病、丝虫病，除霍乱、细菌性和阿米巴性痢疾、伤寒和副伤寒以外的感染性腹泻。

Infectious diseases under Class C are influenza, epidemic parotitis, rubella, acute hemorrhagic conjunctivitis, leprosy, epidemic and endemic typhus, kala-azar, echinococcosis, filariasis. They also include infectious diarrhea other than cholera, bacillary and amebic dysentery, typhoid or paratyphoid.

医疗机构发现甲类传染病时，应当及时采取下列措施：对病人、病原携带者予以隔离治疗，隔离期限根据医学检查结果确定；对疑似病人，确诊前在指定场所单独隔离治疗；对医疗机构内的病人、病原携带者、疑似病人的密切接触者，在指定场所进行医学观察和采取其他必要的预防措施。

When finding an infectious disease under Class A, the medical institution shall immediately take the following measures: isolate the patients and pathogen carriers for treatment, and determine the period of isolation according to the results of medical examination; treat suspected patients separately in isolation at designated places until a definite diagnosis is made; and keep the persons in close contact with the patients, pathogen carriers or suspected patients in medical institutions under medical observation at designated places, and take other necessary preventive measures.

疾病预防控制机构发现传染病疫情或者接到传染病疫情报告时，应当

When finding epidemic situation of infectious diseases or receiving report on

及时采取下列措施：（1）对传染病疫情进行流行病学调查，根据调查情况提出划定疫点、疫区的建议，对被污染的场所进行卫生处理，对密切接触者在指定场所进行医学观察和采取其他必要的预防措施，并向卫生行政部门提出疫情控制方案。

（2）传染病暴发、流行时，对疫点、疫区进行卫生处理，向卫生行政部门提出疫情控制方案，并按照卫生行政部门的要求采取措施。（3）指导下级疾病预防控制机构实施传染病预防、控制措施，组织、指导有关单位对传染病疫情的处理。

such situation, the institutions of disease prevention and control shall timely adopt the following measures：（1）Conduct epidemiological investigation on the epidemic situation of infectious diseases and, on the basis of the findings after such investigation, put forth proposals for the delimitation of epidemic spots and areas, give sanitary treatment to the contaminated places, keep the persons in close contact under medical observation at the designated places and take other necessary preventive measures, and put forth schemes for control of the epidemic situation to health administration departments.

（2）When an infectious disease breaks out and prevails, give sanitary treatment to epidemic spots and areas, put forth schemes for control of epidemic situation to the health administration departments, and take measures in accordance with the requirements of health administration departments. (3) Direct the institutions of disease prevention and control at lower levels in implementing the measures for prevention and control of infectious diseases, and coordinate efforts and direct relevant units in handling the epidemic situation of infectious diseases.

5 口译注释与学习资源

5.1 口译注释

（一）获得性免疫缺陷综合征

获得性免疫缺陷综合征的英语是 acquired immune deficiency syndrome，缩写为 AIDS，一般称为艾滋病，是一种由人类免疫缺陷病毒（human immunodeficiency virus，缩写为 HIV）感染造成的疾病。

（二）感染性疾病（infectious disease）和传染性疾病（communicable disease）

虽然所有传染性疾病都具有感染性，但并非所有感染性疾病都具有传染性。例如，破伤风可引起感染，但不会传染其他人。口语中常说的传染病等同于医学上说的传染性疾病，而口语中说的感染病范围小于医学上说的感染性疾病，常指不具有传染性的感染性疾病，如细菌、真菌感染病。感染性疾病既包含传染病，也包含感染病。当我们做口译或者读英文资料时，看到 infectious disease 要根据语境进行翻译，某些情况下翻译成传染病，某些情况下翻译成感染病，灵活翻译，灵活应对。但其实，在日常医生和普通人交流过程中，当我们说感染性疾病时，都默认是感染病，不具有传染性。

5.2 学习资源

登陆中国大学 MOOC（慕课），学习"医疗口译"课程中"初级卫生保健"的口译实战示范视频。此外还可登录世界卫生组织、中国疾病预防控制中心、英国国民医疗服务体系等组织机构官网学习相关知识。

参考文献

［1］世界卫生组织. 初级卫生保健［EB/OL］.［2021 - 04 - 01］. https://www. who. int/zh/news-room/fact-sheets/detail/primary-health-care.

［2］Pallipedia.（n. d.）. *What is primary health care（PHC）—meaning and definition.* Retrieved November 14，2021，from https://pallipedia. org/primary-health-care-phc/.

［3］NHS.（n. d.）. *General practice.* Retrieved November 14，2021，from https://www. healthcareers. nhs. uk/explore-roles/doctors/roles-doctors/general-practitioner-gp/general-practice-gp.

［4］United Nations Economic and Social Commission for Asia and the Pacific（n. d.）. *Understanding community-based rehabilitation.* Retrieved November 14, 2021, from https://www. dinf. ne. jp/doc/english/intl/z15/z15011un/z1501101. html.

[5] Community Based Rehabilitation (CBR) African Network (CAN). (2019, April 10). *What is CBR?.* Retrieved November 14, 2021, from https://afri-can. org/what-is-cbr/.

[6] Plumb, J., Weinstein, L. C., Brawer, R., & Scott, K. (2012). Community-based partnerships for improving chronic disease management. *Primary Care: Clinics in Office Practice*, 39 (2), 433 - 447. https://doi. org/10. 1016/j. pop. 2012. 03. 011.

[7] Crespo, R., Christiansen, M., Tieman, K., & Wittberg, R. (2020). An emerging model for community health worker-based chronic care management for patients with high health care costs in rural Appalachia. *Preventing Chronic Disease*, 17. https://doi. org/10. 5888/pcd17. 190316.

[8] Chinadaily. com. cn. (2018, March 16). *Hierarchical medical treatment.* Retrieved November 14, 2021, from http://www. chinadaily. com. cn/a/201803/16/WS5aab0546 a3106e7dcc141f40. html.

[9] 北京大学中国卫生发展研究中心简报. 我国城市社区首诊制度研究 [EB/OL]. [2016 - 11 - 30]. https://www. cchds. pku. edu. cn/docs/2018 - 01/201801181805575141 87. pdf.

[10] 中华人民共和国中央人民政府. 卫生部印发重性精神疾病管理治疗工作规范 [EB/OL]. [2012 - 04 - 12]. http://www. gov. cn/gzdt/2012 - 04/12/content_ 2112111. htm.

[11] 冯斯特, 刘素珍. 国内重性精神疾病患者社区管理现状与对策 [J]. 中华护理杂志, 2014, 49 (06): 764 - 768.

[12] 中国人大网. 中华人民共和国传染病防治法 [EB/OL]. [2013 - 10 - 22]. http://www. npc. gov. cn/wxzl/gongbao/2013 - 10/22/content_ 1811005. htm.

第四章

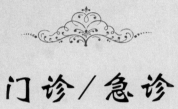

门诊/急诊

1　导读

本章重点为口译技巧之口译笔记（2）和门诊/急诊的 6 篇"口译实战"练习。口译实战练习中英译汉、汉译英各 3 篇，内容涵盖门诊/急诊简介、烧伤、急性中毒、创伤诱发性凝血病、心肺复苏和急性胸痛。请结合本章口译技巧练习 6 篇口译实战文本。

2　口译技巧——口译笔记（2）

本章中，我们将选取 6 篇口译实战练习中的 12 个段落，展示口译笔记（见图 4-1 至图 4-12）。

例 1：Often, one may hear the terms "outpatient" or "inpatient" used when referring to a type of diagnostic or therapeutic procedure. "Inpatient" means that the procedure requires the patient to be admitted to the hospital, primarily so that he or she can be closely monitored during the procedure and afterwards, during recovery. "Outpatient" means that the procedure does not require hospital admission and may also be performed outside the premises of a hospital.

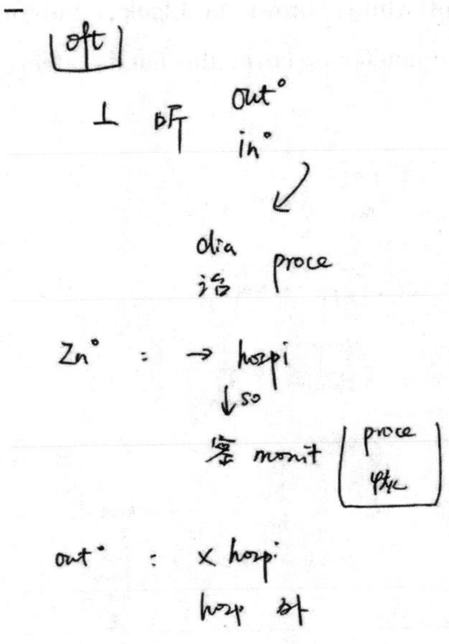

图 4-1　例 1 的口译笔记

例 2：Emergency medicine（EM）is defined by the International Federation for Emergency Medicine in 1991 as "a field of practice based on the knowledge and skills required for the prevention, diagnosis and management of acute and urgent aspects of illness and injury affecting patients of all age groups with a full spectrum of undifferentiated physical and behavioral disorders ...".

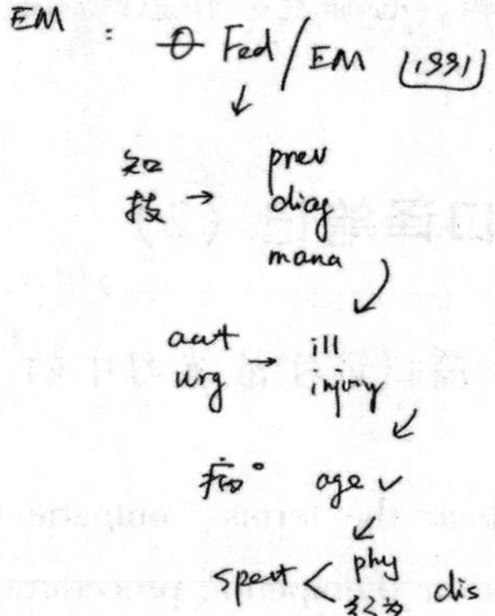

图 4-2　例 2 的口译笔记

例 3：Is it a major or minor burn? Call emergency or seek immediate care for major burns, which are deep, cause the skin to be dry and leathery, may appear charred or have patches of white, brown or black, and/or are larger than 3 inches（about 8 centimeters）in diameter or cover the hands, feet, face, groin, buttocks or a major joint.

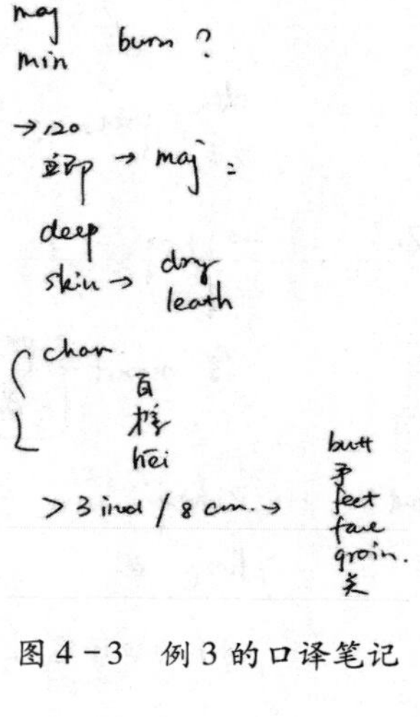

图 4-3　例 3 的口译笔记

例 4：Do not start first aid before ensuring your own safety（switch off electrical current, wear gloves for chemicals, etc.）. Do not apply paste, oil, haldi（turmeric）or raw cotton to the burn. Do not apply ice because it deepens the injury. Avoid prolonged cooling with water because it will lead to hypothermia. Do not open blisters until topical antimicrobials can be applied, such as by a health-care provider. Do not apply any material directly to the wound as it might become infected. Avoid application of topical medication until the patient has been placed under appropriate medical care.

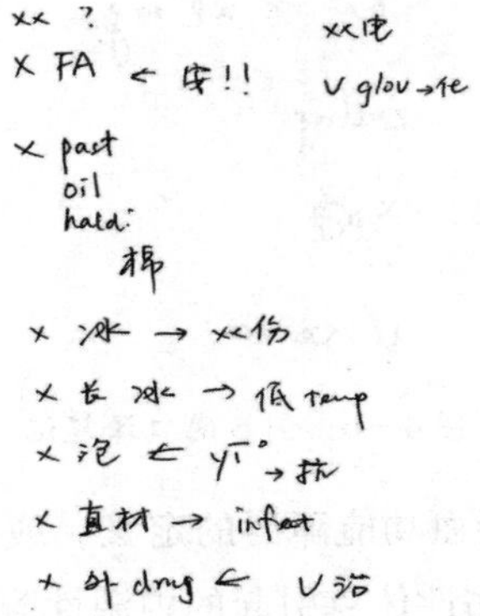

图 4-4　例 4 的口译笔记

例 5：If someone is acutely intoxicated from the effects of volatile substance use （VSU）, there is the possibility of overdose. This can develop from the toxic effects of the substance/s used, mixing with other drugs（particularly other central nervous system depressants such as alcohol, benzodiazepines）, having a low tolerance and not seeking help at the first signs that something is wrong.

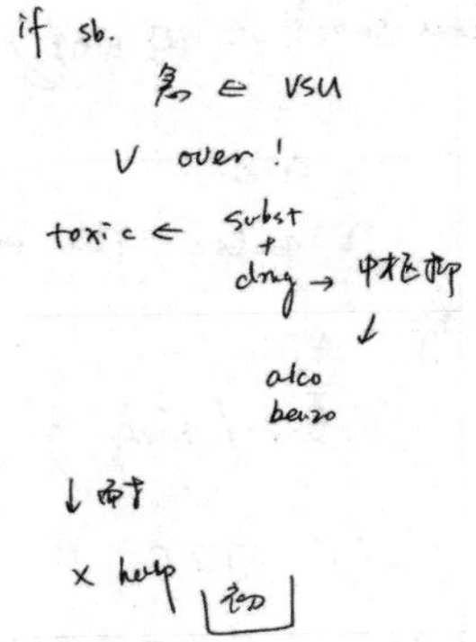

图 4-5　例 5 的口译笔记

例 6: The person should be provided with immediate medical assistance if they are injured, are unconscious or seem to be losing consciousness, have collapsed, are not breathing normally, and/or have a seizure.

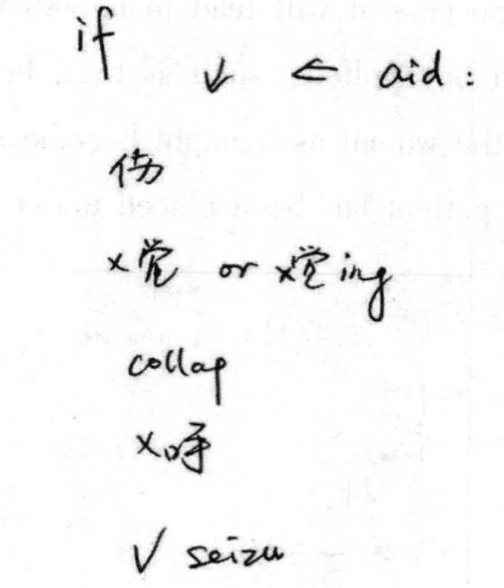

if
　　↓ ← aid :
　　伤
　　X党 or X党ing
　　collap
　　X呼

　　✓ seizu

图 4-6　例 6 的口译笔记

例 7: 尽管对创伤相关凝血功能障碍的定义, 或者说分类和命名的方法尚未达成共识, 但创伤本身和创伤性休克引起的内源性凝血病都被称为急性创伤性凝血病 (ATC)。多因素创伤相关的凝血障碍, 包括急性创伤性凝血病和复苏相关的凝血病, 被认为是创伤诱发性凝血病。

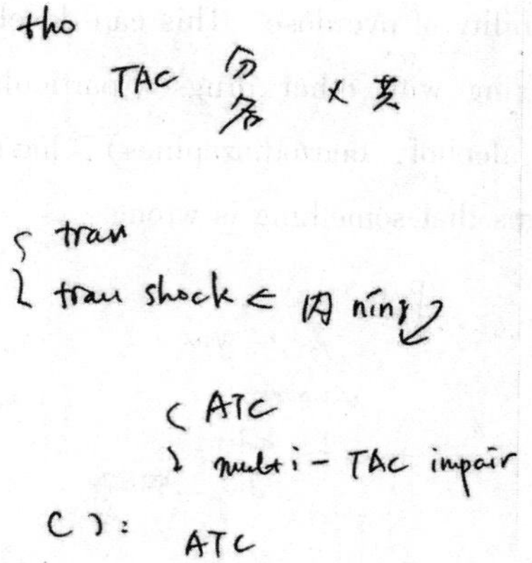

tho
TAC 分类 X名
　　　　名

{ trau
{ trau shock ← 内 ning }

{ ATC
{ multi - TAC impair

( ): ATC
复苏 / ning }

T2C

图 4-7　例 7 的口译笔记

例8：组织损伤和休克协同激发内皮、免疫系统、血小板和凝血活化，而"致命三联征"（凝血病、体温过低和酸中毒）会加剧这些情况。

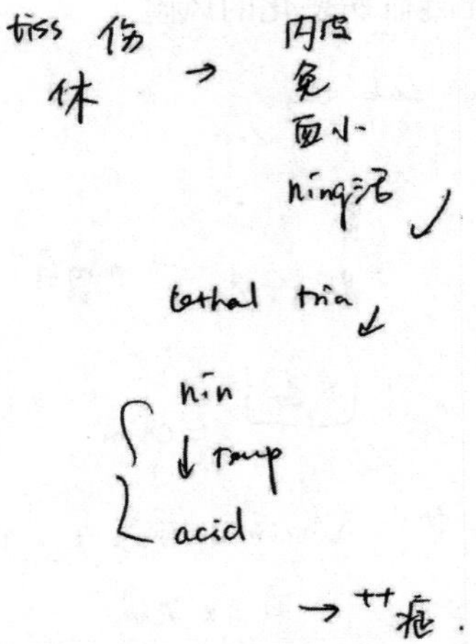

图4-8 例8的口译笔记

例9：自动体外除颤仪用于抢救心脏骤停患者。这通常发生在心脏电活动中断导致危险的快速心跳（室速）或快速且不规则的心跳（室颤）时。如果出现这些不规则的心律之一，心脏便不能有效地泵血，甚至可能停止跳动。

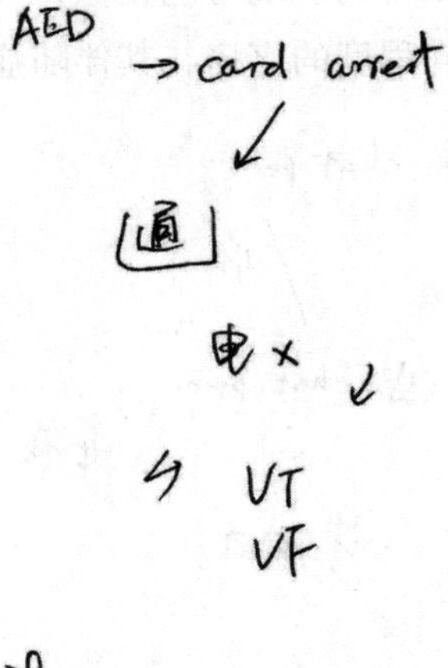

图4-9 例9的口译笔记

例 10：实验室诊断基于常规或黏弹性止血试验检测到的凝血异常；然而，它并不总是与临床状况相匹配。管理重点是通过恢复循环血量来阻止失血和逆转休克，以预防或降低创伤性凝血病恶化的风险。

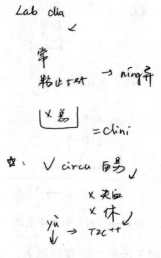

图 4-10 例 10 的口译笔记

例 11：急性胸痛是临床上最常见的症状之一，是以胸痛为主要表现的一组异质性疾病群。不同病因导致的胸痛既可能相似，又可能有不同特征，表现可以是不同部位、不同性质和不同程度的疼痛，其伴随症状亦各不相同。

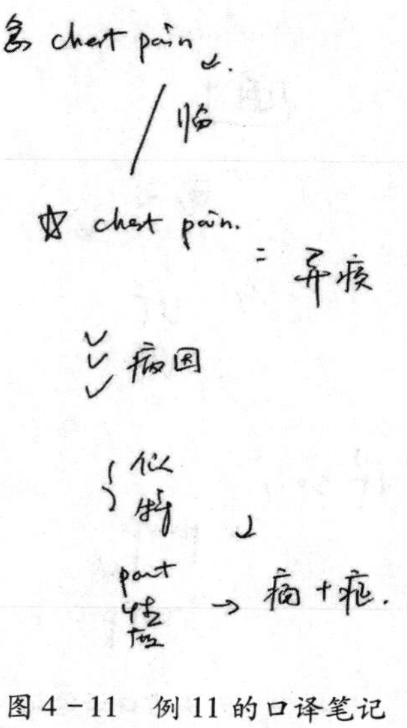

图 4-11 例 11 的口译笔记

例 12：心脏病发作的人可能出现以下症状：胸痛、压迫感或紧绷感，或胸部中央有挤压感或酸痛感；疼痛或不适蔓延到肩部、手臂、背部、颈部、下巴、牙齿，偶尔蔓延到上腹部；恶心、消化不良、胃灼热或腹痛；呼吸急促；头晕、眩晕、昏厥；出汗。

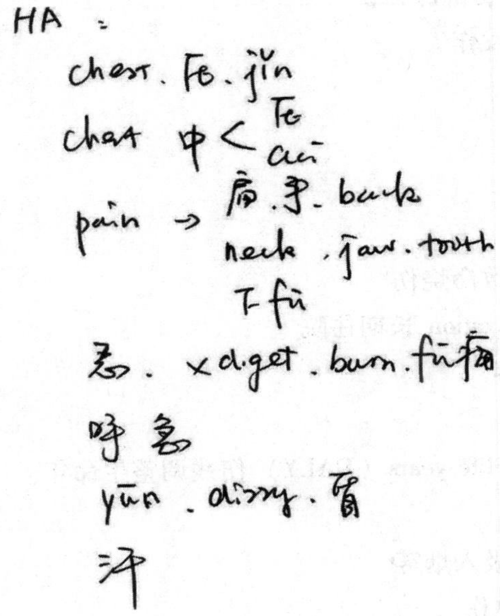

图 4-12 例 12 的口译笔记

3 口译词汇

3.1 英译汉

（一）Outpatient/Emergency Medicine 门诊/急诊

therapeutic procedure 治疗程序

inpatient 住院

overnight monitoring 夜间监测

ambulatory care 门诊服务、非卧床医疗、门诊医疗

pharmacy 药房

emergency department 急诊科

International Federation for Emergency Medicine 国际急诊医学联合会

physical and behavioral disorder 生理和行为紊乱

pre-hospital 院前

in-hospital 院内

loss of consciousness 意识丧失

drug poisoning 药物中毒

epileptic fit 癫痫发作

trauma 外伤

self-harm 自残

（二）Burns 烧伤

death rate 死亡率

non-fatal burn 非致命烧伤

prolonged hospitalization 长期住院

disfigurement 毁容

stigma 歧视

disability-adjusted life-years（DALY）伤残调整生命年

scalding 烫伤

smoke inhalation 吸入烟雾

major burn 严重烧伤

leathery 坚韧

charred 烧焦

minor burn 轻微烧伤

sunburn 晒伤

superficial redness 表面发红

fire-extinguishing liquid 灭火液体

dilute 稀释

electrical current 电流

haldi 姜黄

turmeric 姜黄粉

topical antimicrobial 外敷抗生素

（三）Acute Intoxication 急性中毒

level of tolerance 耐受水平

underlying organic condition 潜在器质性疾病

renal insufficiency 肾功能不全

hepatic insufficiency 肝功能不全

disproportionately 不成比例

transient 短暂的

intensity 强度

complication 并发症

volatile substance use（VSU）使用挥发性物质

central nervous system depressant 中枢神经系统抑制剂

benzodiazepines 苯二氮䓬类药物

seizure 癫痫发作

3.2 汉译英

（一）创伤诱发性凝血病 Trauma-induced Coagulopathy

出血 hemorrhage

急性期死亡 acute-phase mortality

创伤学家 traumatologist

医源性的 iatrogenic

复苏相关 resuscitation-associated

体温过低 hypothermia

代谢性酸中毒 metabolic acidosis

稀释性凝血病 dilutional coagulopathy

范式转变 paradigm shift

创伤性休克 traumatic shock

内源性 endogenous

急性创伤性凝血病 acute traumatic coagulopathy

凝血障碍 coagulation impairment

病理生理学 pathophysiology

低凝状态 hypocoagulability

高凝状态 hypercoagulable state

静脉血栓 thromboembolism

多器官衰竭 multiple organ failure

组织损伤 tissue injury

协同 synergistically

内皮的 endothelial

免疫系统 immune system

血小板 platelet

凝血 clotting

致命三联征 lethal triad

体温过低 hypothermia

酸中毒 acidosis

止血异常 haemostatic abnormality

纤维蛋白原耗竭 fibrinogen depletion

凝血酶生成不足 inadequate thrombin generation

血小板功能受损 impaired platelet function

纤维蛋白溶解失调 dysregulated fibrinolysis

黏弹性止血试验 viscoelastic haemostatic assay

循环血量 circulating blood volume

复苏 resuscitation

（二）心肺复苏 Cardiopulmonary Resuscitation

美国心脏协会 American Heart Association

胸外按压 chest compression

心律 heart rhythm

自动体外除颤仪 automated external defibrillators（AED）

心脏骤停 cardiac arrest

室速 ventricular tachycardia

室颤 ventricular fibrillation

除颤 defibrillation

（三）急性胸痛 Acute Chest Pain

异质性疾病 heterogeneous disease

胃灼热、烧心 heartburn

肺栓塞 pulmonary embolism

挤压感或酸痛感 squeezing or aching sensation

上腹部 upper abdomen

恶心 nausea

消化不良 indigestion

头晕 lightheadedness

眩晕 dizziness

昏厥 fainting

4 口译实战

4.1 英译汉

（一）Outpatient/Emergency Medicine 门诊/急诊[1-2]

Often, one may hear the terms "outpatient" or "inpatient" used when referring to a type of diagnostic or therapeutic procedure. "Inpatient" means that the procedure requires the patient to be admitted to the hospital, primarily so that he or she can be closely monitored during the procedure and afterwards, during recovery. "Outpatient" means that the procedure does not require hospital admission and may also be performed outside the premises of a hospital.

When patients are sick, injured, or require specialized types of testing or treatment but do not require the overnight monitoring or care of a hospital, they often obtain the healthcare they need in an outpatient setting. This is also known as ambulatory care. Primary care physicians, community health clinics, urgent care clinics, specialized outpatient

通常，当提到一种诊断或治疗程序时，人们可能会听到"门诊"或"住院"这两个术语。"住院"是指医疗程序要求患者入院，主要是为了在手术期间和之后的康复期间对其进行密切监测。"门诊"是指医疗程序不需要住院，也可以在院外进行。

当患者生病、受伤或需要特殊类型的测试或治疗但不需要医院的夜间监测和护理时，他们通常会在门诊环境中获得所需的医疗服务。这也称为非卧床医疗。初级保健医生、社区卫生诊所、紧急护理诊所、专科门诊、药房和急诊科都是非卧床医疗环境的例子。

clinics, pharmacies, and the emergency department are examples of outpatient care settings.

Emergency medicine (EM) is defined by the International Federation for Emergency Medicine in 1991 as "a field of practice based on the knowledge and skills required for the prevention, diagnosis and management of acute and urgent aspects of illness and injury affecting patients of all age groups with a full spectrum of undifferentiated physical and behavioral disorders. It further encompasses an understanding of the development of pre-hospital and in-hospital emergency medical systems and the skills necessary for this development."

国际急诊医学联合会在 1991 年将急诊医学定义为"基于专业知识和技能，预防、诊断和管理全年龄段人群重性和急性疾病和伤害的专业领域，诊疗范围覆盖所有身体和行为问题。急诊医学也包括对院前和院内急诊医学体系的最新进展的掌握，需具备相关技能"。

Doctors in EM carry out the immediate assessment and treatment of patients with serious and life-threatening illnesses and injuries. They treat conditions such as loss of consciousness, e. g. from an injury to the head, drug poisoning, an epileptic fit, severe bleeding, damage to the brain or other major organs due to trauma, cardiac arrest (when the pumping action of the heart stops), breathing difficulties, broken bones and mental health problems.

急诊医生对患有严重和危及生命的疾病以及受到严重的危及生命的伤害的患者进行即时评估和治疗。他们会处理以下情况：头部受伤、药物中毒、癫痫发作等导致的意识丧失，严重出血，外伤导致的大脑或其他主要器官受损，心脏骤停（心脏泵血停止），呼吸困难，骨折，以及心理健康问题。

（二）Burns 烧伤[3-5]

Burns are a global public health problem, accounting for an estimated 180,000 deaths annually. The majority of these occur in low- and middle-income countries and almost two thirds occur in the WHO African and South-East Asia regions. In many high-income countries, burn death rates have been decreasing, and the rate of child deaths from burns is currently over 7 times higher in low- and middle-income countries than in high-income countries.

Non-fatal burns are a leading cause of morbidity, including prolonged hospitalization, disfigurement and disability, often with resulting stigma and rejection. Burns are among the leading causes of disability-adjusted life-years（DALY）lost in low- and middle-income countries. In 2004, nearly 11 million people worldwide were burned severely enough to require medical attention. A burn is tissue damage that results from scalding, overexposure to the sun or other radiation, contact with flames, chemicals or electricity, or smoke inhalation.

Is it a major or minor burn? Call

烧伤是一项全球性公共卫生问题，估计每年导致约18万例死亡。其中大部分发生在低收入和中等收入国家，约有三分之二发生在世界卫生组织非洲和东南亚区域。许多高收入国家的烧伤死亡率不断降低。目前低收入和中等收入国家中死于烧伤的儿童比例是高收入国家的七倍以上。

非致命烧伤是一项主要致病因素，造成长期住院、毁容和残疾等，并往往导致患者受到歧视和遭受排斥。烧伤是低收入和中等收入国家中伤残调整生命年减少的主要原因之一。2004年，全世界近1100万人被严重烧伤，需要就医。烧伤是由烫伤，过度暴露于太阳或其他辐射，接触火焰、化学品、电，或吸入烟雾引起的组织损伤。

是严重烧伤还是轻微烧伤？严重

emergency or seek immediate care for major burns, which are deep, cause the skin to be dry and leathery, may appear charred or have patches of white, brown or black, and/or are larger than 3 inches (about 8 centimeters) in diameter or cover the hands, feet, face, groin, buttocks or a major joint. A minor burn that doesn't require emergency care may involve superficial redness similar to a sunburn, pain, blisters, and it is an area no larger than 3 inches (about 8 centimeters) in diameter.

First aid. Stop the burning process by removing clothing and irrigating the burns. Extinguish flames by allowing the patient to roll on the ground, by applying a blanket, or by using water or other fire-extinguishing liquids. Use cool running water to reduce the temperature of the burn. In chemical burns, remove or dilute the chemical agent by irrigating with large volumes of water. Wrap the patient in a clean cloth or sheet and transport to the nearest appropriate facility for medical care.

Do not start first aid before ensuring your own safety (switch off electrical current, wear gloves for chemicals,

烧伤请拨打急救电话或立即寻求治疗。严重烧伤通常很深，会导致皮肤干燥、变韧，可能烧焦或出现白色、棕色、黑色斑块，创面直径大于3英寸（约8厘米），覆盖手、脚、脸、腹股沟、臀部或主要关节。不需要紧急护理的轻微烧伤包括类似于晒伤的表面发红、疼痛、水疱，创面直径不大于3英寸（约8厘米）。

急救。脱去衣物，向烧伤处浇水，终止烧伤过程。在地面翻滚或用毯子包裹，或用水或其他灭火液体扑灭火焰。使用清凉流水降低烧伤部位的温度。发生化学品烧伤时，用大量水冲洗，以清除或稀释化学物质。用干净的布或床单包裹患者，并将其送到最近的合适医疗机构就医。

在确保自身安全（关闭电源、处理化学品时戴手套等）之前，不要开始急救。不要在烧伤处涂抹膏剂、油、

etc.). Do not apply paste, oil, haldi (turmeric) or raw cotton to the burn. Do not apply ice because it deepens the injury. Avoid prolonged cooling with water because it will lead to hypothermia. Do not open blisters until topical antimicrobials can be applied, such as by a health-care provider. Do not apply any material directly to the wound as it might become infected. Avoid application of topical medication until the patient has been placed under appropriate medical care.

姜黄或用棉花覆盖烧伤处。不要敷冰块，因为这会加剧伤害。避免用水降温的时间过长，这可能会导致低温症。在医务人员以及其他人帮助外敷抗生素之前，不要弄破水疱。不要直接在伤口上敷贴任何材料，这可能会引起感染。在接受适当的诊治之前，避免敷用任何外用药物。

(三) Acute Intoxication 急性中毒[6-7]

Intoxication is highly dependent on the type and dose of drug and is influenced by an individual's level of tolerance and other factors. Acute intoxication is usually closely related to dose levels. Exceptions to this may occur in individuals with certain underlying organic conditions (e. g. , renal or hepatic insufficiency) in whom small doses of a substance may produce a disproportionately severe intoxicating effect.

中毒高度取决于药物的类型和剂量，并受个人耐受水平和其他因素的影响。急性中毒通常与剂量密切相关。患有某些潜在器质性疾病（例如肾或肝功能不全）的个体可能出现例外情况，小剂量的某种物质可能会产生不成比例的严重中毒效应。

Acute intoxication is a transient phenomenon. Intensity of intoxication lessens with time, and effects eventually

急性中毒是一种短暂的现象。中毒的强度随着时间的推移而减弱，并且在没有进一步使用该物质的情况下，

disappear in the absence of further use of the substance. Recovery is complete except where tissue damage or another complication has arisen. If someone is acutely intoxicated from the effects of volatile substance use (VSU), there is the possibility of overdose. This can develop from the toxic effects of the substance/s used, mixing with other drugs (particularly other central nervous system depressants such as alcohol, benzodiazepines), having a low tolerance and not seeking help at the first signs that something is wrong.

A person recovering from acute VSU intoxication should be kept safe and be watched until they have fully recovered. If possible, monitor the person in a clinical setting throughout the period of acute intoxication (2 – 4 hours if recovery is uncomplicated or longer if recovery is delayed) if they regularly use volatile substances.

If it is not possible to transfer the person to a medical service, watch them closely and call emergency services if they become unconscious, have a seizure or if their condition becomes worse in any way. The person should be provided with

影响最终会消失。除非出现组织损伤或其他并发症，患者通常可以完全恢复。如果某人因使用挥发性物质引发急性中毒，有可能是使用过量。这可能是由所用物质的毒性作用、与其他药物（特别是其他中枢神经系统抑制剂，如酒精、苯二氮䓬类药物）混合、患者耐受性低以及迹象出现初期不寻求帮助导致。

应确保急性挥发性物质中毒患者康复过程的安全并密切关注其病情，直到他们完全康复。如患者经常使用挥发性物质，条件允许的情况下，在整个急性中毒期间（如果康复情况不复杂，则2~4小时，如果康复延迟则需更长时间）应对患者进行临床监测。

如果无法将患者转移到医疗机构，请密切关注患者，并在其失去知觉、癫痫发作或病情以任何方式恶化时拨打急救电话。如果此人受伤了，失去知觉或似乎正在失去知觉，已经崩溃，呼吸不正常，或是癫痫发作，那么应

immediate medical assistance if they are injured, are unconscious or seem to be losing consciousness, have collapsed, are not breathing normally, and/or have a seizure.

立即为其提供医疗援助。

4.2　汉译英

（一）创伤诱发性凝血病 Trauma-induced Coagulopathy [8-9]

出血是导致创伤患者急性期死亡的最重要因素。此前，创伤学家和研究人员确定了外伤后凝血病出血的医源性和复苏相关原因，包括体温过低、代谢性酸中毒和稀释性凝血病，这些被认为是外伤后出血的主要驱动因素。然而，在过去的 10 年里，危重外伤患者的复苏范式发生了广泛的转变，我们对创伤性凝血病的理解发生了巨大的变化。

Hemorrhage is the most important contributing factor of acute-phase mortality in trauma patients. Previously, traumatologists and investigators identified iatrogenic and resuscitation-associated causes of coagulopathic bleeding after traumatic injury, including hypothermia, metabolic acidosis, and dilutional coagulopathy that were recognized as primary drivers of bleeding after trauma. However, the last 10 years has seen a widespread paradigm shift in the resuscitation of critically injured patients, and there has been a dramatic evolution in our understanding of trauma-induced coagulopathy (TIC).

尽管对创伤相关凝血功能障碍的定义，或者说分类和命名的方法尚未达成共识，但创伤本身和创伤性休克引起的内源性凝血病都被称为急性创伤性凝血病（ATC）。多因素创伤相关的凝血障碍，包括急性创伤性凝血病

Although there is no consensus regarding a definition or an approach to the classification and naming of trauma-associated coagulation impairment, trauma itself and traumatic shock-induced endogenous coagulopathy are both referred

和复苏相关的凝血病，被认为是创伤诱发性凝血病。了解创伤凝血病的病理生理机制非常重要，特别是在为严重创伤患者制定治疗策略的关键问题方面。

在创伤诱发性凝血病（TIC）发展的早期，通常会出现低凝状态，导致出血，而后期创伤性凝血病的特征是与静脉血栓和多器官衰竭相关的高凝状态。组织损伤和休克协同激发内皮、免疫系统、血小板和凝血活化，而"致命三联征"（凝血病、体温过低和酸中毒）会加剧这些情况。创伤性脑损伤在创伤性凝血病中也有明显的作用。止血异常包括纤维蛋白原耗竭、凝血酶生成不足、血小板功能受损和纤维蛋白溶解失调。

实验室诊断基于常规或黏弹性止血试验检测到的凝血异常；然而，它

to as acute traumatic coagulopathy (ATC). Multifactorial trauma-associated coagulation impairment, including ATC and resuscitation-associated coagulopathy is recognized as TIC. Understanding the pathophysiology of TIC is vitally important, especially with respect to the critical issue of establishing therapeutic strategies for patients with severe trauma.

In the early hours of TIC development, hypocoagulability is typically present, resulting in bleeding, whereas later TIC is characterized by a hypercoagulable state associated with venous thromboembolism and multiple organ failure. Tissue injury and shock synergistically provoke endothelial, immune system, platelet and clotting activation, which are accentuated by the "lethal triad" (coagulopathy, hypothermia and acidosis). Traumatic brain injury also has a distinct role in TIC. Haemostatic abnormalities include fibrinogen depletion, inadequate thrombin generation, impaired platelet function and dysregulated fibrinolysis.

Laboratory diagnosis is based on coagulation abnormalities detected by

并不总是与临床状况相匹配。管理重点是通过恢复循环血量来阻止失血和逆转休克，以预防或降低创伤性凝血病恶化的风险。多种血液制品可用于复苏，但是，关于输血成分的最佳组成国际上尚未达成共识。

conventional or viscoelastic haemostatic assays; however, it does not always match the clinical condition. Management priorities are stopping blood loss and reversing shock by restoring circulating blood volume, to prevent or reduce the risk of worsening TIC. Various blood products can be used in resuscitation; however, there is no international agreement on the optimal composition of transfusion components.

（二）心肺复苏 Cardiopulmonary Resuscitation[10-11]

心肺复苏是一种救命技术，在许多紧急情况下都很有用，例如因心脏病发作或溺水，病人的呼吸或心跳停止时。美国心脏协会建议开始心肺复苏时进行剧烈和快速的胸外按压。在通过医疗急救恢复正常心率之前，心肺复苏可以保持富含氧气的血液流向大脑和其他器官。当心脏停止跳动时，身体将无法再获得富含氧气的血液。缺乏富含氧气的血液会在短短几分钟内造成脑损伤。

Cardiopulmonary resuscitation (CPR) is a lifesaving technique that's useful in many emergencies, such as a heart attack or drowning, in which someone's breathing or heartbeat has stopped. The American Heart Association recommends starting CPR with hard and fast chest compressions. CPR can keep oxygen-rich blood flowing to the brain and other organs until emergency medical treatment can restore a normal heart rhythm. When the heart stops, your body no longer gets oxygen-rich blood. The lack of oxygen-rich blood can cause brain damage in only a few minutes.

自动体外除颤仪用于抢救心脏骤停患者。这通常发生在心脏电活动中断导致危险的快速心跳（室速）或快

Automated external defibrillators (AED) are used to revive someone from sudden cardiac arrest. This usually

速且不规则的心跳（室颤）时。如果出现这些不规则的心律之一，心脏便不能有效地泵血，甚至可能停止跳动。发生这种情况时，大脑和其他重要器官无法获得所需的血液和氧气，如果几分钟内不接受治疗，可导致死亡。正常心律恢复得越早，大脑和其他器官免受永久性损伤的可能性就越大。

如果发生室颤或室速，并且附近有自动体外除颤仪，公共场所的旁观者或家庭成员可以使用它恢复心脏正常节律，并可能挽救生命。心脏骤停后做心肺复苏可以在一段时间内让血液流向心脏和大脑。但往往只有除颤才能恢复心脏的正常节律。这些治疗结合在一起可以提高生存机会。

警察和救护人员携带有自动体外

occurs when a disruption in the heart's electrical activity causes a dangerously fast heartbeat (ventricular tachycardia) or a fast and irregular heartbeat (ventricular fibrillation). If you're having one of these irregular heart rhythms, your heart doesn't pump effectively and may even stop. When this happens, your brain and other vital organs don't get the blood and oxygen they need, and you can even die if you don't get treatment within minutes. The sooner your heart's normal rhythm is restored, the greater is the chance that you won't have permanent damage to your brain and other organs.

If you're having ventricular fibrillation or ventricular tachycardia and an AED is nearby, a bystander in a public place or a family member can use it to jolt your heart back to a normal rhythm and possibly save your life. CPR after cardiac arrest can keep blood flowing to your heart and brain for a time. But often only defibrillation can restore the heart's normal rhythm. Together these treatments can improve your chances of survival.

Police and ambulance crews carry

除颤仪，它们在许多公共场所都很常见，包括商场、办公楼、运动场、健身房和飞机。然而，许多心脏骤停都发生在家里，因此拥有一台家用自动体外除颤仪可以节省宝贵的时间，让室颤和室速患者苏醒。

AEDs, and they're commonly available in many public places, including malls, office buildings, sports arenas, gyms and airplanes. However, many cardiac arrests occur at home, so having a home AED can save precious minutes in reviving a person with ventricular fibrillation and ventricular tachycardia.

（三）急性胸痛 Acute Chest Pain[12-13]

急性胸痛是临床上最常见的症状之一，是以胸痛为主要表现的一组异质性疾病群。不同病因导致的胸痛既可能相似，又可能有不同特征，表现可以是不同部位、不同性质和不同程度的疼痛，其伴随症状亦各不相同。

Acute chest pain is one of the most common clinical symptoms, a group of heterogeneous diseases with chest pain as the main manifestation. Chest pain caused by different causes can be similar, but also have different characteristics. Pain occurs in different parts of the body with varied nature, severity and accompanying symptoms.

胸痛的急救取决于病因。胸痛的原因可以从轻微问题，如烧心或情绪压力到严重的医疗紧急情况，如心脏病发作或肺部血栓（肺栓塞）等。很难判断胸痛是由心脏病发作还是其他健康状况引起的，尤其是如果以前从未有过胸痛。不要试图自己诊断原因。如果出现不明原因的持续几分钟以上的胸痛，请寻求紧急医疗帮助。

First aid for chest pain depends on the cause. Causes of chest pain can vary from minor problems, such as heartburn or emotional stress, to serious medical emergencies, such as a heart attack or blood clot in the lungs (pulmonary embolism). It can be difficult to tell if your chest pain is due to a heart attack or other health condition, especially if you've never had chest pain before. Don't try to diagnose the cause yourself.

Seek emergency medical help if you have unexplained chest pain that lasts more than a few minutes.

心脏病发作通常会导致胸痛超过 15 分钟。疼痛可能是轻微的或严重的。有些心脏病会突然发作，但许多人的身体会提前数小时或数天发出警告信号。心脏病发作的人可能出现以下症状：胸痛、压迫感或紧绷感，或胸部中央有挤压感或酸痛感；疼痛或不适蔓延到肩部、手臂、背部、颈部、下巴、牙齿，偶尔蔓延到上腹部；恶心、消化不良、胃灼热或腹痛；呼吸急促；头晕、眩晕、昏厥；出汗。

A heart attack generally causes chest pain for more than 15 minutes. The pain may be mild or severe. Some heart attacks strike suddenly, but many people have warning signs hours or days in advance. Someone having a heart attack may have the following symptoms：chest pain, pressure or tightness, or a squeezing or aching sensation in the center of the chest；pain or discomfort that spreads to the shoulder, arm, back, neck, jaw, teeth or occasionally upper abdomen；nausea, indigestion, heartburn or abdominal pain；shortness of breath；lightheadedness, dizziness, fainting；and sweating.

5 口译注释与学习资源

5.1 口译注释

（一）室颤/室速

有关室颤和室速的详解，请参见参考文献中的相关条目。

（二）非卧床医疗（Ambulatory care）

因为这种医疗服务门诊可以提供，急诊可以提供，社区医院也可以提供，所以称为非卧床医疗。

5.2 学习资源

登陆中国大学 MOOC（慕课），学习"医疗口译"课程中"门诊/急诊"的口译实战示范视频。此外还可登录世界卫生组织、英国国民医疗服务体系、美国妙佑医疗国际等组织机构官网学习相关知识。

参考文献

［1］ NHS. （n. d.）. *Emergency medicine*. Retrieved November 14, 2021, from https：//www. healthcareers. nhs. uk/explore-roles/doctors/roles-doctors/emergency-medicine.

［2］ ACEM. （n. d.）. *What is emergency medicine?*. Retrieved November 14, 2021, from https：// acem. org. au/Content-Sources/About/What-is-emergency-medicine.

［3］ World Health Organization. （n. d.）. *Burns*. Retrieved September 14, 2021, from https：//www. who. int/news-room/fact-sheets/detail/burns?limit = all.

［4］ 世界卫生组织. 烧伤 ［EB/OL］. ［2021 - 08 - 11］. https：//www. who. int/zh/news-room/fact-sheets/detail/burns.

［5］ Mayo Foundation for Medical Education and Research. （2018, January 30）. *First aid for burns*. Retrieved November 14, 2021, from https：//www. mayoclinic. org/first-aid/first-aid-burns/ basics/art - 20056649.

［6］ Pallipedia. （n. d.）. *What is acute intoxication-meaning and definition*. Retrieved November 14, 2021, from https：//pallipedia. org/acute-intoxication/.

［7］ Greene, S. L., Dargan, P. I., & Jones, A. L. （2005, April 1）. Acute poisoning: Understanding 90% of cases in a nutshell. *Postgraduate Medical Journal*. Retrieved November 14, 2021, from https：//pmj. bmj. com/content/81/954/204.

［8］ Kushimoto, S., Kudo, D., & Kawazoe, Y. （2017）. Acute traumatic coagulopathy and trauma-induced coagulopathy: An overview. *Journal of Intensive Care*, 5 （1）. https：//doi. org/ 10. 1186/s40560 - 016 - 0196 - 6.

［9］ Moore, E. E., Moore, H. B., Kornblith, L. Z. et al. （2021）. Trauma-induced coagulopathy. *Nature Reviews Disease Primers*, 7 （30）. https：//doi. org/10. 1038/s41572 - 021 - 00264 - 3.

［10］ Mayo Foundation for Medical Education and Research. （2020, April 16）. *Automated external defibrillators: Do you need an AED?* Retrieved November 14, 2021, from https：//www. mayoclinic. org/diseases-conditions/heart-arrhythmia/in-depth/automated-external-defibrillators/ art - 20043909.

［11］ Mayo Foundation for Medical Education and Research. （2021, May 1）. *Cardiopulmonary resuscitation(CPR): First aid*. Retrieved November 14, 2021, from https：//www. mayoclinic. org/ first-aid/first-aid-cpr/basics/art - 20056600.

［12］ 陈玉国. 急性胸痛急诊诊疗专家共识 ［J］. 中华急诊医学杂志, 2019, 28 （04）：

413 - 420.

[13] Mayo Foundation for Medical Education and Research. (2021, April 21). *Chest pain: First aid.* Retrieved November 14, 2021, from https://www. mayoclinic. org/first-aid/first-aid-chest-pain/basics/art - 20056705.

第五章

呼吸内科

1 导读

本章重点为口译技巧之综述技巧和呼吸内科的6篇"口译实战"练习。口译实战练习中英译汉、汉译英各3篇，内容涵盖呼吸内科介绍、支气管炎、哮喘、肺炎、肺结核和慢性阻塞性肺疾病。请结合本章口译技巧练习6篇口译实战文本。

2 口译技巧——综述技巧

口译中的综述是指对讲话内容进行要点提炼后概括翻译。在口译活动中，尤其是在交替传译中，由于时间安排或者出于其他考虑，讲话人、主办方有时会对译员提出"请你简单翻译一下刚才的内容"一类的要求。此时，口译员一般会按照要求做概要或主旨口译（gist interpreting）。在概要口译中，口译员需注意以下三个方面：（1）听清讲话者意图，抓住逻辑结构；（2）提炼要点重点，去除次要信息；（3）传译用词准确，句式语法简练。

此外，在讲话者逻辑混乱，内容有不必要、非强调性的重复时，可以考虑采取综述的方式帮助听众更好地理解讲话内容。但口译员需要了解综述或者概要口译可能带来漏掉要点、信息不完整等后果。无论是基于自己的判断还是被要求做概要口译，口译员都可能面临违背职业伦理的风险，信息的不完整也可能会对交流结果带来不可逆的影响。因此，如有可能，综述前应向讲话者或主办方简短确认并向听众说明。

通常情况下，口译员**不得综述**，尤其是在医学口译中涉及病情表述、诊疗等与生命安全直接相关的核心信息时。但患者往往会反复提及一些症状，或者在某些影响病人语言表达能力的病情诊疗过程中，口译员可视情况采取概括加强调的方式向医务人员转述病人的话语。

除了口译实战中的概要口译，口译练习中的综述技巧可以帮助口译员筛选主要信息、理清讲话者逻辑。训练口译员的综述能力可以采取从短篇章综述到长篇章综述的循序渐进的方式，具体可以分为两个阶段。

（1）**信息提炼，用原语综述**。听一段演讲，最好是讲话者脱稿的讲话，以原文字数一半的长度，使用原语言写出综述文本。如原文听的是中文，则综述也使用中文，原文是英语，则综述也为英语。此时未增加语言转化和时间限制等压力因素，可训练口译员关键信息提取和压缩的能力。在具备提取关键信息的能力后，可将写出文本改为说的方式，也可逐渐加长原文长度或缩短口头综述的时间。

（2）**语言转换，以译语综述。**此阶段的练习和上一阶段形式一样，唯一区别在于产出时先使用译语（目的语）写出文本，熟练后，可将"写"改为"说"，直接使用目的语说出译文。在加入语言转换负荷后，练习更接近口译中的真实场景，也更具挑战性。

3 口译词汇

3.1 英译汉

（一）Respiratory Medicine 呼吸内科（呼吸病学）

upper respiratory tract 上呼吸道

pharynx 咽部

larynx 喉部

lower respiratory tract 下呼吸道

trachea 气管

bronchus（*pl.* bronchi）支气管

specialist nurse 专科护士

chronic obstructive pulmonary diseases（COPD）慢性阻塞性肺疾病

acute and chronic bronchitis 急性和慢性支气管炎

emphysema 肺气肿

chronic cough 慢性咳嗽

breathlessness 气喘

asthma 哮喘

tuberculosis 肺结核

sarcoidosis 肺结节

lung fibrosis 肺纤维化

idiopathic pulmonary fibrosis 特发性肺间质纤维化

bronchiectasis 支气管扩张

pulmonary embolism 肺栓塞

pneumonia 肺炎

pneumothorax 气胸

bronchoscopy 支气管镜检查

thoracoscopy 胸腔镜检查

pleural and lung ultrasound 胸肺超声波

（二）Bronchitis 支气管炎

inflammation 炎症

flu virus 流感病毒

bronchiole 小支气管

sputum 痰

episode 发作

a heavy feeling in the chest 胸闷

air sac 肺泡

vulnerable group 易感人群

pulmonary rehabilitation 肺康复疗法

mucus clearing device 清痰仪器

（三）Asthma 哮喘

swell 肿胀

wheezing 哮鸣

mucus 黏液

shortness of breath 呼吸短促

chest tightness 胸闷、气紧

viral infection 病毒感染

bacterial infection 细菌感染

exercise-induced asthma 运动型哮喘

occupation-induced asthma 职业型哮喘

allergy-induced asthma 过敏型哮喘

quick relief medicine 快速缓解药

long-term control medicine 长效控制药

inhaled corticosteroid 吸入型皮质类固醇

leukotriene modifier 白三烯调节剂

long-acting beta agonist（LABA）长效 β 激动剂（LABA）

theophylline 茶碱

combination inhaler 组合成分吸入剂

anti-inflammatory drug 抗炎药物

rescue medication 急救用药

short-acting beta agonist 短效 β 激动剂

ipratropium 异丙托胺

oral／intravenous corticosteroid 口服型／静脉注射型皮质类固醇

3.2 汉译英

（一）肺炎 Pneumonia

急性呼吸道感染 acute respiratory infection

肺泡 alveoli

脓液 pus

氧气摄入量 oxygen intake

感染因子 infectious agent

真菌 fungus（*pl.* fungi）

肺炎链球菌 streptococcus pneumoniae

乙型流感嗜血杆菌 haemophilus influenzae type b（Hib）

呼吸道合胞病毒 respiratory syncytial virus

耶氏肺孢子菌 pneumocystis jiroveci

飞沫 droplet

阿莫西林分散片剂 amoxicillin dispersible tablet

肺炎和腹泻综合全球行动计划 Global Action Plan for Pneumonia and Diarrhea（GAPPD）

复方新诺明 cotrimoxazole

预防 prophylaxis

纯母乳喂养 exclusive breastfeeding

辅食喂养 complementary feeding

（二）肺结核 Tuberculosis

结核病 Tuberculosis（TB）

结核分枝杆菌 mycobacterium tuberculosis

细菌 germ

盗汗 night sweat

密切接触 close contact

活动性肺结核 active lung（pulmonary）TB

速诊分子测试 rapid molecular diagnostic test

初步诊断 initial diagnosis

耐药结核病 drug-resistant TB

含量测定 assay

多药耐药 multidrug-resistance

异烟肼 isoniazid

利福平 rifampicin

吡嗪酰胺 pyrazinamide

乙胺丁醇 ethambutol

潜伏性结核病 latent TB

（三）慢性阻塞性肺疾病 COPD

慢性阻塞性肺疾病（也称"慢阻肺"）chronic obstructive pulmonary disease（COPD）

病死率 fatality rate

高血压 hypertension

糖尿病 diabetes

冠心病 coronary heart disease

早检测，早诊断，早干预 early detection, early diagnosis, and early intervention

肺功能检查 pulmonary function test（PFT）

肺活量 forced vital capacity（FVC）

4 口译实战

4.1 英译汉

（一）Respiratory Medicine 呼吸内科[1]

Respiratory medicine involves the management of diseases that occur in the upper respiratory tract（nose, pharynx

呼吸内科是关于上呼吸道（鼻子、咽喉部）和下呼吸道（气管、支气管和肺部）疾病诊治的学科。医生

and larynx) and the lower respiratory tract (trachea , bronchi and lungs). A physician may work closely with specialist nurses or respiratory technicians in the diagnosis and treatment of diseases such as asthma, pneumonia, bronchitis, emphysema and chronic obstructive pulmonary diseases.

Respiratory diseases and disorders can affect your breathing and may cause serious discomfort and pain. They can be serious, so it's important to diagnose them quickly to establish whether you are suffering from an acute or chronic condition. The most common conditions include chronic cough, breathlessness, asthma, chronic obstructive pulmonary disease (previously known as chronic bronchitis and emphysema), lung infections, acute and chronic bronchitis, emphysema, tuberculosis, sarcoidosis, lung fibrosis, idiopathic pulmonary fibrosis, bronchiectasis, lung cancer, pulmonary embolism, pneumonia, pneumothorax, etc.

Investigations may include a bronchoscopy, which is a procedure to look for any problems inside your airways (bronchi) using a flexible telescope, or

与专科护士或呼吸科技术员密切合作，诊断和治疗哮喘、肺炎、支气管炎、肺气肿和慢性阻塞性肺疾病。

呼吸系统疾病会影响呼吸，并可能导致严重的不适和疼痛。这类疾病可能会很严重，因此须快速确诊，以明确病人患的是急性还是慢性疾病。最常见的呼吸系统疾病和症状包括慢性咳嗽、气喘、哮喘、慢性阻塞性肺疾病（以前称为慢性支气管炎和肺气肿）、肺部感染、急性和慢性支气管炎、肺气肿、肺结核、肺结节、肺纤维化、特发性肺间质纤维化、支气管扩张、肺癌、肺栓塞、肺炎、气胸等。

呼吸道疾病的诊断手段包括支气管镜检查和胸腔镜检查。前者使用柔韧的窥视镜检查气道中可能出现的问题；后者使用类似的设备检查胸膜腔

a thoracoscopy, which uses a similar device to examine the pleural cavity (the space between your lung and chest wall). Your doctor may also use a pleural and lung ultrasound, which uses soundwaves to provide a picture of the inside of your body, or an X-ray. They can take biopsies to send to the laboratory if they want to test samples of your body tissue.

（肺和胸腔壁之间的空间）。医生也可以使用胸肺超声波，也就是使用声波形成身体内部的图片，或 X 光片。如果需要检查病人身体组织的样本，可以采取活检的方式。

（二）Bronchitis 支气管炎[2]

Bronchitis is basically an inflammation of the airway passage in the lungs and it can be due to several factors, but most commonly like a cold or even flu viruses. Bronchitis occurs when the bronchioles (air-carrying tubes in the lungs) are inflamed and make too much mucus. There are two basic types of bronchitis:

支气管炎从根本上说是肺部气道的炎症，它可由多种因素引起，但最常见的是普通感冒甚至流感病毒。支气管炎发作是由于支气管（肺部运送空气的管道）肿胀发炎，产生过多的黏液。支气管炎有两种基本类型：

Chronic bronchitis is defined as cough productive of sputum that persists for three months out of a year for at least two consecutive years. The cough and inflammation may be caused by respiratory infection or illness, exposure to tobacco smoke or other irritating substances in the air. Chronic bronchitis can cause airflow obstruction and is grouped under the term chronic

慢性支气管炎是指连续两年每年持续三个月以上的带痰咳嗽。咳嗽和炎症的起因可能是呼吸道感染或疾病、接触香烟的烟雾或空气中的其他刺激性物质。慢性支气管炎可引起气流阻塞，目前被归入慢性阻塞性肺疾病（COPD）。

obstructive pulmonary disease（COPD）.

Acute or short-term bronchitis is more common and usually is caused by a viral infection. Episodes of acute bronchitis can be related to and made worse by smoking. Acute bronchitis could last for 10 to 14 days, possibly causing symptoms for three weeks.

As for symptoms, patients who present with shortness of breath, coughing, lack of energy, are very common. Sometimes the patients will have some chills, low-grade temperatures, and sputum production. Pneumonia and bronchitis may present some similarities, such as cough, fever, fatigue and a heavy feeling in the chest. Bronchitis can sometimes progress to pneumonia. But the two conditions are different.

First, earlier bronchitis is mostly due to the inflammation of the air passageway whereas in a case of pneumonia you will find that the air sacs could be filled with fluids. Second, the symptoms for pneumonia are usually much worse. In addition, pneumonia can be life-threatening, especially to older people and other vulnerable groups.

急性支气管炎更为常见，通常由病毒感染引起。急性支气管炎的发作可能与吸烟有关，吸烟也可造成症状的恶化。急性支气管炎可能持续10至14天，症状持续时间可达3周。

在症状方面，患者常出现呼吸急促、咳嗽、精力不足的情况。有时患者会有寒战、低烧、咳痰的状况。肺炎和支气管炎可能表现出一些相似之处，如咳嗽、发烧、疲劳和胸闷。支气管炎有时也可能发展为肺炎，但这两者有以下差别。

首先，早期的支气管炎更多的是与气道炎症相关，而出现肺炎时肺泡可能会充满积液。其次，肺炎症状通常要严重得多。此外，肺炎可能危及生命，尤其是对老年人和其他易感人群而言。

The treatment for bronchitis depends on what type you have. If you have acute bronchitis, you might not need any treatment, or you might use over-the-counter drugs that break up mucus or that treat fever or pain. If you have a bacterial infection, your doctor might prescribe antibiotics.

If you have chronic bronchitis, treatment will be different. Symptoms can be alleviated by using a variety of methods, including drugs, oxygen therapy, pulmonary rehabilitation, surgery, or a combination of these. Your doctor might prescribe a mucus clearing device, also called an airway clearance device, to help you bring up mucus easily.

支气管炎的治疗方案取决于患者所患支气管炎的类型。急性支气管炎可能不需要任何治疗，可以使用化痰的非处方药或治疗发烧和缓解疼痛的非处方药。如果支气管炎是由细菌感染引起的，医生可能会开抗生素。

慢性支气管炎的治疗有所不同。其症状可以使用各种方法缓解，包括药物疗法、氧气疗法、肺康复疗法、手术或综合疗法。医生可能会使用排痰机，也就是气道清洁仪器，帮助患者轻松排出痰液。

（三）Asthma 哮喘[3-5]

Asthma is a condition in which your airways narrow and swell and may produce extra mucus. This can make breathing difficult and trigger coughing or a whistling sound（wheezing）when you breathe out and are shortness of breath. Typically, the airways are clean and open. There is no swelling. There is no restriction for the air to come in and out

哮喘是使气道变窄、肿胀并且产生额外黏液的疾病。哮喘导致呼吸困难并引发咳嗽，当患者呼气和呼吸急促时，伴有吹哨声（哮鸣音）。通常情况下，气道干净且畅通，没有肿胀。空气进出肺部不会受阻。当哮喘患者接近诱因开始咳嗽时，肺壁开始肿胀，产生黏液，使得气道变窄，肺部气体难以自由流动。

of the lungs. As the patient comes close to a trigger and starts coughing, the lungs' walls start swelling up, building mucus, making the airways narrow and difficult for the air to move freely.

Signs and symptoms for asthma include shortness of breath, chest tightness or pain, wheezing when exhaling, which is a common sign of asthma in children, sleeping trouble which is caused by shortness of breath, coughing or wheezing, and coughing or wheezing attacks that are worsened by a respiratory virus, such as a cold or the flu. Asthma symptoms vary from person to person. The patient may have infrequent asthma attacks, have symptoms only at certain times — such as when exercising — or have symptoms all the time.

Some triggers that can cause an asthma attack are pollen, animal dander, changes in the weather, respiratory infections such as viral or bacterial infections, perfumes, exercise, smoke, etc. To briefly categorize it according to triggers, asthma can be exercise-induced, occupation-induced and allergy-induced.

哮喘症状包括呼吸短促、胸闷或胸痛，儿童哮喘的常见症状还包括呼气时出现哮鸣音，此外还有由呼吸急促、咳嗽或喘息引起的睡眠困难，由感冒或流感等呼吸病毒导致的咳嗽或哮鸣音加重。哮喘症状因人而异。患者可能偶尔哮喘发作，或者只在某些情况下有症状，如锻炼时，也可能随时都有这些症状。

可能导致哮喘发作的诱因有花粉、动物皮屑、天气变化、呼吸道感染（如病毒或细菌感染）、香水、运动、烟雾等。根据触发因素对哮喘进行简要分类，哮喘可分为运动引起的哮喘、职业诱发的哮喘和过敏诱发的哮喘。

Not everyone with asthma takes the same medicine. Some medicines can be inhaled and some can be taken as a pill. Asthma medicines come in two types—quick relief and long-term control. Quick-relief medicines control the symptoms of an asthma attack. Long-term control medicines help you have fewer and milder attacks, but they don't help if you're having an asthma attack.

Long-term asthma control medications need to be taken regularly to control chronic symptoms and prevent asthma attacks, including inhaled corticosteroids, leukotriene modifiers, long-acting beta agonists (LABAs), theophylline, and combination inhalers. Take inhaled corticosteroids for example. These anti-inflammatory drugs are the most effective in reducing swelling and tightening in your airways. For children, long-term use of inhaled corticosteroids can delay their growth slightly. Inhaled corticosteroids don't generally cause serious side effects, so the benefits outweigh its risks.

Quick-relief medications for asthma, also called rescue medications, are taken as needed for rapid, short-term relief of symptoms. These medications include

不是每个哮喘患者都服用同样的药物。有些药物是吸入型的，有些是药片。哮喘药有两种类型：快速缓解药物和长期控制药物。快速缓解药物控制哮喘发作时的症状。长期控制药物可以帮助患者减少哮喘发作次数，降低发作的严重程度，但长期控制药物在哮喘发作时不能帮助患者立即缓解症状。

患者需要定期服用长期控制药物来控制慢性症状和预防哮喘发作。这些药包括吸入型的皮质类固醇、白三烯调节剂、长效β激动剂（LABAs）、茶碱和复方吸入剂。以吸入型皮质类固醇为例，这类抗炎药物是最有效的，可降低气道的肿胀和紧缩状态。对患有哮喘病的儿童来说，长期使用吸入型皮质类固醇会轻微影响其生长发育。吸入型皮质类固醇一般不会有严重的副作用，所以其利大于弊。

哮喘的快速缓解药物，也被称为急救药，可根据患者的需求使用，快速、短期缓解症状。这类药物包括短效β激动剂、异丙托胺、口服型和静

short-acting beta agonists, ipratropium, oral and intravenous corticosteroids, etc. They open the lungs by relaxing airway muscles. They begin working within minutes and are effective for four to six hours, but they're not for daily use.

脉注射型皮质类固醇等。这些药物通过放松气道肌肉打开肺部气道，通常在几分钟内可发挥药效，持续时间四到六个小时，但它们不是日常用药。

4.2 汉译英

（一）肺炎 Pneumonia[6]

肺炎是造成全世界儿童死亡人数最多的感染性疾病。2017 年，肺炎导致 808694 名 5 岁以下儿童死亡，占 5 岁以下儿童死亡总数的 15%。肺炎影响着世界各地的儿童及其背后的家庭，在南亚和撒哈拉以南非洲地区最为流行。

Pneumonia is the single largest infectious cause of death in children worldwide. Pneumonia killed 808,694 children under the age of 5 in 2017, accounting for 15% of all deaths of children under 5 years old. Pneumonia affects children and families everywhere but is most prevalent in South Asia and sub-Saharan Africa.

肺炎是一种影响肺部的急性呼吸道感染。肺部的小气囊被称为肺泡，当健康人呼吸时，肺泡内充满空气。当一个人患肺炎时，肺泡内积聚脓和液体，使呼吸疼痛，也限制了氧气的摄入。肺炎是由多种感染因子引起的，包括病毒、细菌、真菌等。最常见的是肺炎链球菌、乙型流感嗜血杆菌（通常称为 Hib）、呼吸道合胞病毒和耶氏肺孢子菌。

Pneumonia is a form of acute respiratory infection that affects the lungs. The sacs in the lungs are called alveoli. When a healthy person breathes, alveoli are filled with air. When an individual has pneumonia, the alveoli are filled with pus and fluid, which makes breathing painful and limits oxygen intake. Pneumonia is caused by a number of infectious agents, including viruses, bacteria, fungi, etc. The most common are streptococcus pneumoniae, haemophilus influenzae type b which is usually called Hib, respiratory syncytial virus, and pneumocystis jiroveci.

肺炎可以通过多种方式传播。它可以通过咳嗽或打喷嚏时空气中的飞沫传播。此外，肺炎可能在分娩时通过血液传播。肺炎通常情况下使用抗生素治疗。选用的抗生素是阿莫西林分散片剂。大多数肺炎病例仅需口服抗生素。重症肺炎患者才建议住院治疗。

Pneumonia can be spread in several ways. It may spread via air-borne droplets from a cough or sneeze. In addition, pneumonia may spread through blood, especially during and shortly after birth. Pneumonia is commonly treated with antibiotics. The antibiotic of choice is amoxicillin dispersible tablets. Most cases of pneumonia only require oral antibiotics. Hospitalization is recommended only for severe cases of pneumonia.

世界卫生组织和联合国儿童基金会的《肺炎和腹泻全球行动计划》旨在通过采取多种干预措施，预防和治疗儿童肺炎，加快肺炎控制进程。这些措施如下：第一，针对艾滋病暴露儿童，通过接种疫苗、用肥皂洗手、减少家庭空气污染、预防艾滋病病毒和服用复方新诺明来防止感染肺炎。

The WHO and UNICEF integrated Global Action Plan for Pneumonia and Diarrhea (GAPPD) aims to accelerate pneumonia control with a combination of interventions to prevent and treat pneumonia in children, including: Firstly, prevent pneumonia with vaccinations, handwashing with soap, reducing household air pollution, HIV prevention, and cotrimoxazole prophylaxis for HIV-infected and exposed children.

第二，通过提倡纯母乳喂养与适当辅食相结合，保护儿童免受肺炎的侵害。第三，治疗肺炎的重点是确保

Secondly, protect children from pneumonia by promoting exclusive breastfeeding combined with adequate

每个生病的儿童都能获得正确的护理。患儿的护理可由社区医院卫生工作人员提供。在肺炎严重时，需送往医疗卫生机构，以确保儿童能够获得治病所需的抗生素和氧气，以恢复健康。

complementary feeding. Thirdly, treat pneumonia with a focus on making sure that every sick child has access to the right kind of care—either from a community-based health worker or in a health facility if the disease is severe—and can get the antibiotics and oxygen they need to get well.

（二）肺结核 Tuberculosis[7-9]

结核病（TB）是由细菌（结核分枝杆菌）引起的，通常影响肺部。结核病是可以预防和治愈的。结核病可以通过空气人传人。当结核患者咳嗽、打喷嚏或吐痰时，结核分枝杆菌就会被排到空气中。即便其他人吸入少量细菌也会被感染。

Tuberculosis (TB) is caused by bacteria (mycobacterium tuberculosis) that most often affect the lungs. Tuberculosis is preventable and curable. TB is spread from person to person through the air. When people with lung TB cough, sneeze, or spit, they propel the TB germs into the air. Even when a person inhales only a few of these germs he or she will become infected.

当一个人患上活动性肺结核时，其症状（如咳嗽、发烧、盗汗或体重减轻）在数月中都可能比较轻微。这会延误其就医，并造成人际传播。活动性肺结核患者可在一年内通过密切接触感染5至15人。

When a person develops active lung TB, the symptoms (such as cough, fever, night sweats, or weight loss) may be mild for many months. This can lead to delays in seeking care and results in the transmission of the bacteria to others. People with active lung TB can infect 5 – 15 other people through close contact over the course of a year.

活动性肺结核的常见症状包括咳痰、咳血、胸痛、虚弱、体重减轻、发烧和盗汗。世界卫生组织建议对有结核病症状和体征的人群使用快速分子诊断测试来初步诊断结核，因为这种检测方法具有高诊断准确度，有助于结核病和耐药结核病的早期发现。世界卫生组织建议的快速检测有 Xpert MTB/RIF、Xpert Ultra 和 Truenat 含量测定。诊断耐多药和其他耐药形式的结核病以及与艾滋病病毒相关的结核病则更为复杂且费用高昂。

结核病是一种可治愈的疾病。结核病的治疗通常涉及连续几个月服用抗生素。如果患者被诊断为活动性肺结核且已有症状，肺部受损，则至少会开 6 个月的联合抗生素治疗。通常的治疗方案是：2 种抗生素（异烟肼和利福平）治疗 6 个月，前 2 个月增加 2 种抗生素（吡嗪酰胺和乙胺丁醇）。

肺外结核病，即发生在肺部以外

Common symptoms of active lung TB are cough with sputum and blood at times, chest pains, weakness, weight loss, fever, and night sweats. WHO recommends the use of rapid molecular diagnostic tests as the initial diagnostic test in all persons with signs and symptoms of TB as they have high diagnostic accuracy and will lead to major improvements in the early detection of TB and drug-resistant TB. Rapid tests recommended by WHO are the Xpert MTB/RIF, Xpert Ultra, and Truenat assays. Diagnosing multidrug-resistant and other resistant forms of TB, as well as HIV-associated TB, can be complex and expensive.

TB is a treatable and curable disease. Treatment for TB usually involves taking antibiotics for several months. You'll be prescribed at least a 6-month course of a combination of antibiotics if you're diagnosed with active pulmonary TB, where your lungs are affected and you have symptoms. The usual treatment is: 2 antibiotics (isoniazid and rifampicin) for 6 months, and 2 additional antibiotics (pyrazinamide and ethambutol) for the first 2 months of the 6-month treatment period.

Extrapulmonary TB, which is TB

的结核病，可以使用治疗肺结核的联合抗生素疗法进行治疗。耐多药结核病则需要更长的抗生素疗程，一般在9至24个月，视具体情况而定。耐多药结核病的治疗效果往往比普通结核病差。

潜伏性结核是指机体感染结核分枝杆菌后没有任何明显感染症状。如果您是结核分枝杆菌携带者，并且年龄在65岁及以下，通常建议要么连续服用利福平搭配异烟肼3个月，要么单独服用异烟肼6个月。如果潜伏性结核具有耐药性，也并不总是会采取治疗措施。

（三）慢性阻塞性肺疾病 COPD [10]

慢性阻塞性肺疾病是中国和世界范围内的常见病。世界卫生组织预测，从2010年到2030年，慢性阻塞性肺疾病将成为排名第三的致死性疾病和排名第五的致残性疾病。据初步统计，现在我国四十岁以上的人群有8.2%患有慢性阻塞性肺疾病。换句话说，我们国家有四千万人患慢性阻塞性肺疾病。而且慢性阻塞性肺疾病的一个很大问题是它的病死率高。2000年，

that occurs outside the lungs, can be treated using the same combination of antibiotics as those used to treat pulmonary TB. Multidrug-resistant TB requires a much longer course of antibiotics from 9 to 24 months, depending on the strain. Multidrug-resistant TB tends to have less favorable outcomes than standard TB.

Latent TB is where you've been infected with the TB bacteria, but do not have any symptoms of active infection. If you have latent TB and are aged 65 or under, treatment is usually recommended: either taking a combination of rifampicin and isoniazid for 3 months or isoniazid on its own for 6 months. Latent TB is also not always treated if it's thought to be drug-resistant.

Chronic obstructive pulmonary disease (COPD) is a common disease in China and the world. WHO predicts that COPD will be the third leading cause of death and the fifth leading cause of disability over the course from 2010 to 2030. At present in China, it's preliminarily estimated that 8.2% of people over the age of 40 have COPD. In other words, there are 40 million people with COPD nationwide. A

慢性阻塞性肺疾病的死亡人数为 128 万，也就是说每分钟有 2.5 个人死于慢性阻塞性肺疾病。

从学术定义来说，第一秒钟呼气量小于正常肺容量的 70% 的时候，我们就把它定义为慢性阻塞性肺疾病，这个是在医学上的定义。在早期，慢性阻塞性肺疾病没有明显的症状，但是随着病程的进展，主要的临床表现就是咳痰，特别是所谓的喘，或者说气促、气紧、气急，在不同的地方有不同的命名。当患者出现气促症状时，特别是在稍微活动后症状加重，往往就会去看医生。继续发展的话，开始是赶公共汽车或上楼梯觉得气紧，后来日常生活中也会出现气紧，比如洗澡，甚至刷牙时，最后坐着时都会觉得喘不过气来。这时，病情就已经发展到比较晚期了。

刚才我们讲了慢性阻塞性肺疾病是如何发展的。我们知道它是一个进

big problem with COPD is its high fatality rate. In 2000, there were 1.28 million deaths. In other words, 2.5 people die of COPD every minute.

In academic definition, when the volume that the lungs exhale in the first second is less than 70% of the normal volume, it is defined as COPD. That's the standard in the medical definition. There are no obvious early symptoms, but as COPD develops, the main clinical feature is sputum, especially the so-called wheezing, or in other words, shortness of breath, tight breath, or fast breath. It has different names in different places. When patients with shortness of breath feel the symptoms exacerbating after a moderate exercise, they often go to the doctor. As the disease develops, patients will start to feel a tight breath when catching the bus or climbing the stairs. Then gradually, they wheeze in daily life, when taking a bath or even just brushing the teeth. At last, they might feel out of breath only sitting up. At this point, the disease has already developed into the late phase.

We just talked about how COPD develops. We know it's a progressive

展性的疾病。所以慢性阻塞性肺疾病与高血压、糖尿病、冠心病等其他疾病一样，需要注意早检测，早诊断，早干预。早期发现和诊断慢性阻塞性肺疾病的主要方法有哪些？主要是靠肺功能检查。肺功能检查不贵，也不复杂。用力吹一口气，发现你在第一秒的呼气容积小于用力肺活量的70%，你就可能被诊断有慢性阻塞性肺疾病。所以这个肺功能检查是非常简单的。

disease. Therefore, for COPD, like other diseases, such as hypertension, diabetes, and coronary heart disease, attention needs to be paid to early detection, early diagnosis, and early intervention. What can be the major methods to discover and diagnose COPD in its early phase? It is mainly by pulmonary function test (PFT). This test is not expensive or complicated. If you blow hard and find that the air you blow out in the first second is less than 70% of the forced vital capacity (FVC), you are likely to be diagnosed with COPD. So, we can say that PFT is very simple.

5 口译注释与学习资源

5.1 口译注释

（一）"支气管炎""肺气肿"的翻译

支气管炎和肺气肿早期无气流受限，因此不能诊断为慢性阻塞性肺疾病。只有当支气管炎和肺气肿发展到肺功能检查发现气流受限的地步时，方可诊断为慢性阻塞性肺疾病。因此，上文在翻译时将支气管炎、肺气肿与慢性阻塞性肺疾病并列。

（二）"发作"的翻译

（1）**attack** 在医学英语中常常翻译为"突发""发作""侵害""感染"而非"袭击"，可以做名词或者动词使用。

如：本章"口译实战"英译汉第三篇中的"Long-term control medicines help you have fewer and milder **attacks**, but they don't help if you're having an asthma **attack**."，两处 attack 均译为"发作"。

又如：heart **attack** 突发心脏病。

再如：The virus seems to have **attacked** his throat. 病毒似乎已侵害到他的咽喉。

（2）**episode** 在医学英语中也表示"发作"而非"（电视的）剧集"，如英译汉第二篇中"**Episodes** of acute bronchitis can be related to and made worse by smoking"译为"急性支气管炎的发作可能与吸烟有关，吸烟也可造成症状的恶化"。

（三）肺孢子菌肺炎

肺孢子菌肺炎（pneumocystis pneumonia，PCP），又称为耶氏肺孢子菌肺炎（pneumocystis jirovecii pneumonia，PJP），是由耶氏肺孢子菌（pneumocystis jirovecii）引起的，它曾经被命名为卡氏肺孢子菌（pneumocystis carinii）。

5.2 学习资源

登录中国大学 MOOC（慕课），学习"医疗口译"课程中"呼吸内科"的口译实战示范视频。

参考文献

［1］NHS. （n. d.）. *Respiratory medicine.* Retrieved November 13，2021，from https：//www. healthcareers. nhs. uk/explore-roles/doctors/roles-doctors/medicine/respiratory-medicine.

［2］Cleveland Clinic. （n. d.）. *Bronchitis symptoms & treatment.* Retrieved November 13，2021，from https：//my. clevelandclinic. org/health/diseases/3993 − bronchitis.

［3］Mayo Foundation for Medical Education and Research. （2020，August 11）. *Asthma.* Retrieved November 13，2021，from https：//www. mayoclinic. org/diseases-conditions/asthma/symptoms-causes/syc − 20369653.

［4］Mayo Foundation for Medical Education and Research. （2020，June 19）. *Asthma medications: Know your options.* Retrieved November 13，2021，from https：//www. mayoclinic. org/diseases-conditions/asthma/in-depth/asthma-medications/art − 20045557.

［5］Centers for Disease Control and Prevention. （2018，January 30）. *Asthma-management and treatment.* Retrieved November 13，2021，from https：//www. cdc. gov/asthma/management. html #how.

［6］World Health Organization. （n. d.）. *Pneumonia.* Retrieved November 13，2021，from https：//www. who. int/news-room/fact-sheets/detail/pneumonia.

［7］ NHS. (n. d.). *Tuberculosis*. Retrieved November 13，2021，from https://www. nhs. uk/ conditions/tuberculosis-tb/treatment/.

［8］ World Health Organization. (n. d.). *Tuberculosis (TB)*. Retrieved November 13，2021，from https://www. who. int/news-room/fact-sheets/detail/tuberculosis.

［9］ 原创力文档网. 肺结核知识读本［EB/OL］. ［2021 - 09 - 10］. https://max. book118. com/html/2021/1030/8141070052004027. shtm.

［10］ 钟南山. 钟南山院士为你讲授慢阻肺的医学知识［EB/OL］. ［2020 - 06 - 18］. https:// www. bilibili. com/video/BV19f4y1y75M? from = search&seid = 6507878605804789638.

第六章

消化内科

1 导读

本章的重点为口译技巧"抓关键词"和消化内科的6篇"口译实战"练习。口译实战练习中英译汉、汉译英各3篇，内容涵盖消化内科、消化性溃疡、肝硬化、胃炎、酒精性肝病与非酒精性脂肪性肝病和上消化道内镜。请结合本章口译技巧练习6篇口译实战文本。

2 口译技巧——意义听辨（1）：抓关键词

口译信息加工过程的第一步和最重要的一步正是意义听辨。没有对信息的听、辨、析、解，就没有正确的传译和表达可言。关键词是意义传递的关键节点。在传递意图时，讲话者的一句话或者一段话中各个单词的重要程度并不相同，其中最重要的词才是关键词。抓关键词对于高效的口译听辨至关重要。

2.1 何为关键词

（1）实词，包括下面"口译词汇"部分的名词术语、任何一句话中的行为动词、人称代词和指涉代词、数字和日期等。

（2）词组，包括固定搭配和常见搭配，通常由2~7个词语组成，但是这几个词可以作为一个关键点来记，如difficulty in swallowing, inflammatory bowel disease（IBD），Non-alcoholic fatty liver disease（NAFLD）等。

2.2 如何练习判断关键词

（1）读：读完一句话之后暂停，强迫自己在这句话中选出3个关键词。不管这句话有多长，都只能选3个关键词或词组，然后根据关键词或词组复述出整句话，最好能够做到一字不差。练习时可以先选择短一点的句子，然后逐渐挑战长句和难句。

（2）听：按上面的步骤，但是输入方式由"读"（视觉输入）变为"听"（听觉输入）。

3 口译词汇

3.1 英译汉

（一）Gastroenterology 消化内科（消化科/胃肠科/胃肠病学）

gastroenterologist 消化科医生，胃肠病学家

esophagus 食管

stomach，intestines，liver 胃、肠、肝

small intestine，colon and rectum 小肠、结肠和直肠

gallbladder，bile ducts，pancreas 胆囊、胆道、胰腺

physiology 生理学

motility 动力学

gastroesophageal reflux 胃食管反流

esophageal cancer 食管癌

gastritis 胃炎

gastric cancer 胃癌

inflammatory bowel disease（IBD）炎症性肠病

Irritable Bowel Syndrome（IBS）肠易激综合征

colorectal cancer 大肠癌

enteritis 小肠炎

colitis 结肠炎

pancreatitis 胰腺炎

pancreatic cancer 胰腺癌

colon polyps and cancer 结肠息肉和癌症

biliary tract disease 胆道疾病

internal medicine residency 内科住院医师培训

fellowship 专科医师培训

upper endoscopy 上消化道内镜检查

colonoscopy 结肠镜检查

sigmoidoscopy 乙状结肠镜检查

perform advanced endoscopic procedures 进行高级内镜操作

polypectomy 息肉切除术

esophageal and intestinal dilation 食道和肠道扩张

hemostasis 止血

cautery 烧灼

injection or cautery to stop bleeding 注射或烧灼止血

conditions 病症，病情

endoscopic biliary examination 内镜胆道检查

endoscopic retrograde cholangiopancreatography（ERCP）内镜逆行胰胆管造影术

endoscopic mucosal resection（EMR）内镜黏膜切除术

placement of internal drainage tubes（stents）内部引流管放置（支架）

endoscopic ultrasound（EUS）内镜超声

（二）Peptic Ulcers 消化性溃疡

gastric ulcer 胃溃疡

duodenal ulcer 十二指肠溃疡

the upper portion of the small intestine（duodenum）小肠上部（十二指肠）

open ulcer 开放性溃疡

digestive tract 消化道

stomach acid 胃酸

mucous layer 黏膜层

gastrointestinal（GI）bleeding 消化道出血

nausea 恶心

burning stomach pain 胃灼痛

feeling of fullness 饱胀感

bloating or belching 腹胀或嗳（ǎi）气（打嗝）

intolerance to fatty foods 高脂肪食物不耐受

vomiting 呕吐

acid reflux 反酸

heartburn 烧心，胃灼热

loss of appetite 食欲不振

dysphagia 吞咽困难

ascites 腹水

constipation 便秘

hematochezia 便血

melena 黑便

hematemesis 呕血

jaundice 黄疸

foods that buffer stomach acid 缓冲胃酸的食物

acid-reducing medication 降酸药物

black or tarry stools 黑便或柏油样便

abdominal distension（bloating）腹胀

unexplained weight loss and appetite changes 不明原因的体重减轻和食欲改变

Helicobacter pylori（H. pylori）幽门螺杆菌

over-the-counter（OTC）and prescription pain medications 非处方药和处方止痛药

nonsteroidal anti-inflammatory drugs（NSAID）非甾（zāi）体抗炎药

ibuprofen, naproxen sodium, ketoprofen 布洛芬、萘普生钠、酮洛芬

steroids, anticoagulants, low-dose aspirin, selective serotonin reuptake inhibitors（SSRIs）类固醇、抗凝剂、低剂量阿司匹林和选择性血清素再摄取抑制剂

proton pump inhibitors（PPIs）, histamine receptor blockers and protectants 质子泵抑制剂、组胺受体阻滞剂和保护剂

（三）Cirrhosis 肝硬化

scarring（fibrosis）of the liver 肝脏瘢痕形成（纤维化）

chronic alcoholism 慢性酒精中毒/长期酗酒

scar tissue 瘢痕组织

chronic hepatitis 慢性肝炎

alcoholic liver disease 酒精性肝病

primary liver cancer 原发性肝癌

hepatic encephalopathy 肝性脑病

decompensated cirrhosis 失代偿性肝硬化

advanced cirrhosis 晚期肝硬化

swelling in your legs, feet or ankles（edema）腿、脚或脚踝肿胀（水肿）

yellow discoloration in the skin and eyes（jaundice）皮肤和眼睛发黄（黄疸）

fluid accumulation in your abdomen（ascites）腹膜腔积液（腹水）

spiderlike blood vessels on your skin 皮肤上的蜘蛛状血管

absent or loss of periods not related to menopause for women 女性与更年期无关的月经消失或减少

loss of sex drive, breast enlargement (gynecomastia) or testicular atrophy for men 性欲减退、男性乳房增大 (男性乳房发育症) 或睾丸萎缩

chronic viral hepatitis (hepatitis B, C and D) 慢性病毒性肝炎 (乙型、丙型和丁型肝炎)

fat accumulating in the liver (non-alcoholic fatty liver disease) 肝脏中的脂肪堆积 (非酒精性脂肪性肝病)

iron build-up in the body (hemochromatosis) 体内铁积聚 (血色素沉着症)

cystic fibrosis 囊性纤维化

copper accumulated in the liver (Wilson's disease) 肝脏中铜积聚 (威尔逊病)

poorly formed bile ducts (biliary atresia) 胆管形成不良 (胆道闭锁)

Alpha-1 antitrypsin deficiency α-1 抗胰蛋白酶缺乏症

inherited disorders of sugar metabolism (galactosemia or glycogen storage disease) 遗传性糖代谢紊乱 (半乳糖血症或糖原贮积病)

genetic digestive disorder (Alagille syndrome) 遗传性消化系统疾病 (阿拉吉勒综合征)

autoimmune hepatitis 自免疫性肝炎

destruction of the bile ducts (primary biliary cirrhosis) 胆管破坏 (原发性胆汁性肝硬化)

hardening and scarring of the bile ducts (primary sclerosing cholangitis) 胆管硬化和瘢痕形成 (原发性硬化性胆管炎)

syphilis or brucellosis 梅毒或布鲁氏菌病

methotrexate or isoniazid 甲氨蝶呤或异烟肼

non-alcoholic steatohepatitis (NASH) 非酒精性脂肪性肝炎

3.2 汉译英

(一) 胃炎 Gastritis

急性胃炎 acute gastritis

慢性、长期胃炎 chronic, long-term gastritis

黏膜 mucosa

幽门螺杆菌 Helicobacter pylori（H. pylori）

消化不良 indigestion（dyspepsia）

黏膜修复的新陈代谢 metabolism of mucosal repair

社会经济地位较低的群体 lower socioeconomic groups

侵蚀性胃炎 erosive gastritis

非侵蚀性胃炎 non-erosive gastritis

胃壁炎症 inflammation of the stomach lining

皮质类固醇 corticosteroids

抗酸剂 antacids

减少胃酸暴露 reduce stomach acid exposure

碳酸钙药物 calcium carbonate medications

西咪替丁、雷尼替丁 cimetidine，ranitidine

奥美拉唑、埃索美拉唑 omeprazole，esomeprazole

胃食管反流病 gastroesophageal reflux disease

（二）酒精性肝病与非酒精性脂肪性肝病 ALD and NAFLD

酒精性肝病 alcoholic liver disease（ALD）

非酒精性脂肪性肝病 nonalcoholic fatty liver disease（NAFLD）

肝脏肿大和压痛 liver enlargement（hepatomegaly）and pressure pain

上消化道出血 upper gastrointestinal bleeding

肝细胞坏死 liver cell necrosis

肝功能衰竭 liver failure

流行病学调查 epidemiological research

发病率 prevalence

阈值效应 threshold effect

剂量－效应关系 dose-effect relationship

晚期瘢痕肝（肝硬化）advanced scarring liver（cirrhosis）

酒精介导的肝毒性 alcohol-mediated liver toxicity

右上腹不适 discomfort in the upper right abdomen

胰岛素抵抗/耐受 insulin resistance

胰岛素激素 hormone insulin

高血糖 high blood sugar（hyperglycemia）

糖尿病前期或 2 型糖尿病 prediabetes or type 2 diabetes

甘油三酯 triglyceride

（三）上消化道内镜 Upper Endoscopy

食管胃十二指肠镜 esophagogastroduodenoscopy（EGD）

管腔内壁 the inner lining of the lumen

食管镜 esophagoscopy

胃镜 gastroscopy

十二指肠镜 duodenoscopy

抗凝药物（如香豆素、肝素）anti-coagulant medication（i. e., Coumadin, Heparin）

泰诺（对乙酰氨基酚）Tylenol（acetaminophen）

美林、雅维（布洛芬）Motrin, Advil（ibuprofen）

萘普生、努普林 Naprosyn, Nuprin

做剧烈运动 do strenuous exercise

4　口译实战

4.1　英译汉

（一）Gastroenterology 消化内科（消化科/胃肠科/胃肠病学）[1]

Gastroenterology is the study of the normal function and diseases of the esophagus, stomach, small intestine, colon and rectum, pancreas, gallbladder, bile ducts and liver. It involves a detailed understanding of the normal action（physiology）of the gastrointestinal organs including the movement of material through the stomach and intestine（motility）, the digestion and absorption of nutrients into the body, removal of waste from the system, and the function of the liver as a

胃肠病学是研究食道、胃、小肠、结肠和直肠、胰腺、胆囊、胆管和肝脏的正常功能及疾病的学科，涉及对胃肠器官正常功能（生理学）的详细理解，其中包括物质通过胃肠的运动（动力学）、营养物质在人体的消化和吸收、废物清除以及肝脏作为消化器官的功能。

digestive organ.

It includes common and important conditions such as colon polyps and cancer, hepatitis, gastroesophageal reflux (heartburn), peptic ulcer, colitis, gallbladder and biliary tract disease, nutritional problems, Irritable Bowel Syndrome (IBS), and pancreatitis. In essence, all normal activity and disease of the digestive organs is part of the study of gastroenterology.

A gastroenterologist must first complete a three-year Internal Medicine residency and is then eligible for additional specialized training (fellowship) in gastroenterology. This fellowship is generally 2 - 3 years long, so by the time gastroenterologists have completed their training, they have had 5 - 6 years of additional specialized education following medical school.

Gastroenterologists also receive dedicated training in endoscopy (upper endoscopy, sigmoidoscopy, and colonoscopy). Endoscopy is the use of narrow, flexible lighted tubes with built-in video cameras, to visualize the inside of the intestinal tract. This specialized training includes detailed and intensive

常见的主要病症包括结肠息肉和结肠癌、肝炎、胃食管反流（胃灼热）、消化性溃疡、结肠炎、胆囊和胆道疾病、营养性疾病、肠易激综合征、胰腺炎等。从本质上讲，消化器官的所有正常活动和疾病都属于胃肠病学研究的范畴。

消化科医生必须首先完成为期三年的内科住院医师培训，然后才有资格接受额外的消化科专科医师培训。专科医师培训通常为期2~3年，因此当消化科医生完成培训时，他们在离开医学院之后又接受了5~6年的额外专业教育。

消化科医生还要接受专门的内镜培训（上消化道内镜检查、乙状结肠镜检查和结肠镜检查）。内镜检查使用细小、灵活、带有内置摄像头的灯管来观察肠道内部。这一专业培训的内容包括详细而深入地学习何时以及如何进行内镜检查、安全有效地开展检查的最佳方法，以及如何使用镇静

study of how and when to perform endoscopy, optimal methods to complete these tests safely and effectively, and the use of sedating medications to ensure the comfort and safety of patients.

Gastroenterology trainees also learn how to perform advanced endoscopic procedures such as polypectomy (removal of colon polyps), esophageal and intestinal dilation (stretching of narrowed areas), and hemostasis (injection or cautery to stop bleeding). Importantly, gastroenterologists learn how to properly interpret the findings and biopsy results of these studies in order to make appropriate recommendations to treat conditions and/or prevent cancer.

Some gastroenterologists also receive directed training in advanced procedures using endoscopes such as endoscopic biliary examination (endoscopic retrograde cholangiopancreatography or ERCP), removal of tumors without surgery (endoscopic mucosal resection or EMR), placement of internal drainage tubes (stents) and endoscopic ultrasound (EUS). This provides them with the training necessary to non-surgically remove stones in the bile ducts, evaluate and treat

药物来确保患者的舒适度和安全。

医学生在消化科还要学习如何进行高级内镜操作，如息肉切除（切除结肠息肉）、食道和肠道扩张（狭窄区域的扩张）、止血（注射或烧灼止血）。重要的是，消化科医生要学习如何正确理解检查结果和活检结果，以便为治疗病症和预防癌症提出适当的建议。

有些消化科医生还接受了内镜高级操作的定向培训，例如内镜胆道检查（内镜逆行胰胆管造影术，又称ERCP）、无开放手术肿瘤切除（内镜黏膜切除术或 EMR）、内部引流管放置（支架）和内镜超声（EUS）。这些培训可使医生们学会以非手术的方式切除胆管结石，评估和治疗胃肠道及肝脏肿瘤，并为一些患者提供开放手术之外的微创方案。

tumors of the gastrointestinal tract and liver, and provide minimally invasive alternatives to surgery for some patients.

The most critical emphasis during the training period is attention to detail and incorporation of their comprehensive knowledge of the entire gastrointestinal tract to provide the highest quality endoscopy and consultative services. The final product is a highly trained specialist with a unique combination of broad scientific knowledge, general Internal Medicine training, superior endoscopic skills and experience, and the ability to integrate these elements to provide optimal health care for patients.

培训的关键点是强调细节和全面学习胃肠道知识，以提供最高质量的内镜和咨询服务。最终，医生们将成为训练有素的专家，拥有丰富的科学知识，接受过系统的内科培训，具有卓越的内镜技术和经验，以及整合这些要素为患者提供最佳医疗服务的能力。

（二）Peptic Ulcers 消化性溃疡[2]

Peptic ulcers occur when acid in the digestive tract eats away at the inner surface of the stomach or small intestine. The acid can create a painful open sore that may bleed. Your digestive tract is coated with a mucous layer that normally protects against acid. But if the amount of acid is increased or the amount of mucus is decreased, you could develop an ulcer. Peptic ulcers include gastric ulcers that occur on the inside of the stomach and duodenal ulcers that occur

当消化道中的酸侵蚀胃或小肠的内表面时，就会发生消化性溃疡。酸会导致出现开放性溃疡，带来疼痛，并可能造成出血。通常消化道内有一层可以抵御酸腐蚀的黏液层。但如果酸量增加或黏液量减少，就可能会产生溃疡。消化性溃疡包括发生在胃内部的胃溃疡和发生在小肠上段（十二指肠）内部的十二指肠溃疡。

on the inside of the upper portion of your small intestine (duodenum).

Symptoms include burning stomach pain, feeling of fullness, bloating or belching, intolerance to fatty foods, heartburn and nausea. The most common peptic ulcer symptom is burning stomach pain. Stomach acid makes the pain worse, as does having an empty stomach. The pain can often be relieved by eating certain foods that buffer stomach acid or by taking an acid-reducing medication, but then it may come back. The pain may be worse between meals and at night.

Many people with peptic ulcers don't even have symptoms. Less often, ulcers may cause severe symptoms such as vomiting or vomiting blood (hematemesis), blood in stools (hematochezia), or stools that are black or tarry (melena), trouble breathing, feeling faint, unexplained weight loss and appetite changes.

Common causes include bacteria, regular use of certain pain relievers and other medications. Helicobacter pylori bacteria commonly live in the mucous layer that covers and protects tissues that

症状包括胃灼痛、饱胀感、腹胀或嗳气、高脂肪食物不耐受、烧心和恶心。最常见的消化性溃疡症状是胃灼痛。胃酸会使疼痛加剧，空腹时胃痛也会加剧。通常可以通过进食某些缓冲胃酸的食物或服用降酸药物来缓解疼痛，但随后可能复发。两餐之间和夜晚疼痛可能会加重。

许多患有消化性溃疡的人甚至没有症状。少数情况下，溃疡可能会导致严重症状，例如呕吐或吐血（呕血）、便血、黑色或柏油样大便（黑便）、呼吸困难、感觉虚弱、不明原因的体重减轻和食欲改变。

消化性溃疡常由细菌以及经常使用某些止痛药和其他药物引起。幽门螺杆菌通常生活在覆盖并保护胃和小肠的黏液层中。很多时候幽门螺杆菌不会引起任何问题，但它也可能导致

line the stomach and small intestine. Often, H. pylori causes no problems, but it can cause inflammation of the stomach's inner layer, producing an ulcer. It's not clear how H. pylori infection spreads. It may be transmitted from person to person by close contact. People may also contract H. pylori through food and water.

胃内层发炎，从而产生溃疡。目前尚不清楚幽门螺杆菌如何传播。它可能通过人与人之间的密切接触传播。人也可能在吃东西和喝水的过程中感染幽门螺杆菌。

Taking aspirin, as well as certain over-the-counter and prescription pain medications called nonsteroidal anti-inflammatory drugs（NSAIDs）, can irritate or inflame the lining of your stomach and small intestine. These medications include ibuprofen, naproxen sodium, ketoprofen and others. They do not include acetaminophen. Taking certain other medications along with NSAIDs, such as steroids, anticoagulants, low-dose aspirin, selective serotonin reuptake inhibitors（SSRIs）, can also greatly increase the chance of developing ulcers.

服用阿司匹林以及某些称为非甾体抗炎药的非处方药和处方止痛药会刺激胃和小肠内壁或使之发炎。这些药物包括布洛芬、萘普生钠、酮洛芬等，不包括对乙酰氨基酚。与非甾体抗炎药一起服用的其他药物，如类固醇、抗凝剂、低剂量阿司匹林和选择性血清素再摄取抑制剂，也会大大增加发生溃疡的机会。

If NSAIDs are causing your peptic ulcer and you don't have an H. pylori infection, your doctor may tell you to stop taking the NSAID, reduce how much of the NSAID you take or switch to another medicine that won't cause a

如果非甾体抗炎药导致了消化性溃疡并且患者没有感染幽门螺杆菌，那么医生可能会让患者停用非甾体抗炎药，减少服用量或改用另一种不会引起消化性溃疡的药物。医生也可能会开些药物来减少胃酸和缓解消化性

peptic ulcer. Your doctor may also prescribe medicines to reduce stomach acid and coat and protect your peptic ulcer. Proton pump inhibitors, histamine receptor blockers, and protectants can help relieve pain and help your ulcer heal.

溃疡。质子泵抑制剂、组胺受体阻滞剂和保护剂可以帮助缓解疼痛，使溃疡愈合。

（三）Cirrhosis 肝硬化 [3-4]

Cirrhosis is a late stage of scarring （fibrosis） of the liver caused by many forms of liver diseases and conditions, such as hepatitis and chronic alcoholism. Each time your liver is injured — whether by disease, excessive alcohol consumption or another cause — it tries to repair itself. In the process, scar tissue forms. As cirrhosis progresses, more and more scar tissue forms, making it difficult for the liver to function （decompensated cirrhosis）. Advanced cirrhosis is life-threatening.

肝硬化是肝脏瘢痕形成（纤维化）的晚期，由多种肝脏病症引起，例如肝炎和慢性酒精中毒。每次肝脏受伤时，无论是由于疾病、过度饮酒还是其他原因，它都会尝试自我修复。瘢痕组织会在这个过程中形成。在肝硬化的进程中，会有越来越多的瘢痕组织形成，使肝脏难以发挥作用（失代偿性肝硬化）。晚期肝硬化会危及生命。

The liver damage done by cirrhosis generally can't be undone. But if liver cirrhosis is diagnosed and treated early, further damage can be limited and, rarely, reversed. Cirrhosis often has no signs or symptoms until liver damage is extensive.

肝硬化造成的肝损伤通常无法逆转。但是，如果肝硬化得到及早诊断和治疗，进一步损伤可以被阻止，肝损伤可能会逆转，虽然这种情况较为罕见。在肝脏受损严重之前肝硬化通常不会导致任何体征或症状。

When signs and symptoms do occur, they may include fatigue, easy bleeding or bruising, loss of appetite, nausea, swelling in your legs, feet or ankles (edema), weight loss, itchy skin, yellow discoloration in the skin and eyes (jaundice), fluid accumulation in your abdomen (ascites), spiderlike blood vessels on your skin, redness in the palms of the hands, absent or loss of periods not related to menopause for women and loss of sex drive, breast enlargement (gynecomastia) or testicular atrophy for men, and confusion, drowsiness and slurred speech (hepatic encephalopathy).

A wide range of diseases and conditions can damage the liver and lead to cirrhosis. Some of the causes include chronic alcohol abuse, chronic viral hepatitis (hepatitis B, C and D), fat accumulating in the liver (nonalcoholic fatty liver disease), iron buildup in the body (hemochromatosis), cystic fibrosis, copper accumulated in the liver (Wilson's disease) and poorly formed bile ducts (biliary atresia).

Other causes are Alpha-1 antitrypsin deficiency, inherited disorders of sugar

可能的体征和症状包括疲劳、易出血或瘀伤、食欲不振、恶心、腿脚或脚踝肿胀（水肿）、体重减轻、皮肤瘙痒、皮肤和眼睛发黄（黄疸）、腹膜腔积液（腹水）、皮肤上的蜘蛛状血管、手掌发红、女性与更年期无关的月经消失、男性性欲减退及乳房增大（男性乳房发育症）或睾丸萎缩、意识模糊、嗜睡和言语不清（肝性脑病）。

许多疾病和状况也会损害肝脏并导致肝硬化。病因包括慢性酒精滥用、慢性病毒性肝炎（乙型、丙型和丁型肝炎）、肝脏脂肪堆积（非酒精性脂肪性肝病）、体内铁积聚（血色素沉着症）、囊性纤维化、肝脏中铜积聚（威尔逊病）和胆管形成不良（胆道闭锁）。

病因还有 α-1 抗胰蛋白酶缺乏症、遗传性糖代谢紊乱（半乳糖血症

metabolism （ galactosemia or glycogen storage disease ） and genetic digestive disorder （ Alagille syndrome ）, liver disease caused by your body's immune system （ autoimmune hepatitis ）, destruction of the bile ducts （primary biliary cirrhosis）, hardening and scarring of the bile ducts （primary sclerosing cholangitis）, infection （such as syphilis or brucellosis ） and medications （including methotrexate or isoniazid）.

或糖原贮积病）和遗传性消化系统疾病（阿拉吉勒综合征）、由免疫系统引起的肝病（自身免疫性肝炎）、胆管破坏（原发性胆汁性肝硬化）、胆管硬化和瘢痕形成（原发性硬化性胆管炎）、感染（如梅毒或布鲁氏菌病）和药物（包括甲氨蝶呤或异烟肼）。

4.2　汉译英

（一）胃炎 Gastritis[5]

你的胃有一层黏液保护层，称为黏膜。这种内衬可以保护胃免受消化食物的强烈胃酸的影响。当某些东西损坏或削弱这种保护层时，黏膜就会发炎，导致胃炎。幽门螺杆菌是导致胃炎的最常见细菌。其他诱发因素还包括酗酒、自身免疫性疾病、胆汁反流、药物、身体压力、严重疾病或受伤、严重烧伤和脑损伤。

Your stomach has a protective lining of mucus called the mucosa. This lining protects your stomach from the strong stomach acid that digests food. When something damages or weakens this protective lining, the mucosa becomes inflamed, causing gastritis. Helicobacter pylori is the most common bacterial cause of gastritis. Other triggers include alcohol abuse, autoimmune disease, bile reflux, medications, physical stress, severe illness or injury, severe burns and brain injuries.

胃炎症状可与消化不良症状相仿。消化不良是与消化食物困难相关的胃部疼痛或不适。可能引起下肋之间的灼烧感。每 1 000 人中大约有 8 人受

Gastritis symptoms can mimic indigestion symptoms. Indigestion or dyspepsia is pain or discomfort in the stomach associated with difficulty in

到急性胃炎的影响。慢性、长期胃炎不太常见，会影响大约每 10 000 人中的 2 人。

患胃炎的风险会随着年龄的增长而增加。老年人的胃壁较薄，血液循环减少，黏膜修复的新陈代谢较慢。老年人也更有可能服用导致胃炎的药物，如非甾体抗炎药（NSAIDs）。世界上大约三分之二的人口感染了幽门螺杆菌。幸运的是，这在美国不太常见。在美国，幽门螺杆菌在老年人和社会经济地位较低的群体中更常见。

胃炎有两种主要类型：侵蚀性和非侵蚀性。侵蚀性胃炎会导致胃壁炎症和糜烂。这种情况也称为反应性胃炎。病因包括酒精、吸烟、非甾体抗炎药、皮质类固醇、病毒或细菌感染以及疾病或受伤造成的压力。非侵蚀性胃炎就是胃壁炎症，但没有侵蚀或损害胃壁。

digesting food. It may be a feeling of burning between your lower ribs. Acute gastritis affects about 8 out of every 1, 000 people. Chronic, long-term gastritis is less common. It affects approximately 2 out of every 10, 000 people.

Your risk of developing gastritis goes up with age. Older adults have thinner stomach linings, decreased circulation and a slower metabolism of mucosal repair. Older adults are also more likely to be on medications such as nonsteroidal anti-inflammatory drugs （NSAIDs） that can cause gastritis. About two-thirds of the world's population is infected with H. pylori. Fortunately, it is less common in the United States. In the United States, H. pylori is found more often in older adults and lower socioeconomic groups.

There are two main types of gastritis: erosive and non-erosive. Erosive gastritis causes both inflammation and erosion of the stomach lining. This condition is also known as reactive gastritis. Causes include alcohol, smoking, NSAIDs, corticosteroids, viral or bacterial infections and stress from illnesses or injuries. Non-erosive gastritis is inflammation of the stomach lining without erosion or compromising the stomach lining.

胃炎的治疗因病因而异。某些药物可杀死细菌，而另一些药物可缓解消化不良症状。你的医疗服务提供者可能会推荐抗生素、抗酸剂、组胺（H2）阻滞剂和质子泵抑制剂。抗生素可以治疗细菌感染。可能需要在几周内服用不止一种抗生素。

Treatment for gastritis varies depending on the cause. Certain medications kill bacteria, while others alleviate indigestion-type symptoms. Your healthcare provider might recommend antibiotics, antacids, histamine (H2) blockers and proton pump inhibitors. Antibiotics can treat the bacterial infection. You may need to take more than one type of antibiotic for couple of weeks.

碳酸钙药物可减少胃酸暴露，可帮助缓解炎症。抗酸剂也可治疗胃灼热。西咪替丁、雷尼替丁和类似药物可减少胃酸的产生。奥美拉唑和埃索美拉唑等药物可减少胃酸产量。质子泵抑制剂还可以治疗胃溃疡和胃食管反流病。

Calcium carbonate medications reduce stomach acid exposure. They can help relieve inflammation. Antacids also treat heartburn. Cimetidine, ranitidine and similar medications decrease the production of stomach acid. Medications such as omeprazole and esomeprazole reduce the amount of acid your stomach produces. Proton pump inhibitors can also treat stomach ulcers and gastroesophageal reflux disease.

（二）酒精性肝病与非酒精性脂肪性肝病 ALD and NAFLD[6-7]

酒精性肝病（ALD）是由长期大量饮酒导致的肝病。初期通常表现为

Alcoholic liver disease or ALD occurs after years of heavy drinking. The

脂肪肝，进而可发展成酒精性肝炎、肝纤维化和肝硬化。症状包括恶心、呕吐、黄疸、肝脏肿大和压痛。并发症包括肝功能衰竭和上消化道出血等。严重酒精中毒可诱发大量肝细胞坏死，甚至肝功能衰竭。

在北美、欧洲等发达地区，非酒精性肝病是肝硬化的首要病因。我国目前尚无全国性非酒精性肝病发病率的流行病学调查。地区性的流行病学调查结果显示，我国饮酒人群比例呈现上升趋势。华北地区流行病学调查结果显示，从20世纪80年代初到90年代初，嗜酒者在一般人群中的比例从0.21%升至14.3%。21世纪初，东北地区流行病学调查结果显示，酗酒比例高达26.98%。多项研究证实，非酒精性肝病疾病谱中肝硬化和肝衰竭的比例也不断提升，酒精已成为我国继病毒性肝炎后导致肝损害的第二大病因。

initial stage usually manifests as fatty liver, which can then develop into alcoholic hepatitis, liver fibrosis and cirrhosis. Symptoms include nausea, vomiting, jaundice, liver enlargement and pressure pain. It can also be complicated by liver failure and upper gastrointestinal bleeding. Severe alcoholism can induce extensive liver cell necrosis and even liver failure.

In developed regions such as North America and Europe, ALD is the leading cause of liver cirrhosis. No epidemiological research is available on ALD prevalence in China. Regional surveys show that the proportion of alcoholic drinkers is showing an upward trend in China. The epidemiological results in North China showed that from the early 1980s to the early 1990s, the proportion of alcoholics in the general population rose from 0.21% to 14.3%. At the beginning of the 21st century, the proportion of excessive drinking was as high as 26.98% in Northeast China. Multiple studies have confirmed that the proportion of liver cirrhosis and liver failure is also increasing in the ALD disease spectrum. Alcohol has become the second leading cause of liver damage

酒精所造成的肝损伤是有阈值效应的，即达到一定饮酒量或饮酒年限，肝损害风险就会呈指数增加。然而，由于个体差异较大，也有研究显示饮酒与肝损害的剂量 – 效应关系并不十分明确。

非酒精性脂肪性肝病是用于描述一系列会影响很少饮酒或不饮酒人群的肝病的总称术语。非酒精性脂肪性肝病的主要特征是肝细胞中储存了过多的脂肪。非酒精性脂肪性肝病在世界各地越来越普遍，尤其是在西方国家。在美国，它是最常见的慢性肝病，影响大约四分之一的人口。

(三) 上消化道内镜 Upper Endoscopy [8-9]

食管胃十二指肠镜检查，也称为EGD 或上消化道内镜检查，是医生对食道、胃和十二指肠内部的检查。一根称为内镜的柔软发光细管，被导入口腔和喉咙，然后进入食道、胃和十二指肠。内镜可使医生查看管腔内壁，以及通过内镜插入仪器以取出组织样

after viral hepatitis in China.

Above a certain volume or duration of alcoholic consumption, the risk of liver damage caused by alcohol increases exponentially, i. e. a threshold effect. However, due to the large individual differences, the dose-effect relationship between alcohol consumption and liver damage is not clear in some studies.

Nonalcoholic fatty liver disease (NAFLD) is an umbrella term for a range of liver conditions affecting people who drink little to no alcohol. The main characteristic of NAFLD is too much fat stored in liver cells. NAFLD is increasingly common around the world, especially in Western nations. In the United States, it is the most common form of chronic liver disease, affecting about one-quarter of the population.

An esophagogastroduodenoscopy, also called EGD or upper endoscopy, is a procedure that allows the doctor to examine the inside of the esophagus, stomach, and duodenum. A thin, flexible, lighted tube, called an endoscope, is guided into the mouth and

本进行活检。

如果你正在服用抗凝药物，如香豆素、肝素，请务必告诉你的医生。在内镜检查前 7 天，停止服用铁剂、阿司匹林或阿司匹林产品。请注意，泰诺（对乙酰氨基酚）不会干扰该检查。如果对药物有任何疑问，请咨询医生。

在做内镜检查前 5 天，停止服用非甾体抗炎药，例如美林、雅维（布洛芬）、萘普生、努普林等。在内镜检查前 1 天，在手术前一晚午夜后不要吃任何固体食物。在做内镜检查当天，检查前至少 8 小时不要进食或饮水。可以在检查前 4 小时用少量水服用药物。

穿宽松舒适的衣服。在手术过程中，你可以在我们提供的长袍下穿短

throat, then into the esophagus, stomach, and duodenum. The endoscope allows the doctor to view the inner lining of the lumen, as well as to insert instruments through a scope for the removal of a sample of tissue for biopsy.

If you are taking any anti-coagulant medication, e. g. Coumadin and Heparin, please be sure to notify your doctor. 7 days before endoscopy, stop taking iron, aspirin or aspirin products. Please note that Tylenol (acetaminophen) does not interfere with the procedure. Please consult your doctor if you have any questions about your medication.

5 days before endoscopy, stop taking non-steroidal anti-inflammatories, e. g. Motrin, Advil (ibuprofen), Naprosyn, and Nuprin. 1 day before endoscopy, do not eat any solid food after midnight, the night before the procedure. On the day of endoscopy, nothing to eat or drink at least 8 hours before the procedure. Medication can be taken 4 hours before examination with little sips of water.

Wear loose comfortable clothing. You may keep short sleeve clothing on

袖衣服。手术室可能很冷，所以你也可以带上袜子。在检查当天让人开车送你回家。由于镇静剂的作用，你不能自行开车。建议在手术后 24 小时内不要马上工作、做任何剧烈运动、开车或签署任何法律文件。

during the procedure under the gown we provide. The procedure room can be cold, so you can bring socks too. Have someone drive you home the day of the procedure. Due to the sedation, you will not be allowed to drive yourself. It is recommended that you do not go back to work, do any strenuous exercise, drive, or sign any legal documents for 24 hours after the procedure.

5 口译注释与学习资源

5.1 口译注释

剂量效应

The dose effect, or dose-response relationship, or exposure-response relationship, describes the magnitude of the response of an organism, as a function of exposure (or doses) to a stimulus or stressor (usually a chemical) after a certain exposure time. Studying dose response is central to determining "safe", "hazardous" and "beneficial" levels and dosages for drugs, alcohol and other substances to which humans or other organisms are exposed. 剂量效应，也称剂量-反应关系，或暴露-反应关系，描述在一定暴露时间后，生物体在刺激或应激物（通常为化学物质）暴露（或剂量）下的反应程度。研究剂量-反应对于确定人类或其他生物所接触的药物、酒精和其他物质的"安全""危险"和"有益"水平及剂量至关重要。

5.2 学习资源

登录中国大学 MOOC（慕课），学习"医疗口译"课程中"消化科"的口译实战示范视频。另外可以学习中华人民共和国国家卫生健康委员会（National Health Commission, NHC）、美国胃肠病学会（American College of Gastroenterology, ACG）、美国国立卫生研究院（National Institutes of Health, NIH）、妙佑医疗国际（Mayo Clinic）、克利夫兰诊所（Cleveland Clinic）以及斯坦福医疗（Stanford Healthcare）等机构官网相关内容。

参考文献

［1］ American College of Gastroenterology. (2019, September 9). *What is a gastroenterologist?*. Retrieved November 8, 2021, from https: //gi. org/patients/gi-health-and-disease/what-is-a − gastroenterologist/.

［2］ Mayo Foundation for Medical Education and Research. (2020, August 6). *Peptic ulcer*. Retrieved November 8, 2021, from https: //www. mayoclinic. org/diseases-conditions/peptic-ulcer/symptoms-causes/syc.

［3］ Mayo Foundation for Medical Education and Research. (2021, February 6). *Cirrhosis*. Retrieved November 8, 2021, from https: //www. mayoclinic. org/diseases-conditions/cirrhosis/symptoms-causes/syc − 20351487.

［4］ Liver Institute PLLC. (n. d.). *Facts about cirrhosis*. Retrieved November 8, 2021, from https: //www. liverinstitutepllc. org/facts-about-cirrhosis.

［5］ Cleveland Clinic. (n. d.). *Gastritis: Indigestion, symptoms, causes, treatment, diagnosis*. Retrieved November 8, 2021, from https: //my. clevelandclinic. org/health/diseases/10349 − gastritis.

［6］ Johns Hopkins Medicine. (n. d.). *Alcoholic liver disease*. Retrieved November 8, 2021, from https: //www. hopkinsmedicine. org/health/conditions-and-diseases/alcoholinduced-liver-disease.

［7］ 中华医学会，中华医学会杂志社，中华医学会消化病学分会，等. 酒精性肝病基层诊疗指南（2019 年）［J］. 中华全科医师杂志，2020，19（11）：990 − 996.

［8］ MUSC Health (n. d.). *Upper Endoscopy(EGD)*. Retrieved November 8, 2021, from https: //muschealth. org/medical-services/ddc/patients/gi-procedures/upper-endoscopy.

［9］ Stanford Health Care（SHC）−Stanford Medical Center. (2017, September 12). *Preparing for the procedure*. Retrieved November 8, 2021, from https: //stanfordhealthcare. org/medical-tests/e/egd/what-to-expect/before-procedure. html.

第七章

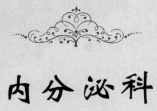

内分泌科

1　导读

本章的重点为"听词取意"这一口译技巧和内分泌科的 6 篇"口译实战"练习。口译实战练习中英译汉、汉译英各 3 篇，内容涵盖内分泌科介绍，糖尿病与运动，代谢综合征，低血糖，人类生长激素与衰老，以及围绝经期、更年期和绝经后。请结合本章口译技巧练习 6 篇口译实战文本。

2　口译技巧——意义听辨（2）：听词取意

口译听辨的主要目的是通过捕捉关键词来"听词取意"。"听词取意"的前期练习为"抓关键词"（见第六章），同时与"双语转换"密不可分（见第十三章和第十四章）。

口译的"听"与外语学习的"听"并不相同。普通外语学习的"听"可能是为了听写、填空或判断对错等，不涉及语言转换和文化调解；但口译的"听"是听辨和判断讲话人希望表达的信息与意图，译员还要将此信息与意图以清晰的译语传递给目的文化的听众。因此，口译"听辨"的关键并非听取字词，而是得"意"忘"形"。

口译初学者往往是听到了字词，但遗漏了讲话者意图，往往只关注表层的语言结构而忽略了深层的意义结构，结果导致未解其意，不得要领，翻译腔重，逐词对应，硬译、死译，让听众"见树不见林"，听起来十分吃力。

在掌握"抓关键词"和"听词取意"等意义听辨技巧和原则之后，就能减少语言外壳对口译中意义传译的影响，生成更为地道自然的译语。

3　口译词汇

3.1　英译汉

（一）Endocrinology 内分泌科/内分泌学
endocrinologist 内分泌科医生，内分泌学家
endocrine glands 内分泌腺
diabetes，metabolic and nutritional disorders 糖尿病、新陈代谢和营养性疾病

pituitary diseases 垂体疾病

menstrual and sexual problems 月经和性疾病

endocrine organs 内分泌器官

pituitary, thyroid, adrenals, ovaries, testes, and pancreas （脑）垂体、甲状腺、肾上腺、卵巢、睾丸和胰腺

pediatrics, internal medicine, and obstetrics and gynecology 儿科、内科和妇产科

MD or an analogous medical degree 医学博士或类似的医学学位

PhD degree 哲学博士学位

thyroid disease, osteoporosis, infertility, and disorders of the pituitary and adrenal glands 甲状腺疾病、骨质疏松症、不孕症、垂体和肾上腺疾病

laboratory tests, tissue sampling, genetic analysis and high-resolution medical imaging 实验室检查、组织取样、基因分析和高分辨率医学影像

stimulate or inhibit hormonal pathways 刺激或抑制激素通路

bone mineral density tests 骨矿物质密度检查

thyroid ultrasonography and ultrasound-guided fine needle aspiration biopsies 甲状腺超声检查和超声引导下的细针穿刺活检

radiopharmaceutical agents 放射性药物

outpatient department 门诊部

inpatient department 住院部

（二）Diabetes and Physical Activity 糖尿病与运动

insulin 胰岛素

glucose 葡萄糖

blood glucose 血糖

type 1, type 2, and gestational diabetes 1 型、2 型和妊娠期糖尿病

blood sugar/glucose level 血糖水平

nerve damage 神经损伤

dehydration 脱水

carbohydrate 碳水化合物

glucose tablets 葡萄糖片

low blood sugar（hypoglycemia）低血糖

high blood sugar（hyperglycemia）高血糖

ketones 酮类物质，尿酮

ketoacidosis 酮症酸中毒

complication 并发症

diabetic ketoacidosis 糖尿病酮症酸中毒

hyperglycemic hyperosmolar syndrome 高血糖高渗综合征

sores 疮口

blisters 水疱

irritation，cuts 刺激，割伤

（三）Metabolic Syndrome 代谢综合征

waistline 腰围

abdominal obesity or "having an apple shape" 腹部肥胖或"苹果身材"

triglyceride 甘油三酯

pump blood 泵血

plaque buildup 斑块堆积

insulin resistance 胰岛素抵抗

high-density lipoprotein （HDL）：高密度脂蛋白

low-density lipoprotein （LDL）：低密度脂蛋白

3.2　汉译英

（一）低血糖 Hypoglycemia

分升 deciliter （dL）

空腹血糖 fasting blood sugar

毫摩尔 millimole

刺痛 tingling

体征和症状 signs and symptoms

癫痫发作 seizures

糖原 glycogen

胰腺 pancreas

肾衰竭患者 people with kidney failure

奎宁 quinine

疟疾 malaria

重型肝炎或肝硬化 severe hepatitis or cirrhosis

神经性厌食症 anorexia nervosa

胰腺肿瘤（胰岛素瘤）tumor of the pancreas（insulinoma）

肾上腺 adrenal gland

垂体瘤疾病 pituitary tumor disorders

生长激素 growth hormone（GH）

（二）人类生长激素与衰老 Human Growth Hormone and Aging

青春之泉 fountain of youth

胡安·庞塞·德莱昂 Juan Ponce de Leon

脑下垂体 pituitary gland

下丘脑 hypothalamus

肠道 intestinal tract

软骨 cartilage

胰岛素样生长因子－1（IGF－1）insulin-like growth factor-1（IGF-1）

处方药 prescription drug

液体潴留 fluid retention

（三）围绝经期、更年期和绝经后 Perimenopause，Menopause and Postmenopause

围绝经期（更年期过渡期）perimenopause（menopause transition）

更年期 menopause

绝经后 postmenopause

雌激素 estrogen

经期 menstrual cycles

骨质疏松症 osteoporosis

4　口译实战

4.1　英译汉

（一）Endocrinology 内分泌科[1]

An endocrinologist is an internist who concentrates on disorders of the endocrine glands. This specialist also deals with

内分泌科医生是专注于内分泌腺功能紊乱的内科医生，还处理糖尿病、代谢和营养性疾病、肥胖、垂体疾病

disorders such as diabetes, metabolic and nutritional disorders, obesity, pituitary diseases, and menstrual and sexual problems. Endocrinology is the specialty of medicine that deals with the problems, diseases and medical conditions of the endocrine system.

The endocrine organs include the pituitary, thyroid, adrenals, ovaries, testes, and pancreas. Because endocrinologists rely on laboratory tests to assist in determining the disorders of their patients, many have backgrounds in biochemistry. In addition, endocrinologists usually have background training in one of a number of different medical fields such as pediatrics, internal medicine, and obstetrics and gynecology. All medical endocrinologists have an MD or an analogous medical degree and some also have a PhD or another advanced science degree.

Endocrinologists typically evaluate, diagnose and treat people with diabetes, thyroid disease, osteoporosis, infertility, and disorders of the pituitary and adrenal glands, as well as diseases that can affect growth, development and metabolism. These are done through the use of

以及月经和性问题。内分泌科是处理内分泌系统问题、疾病和状况的医学专科。

内分泌器官主要包括脑垂体、甲状腺、肾上腺、卵巢、睾丸和胰腺。由于内分泌科医生依靠实验室检查来帮助确诊患者的疾病,许多内分泌科医生都有生物化学背景。此外,内分泌科医生往往在许多不同的医学科室接受过基础培训,例如儿科、内科和妇产科。所有内分泌科医生都拥有医学博士或类似的医学学位,有些还拥有哲学博士学位或其他高级科学学位。

内分泌科医生评估、诊断和治疗的病人通常患有糖尿病、甲状腺疾病、骨质疏松症、不孕症、垂体和肾上腺疾病以及可能影响生长、发育和新陈代谢的疾病。内分泌科医生的工作借助实验室检查、组织取样、基因分析和高分辨率医学影像来完成。内分泌

laboratory tests, tissue sampling, genetic analysis and high-resolution medical imaging. Endocrinologists frequently perform dynamic endocrine testing to stimulate or inhibit hormonal pathways to diagnose various conditions.

They can perform and interpret bone mineral density tests in the evaluation of people with metabolic bone disease and may perform thyroid ultrasonography and ultrasound-guided fine needle aspiration biopsies in the evaluation of patients with thyroid conditions. Some endocrinologists attain special certification to use radiopharmaceutical agents in the diagnosis and treatment of various endocrine conditions. Although endocrinologists spend most of their time taking care of patients in an outpatient setting, some may perform inpatient consultations as well.

There are few emergencies in the field of endocrinology, so many endocrinologists are able to balance the demands of work and family quite easily. Because endocrinologists are in high demand in urban, suburban and rural settings, many have the ability to set schedules to suit personal and

科医生经常进行动态的内分泌检查，以刺激或抑制激素通路来诊断各种疾病。

他们可以做骨矿物质密度检查并对结果进行解读，对代谢性骨病患者进行评估，也能进行甲状腺超声检查和超声引导下的细针穿刺活检，对甲状腺疾病患者进行评估。一些内分泌科医生还拥有使用放射性药物来诊断和治疗各种内分泌疾病的特殊资质。尽管内分泌科医生大部分时间都在门诊上诊治患者，但有些也会进行住院咨询。

内分泌科的急症很少，所以很多内分泌科医师能轻松平衡工作和家庭。由于城市、郊区和农村地区对内分泌科医生的需求很大，许多人能够根据个人和专业需求设定时间表，并在需要时兼职。内分泌科医生可以选择在不同单位工作，包括医院、学术医疗中心、门诊和私人诊所。

professional needs as well as work part time if desired. Endocrinologists have the option of working in many different environments, including hospitals, academic medical centers, clinics and private practice.

（二）Diabetes and Physical Activity 糖尿病与运动[2-3]

Diabetes is a disease that occurs when your blood glucose is too high. Blood glucose is your main source of energy and comes from the food you eat. Insulin, a hormone made by the pancreas, helps glucose from food get into your cells to be used for energy. Sometimes your body doesn't make enough—or any—insulin or doesn't use insulin well. Glucose then stays in your blood and doesn't reach your cells.

Over time, having too much glucose in your blood can cause health problems. Although diabetes has no cure, you can take steps to manage your diabetes and stay healthy. The most common types of diabetes are type 1, type 2, and gestational diabetes. If you have type 1 diabetes, your body does not make insulin. Your immune system attacks and destroys the cells in your pancreas that make insulin. Type 1 diabetes is

糖尿病是血糖过高时发生的疾病。血糖是主要的能量来源，来自所吃的食物。胰岛素是由胰腺制造的激素，可帮助食物中的葡萄糖进入细胞供能。身体有时不能制造足够的胰岛素，完全不能产生胰岛素，或是不能很好地利用胰岛素。这会导致葡萄糖滞留在血液中，无法到达细胞。

随着时间推移，血液中葡萄糖过量会带来健康问题。尽管糖尿病无法治愈，但可采取措施来管理糖尿病并保持健康。最常见的糖尿病类型是1型、2型和妊娠期糖尿病。如果患上1型糖尿病，那身体不会产生胰岛素，免疫系统会攻击并破坏胰腺中制造胰岛素的细胞。尽管1型糖尿病能出现在任何年龄段，但常见于儿童和年轻人。1型糖尿病患者需要每天注射胰岛素以维持生命。

usually diagnosed in children and young adults, although it can appear at any age. People with type 1 diabetes need to take insulin every day to stay alive.

If you have type 2 diabetes, your body does not make or use insulin well. You can develop type 2 diabetes at any age, even during childhood. However, this type of diabetes occurs most often in middle-aged and older people. Type 2 is the most common type of diabetes. Gestational diabetes develops in some women when they are pregnant. Most of the time, this type of diabetes goes away after the baby is born. However, if you've had gestational diabetes, you have a greater chance of developing type 2 diabetes later in life. Sometimes diabetes diagnosed during pregnancy is actually type 2 diabetes.

If you have diabetes, being active makes your body more sensitive to insulin, which helps manage your diabetes. Physical activity also helps control blood sugar levels and lowers your risk of heart disease and nerve damage. But before starting any physical activity, check with your health care provider to know the best physical activities for you. Be sure to

如果患有 2 型糖尿病，身体就不能很好地制造或使用胰岛素。任何年龄的人都有可能患上 2 型糖尿病，即使是儿童，但 2 型糖尿病在中老年群体中最常见。2 型糖尿病是最常见的糖尿病类型。一些女性在怀孕时会患上妊娠期糖尿病。大多数情况下，这种糖尿病会在婴儿出生后消失。但如果患上妊娠期糖尿病，那以后患 2 型糖尿病的概率就更大。有时在怀孕期间诊断出的糖尿病实际上就是 2 型糖尿病。

如果患上糖尿病，积极运动会使身体对胰岛素更加敏感，有助于控制病情。运动还有助于控制血糖水平，降低心脏病和神经损伤的风险。但在开始运动之前，请咨询医生，了解最适合的运动。一定要和医生讨论自己喜欢什么活动，该如何准备，以及该避免什么。在运动时多喝水，以防止脱水。

discuss which activities you like, how to prepare, and what you should avoid. Drink plenty of fluids while being physically active to prevent dehydration.

Make sure to check your blood sugar before being physically active, especially if you take insulin. If it's below 100 mg/dL, you may need to eat a small snack containing 15－30 grams of carbohydrates, such as 2 tablespoons of raisins or half a cup of fruit juice or regular soda (not diet), or glucose tablets so your blood sugar doesn't fall too low while being physically active. Low blood sugar or hypoglycemia can be very serious.

If it's above 240 mg/dL (13.3 mmol/L), your blood sugar may be too high (hyperglycemia) to be active safely. During exercise, very high blood sugar levels can lead to life-threatening complications, such as diabetic ketoacidosis or hyperglycemic hyperosmolar syndrome.

Test your urine for ketones. The presence of ketones indicates that your body doesn't have enough insulin to control your blood sugar. If you are physically active when you have high ketone levels, you risk ketoacidosis—a serious diabetes

在运动前一定要检查血糖，尤其是如果你在注射胰岛素的话。如果血糖低于 100 毫克/分升，那就要吃点东西，如 15～30 克碳水化合物、2 汤匙葡萄干、半杯果汁、普通苏打水（非节食型）或葡萄糖片，这样在运动时血糖才不会太低。低血糖会导致非常严重的后果。

如果血糖超过 240 毫克/分升（13.3 毫摩尔/升），此时血糖水平太高，会使运动不安全。运动中，过高的血糖水平会导致危及生命的并发症，例如糖尿病酮症酸中毒或高血糖高渗综合征。

测试尿液中的酮类物质。尿酮的存在表明身体没有足够的胰岛素来控制血糖。如果在尿酮水平很高的时候运动，就会有酮症酸中毒的危险，这是一种严重的糖尿病并发症，需要立即治疗。进行体育锻炼时，应穿着合

complication that needs immediate treatment. When you're physically active, wear cotton socks and athletic shoes that fit well and are comfortable. After your activity, check to see how it has affected your blood glucose level. After being physically active, check your feet for sores, blisters, irritation, cuts, or other injuries.

身舒适的棉袜和运动鞋。在运动后，检查一下运动对血糖水平的影响。运动后，检查足部是否有疮口、水疱、发炎、割伤或其他损伤。

（三）Metabolic Syndrome 代谢综合征[4]

Metabolic syndrome is the name for a group of risk factors that raises your risk for heart disease and other health problems, such as diabetes and stroke. The five conditions described below are metabolic risk factors. You can have any one of these risk factors by itself, but they tend to occur together. You must have at least three metabolic risk factors to be diagnosed with metabolic syndrome.

代谢综合征是一组风险因素的统称，这些因素会增加患心脏病和出现其他健康问题的风险，比如糖尿病和中风。下面描述的五种情况是代谢风险因素。你也许只具有其中一个风险因素，但这些风险因素往往会一同出现。必须至少出现三个代谢风险因素才能被诊断为代谢综合征。

(1) A large waistline. This is also called abdominal obesity or "having an apple shape". Excess fat in the stomach area is a greater risk factor for heart disease than excess fat in other parts of the body, such as on the hips. (2) A high triglyceride level. Triglycerides are a type of fat found in the blood. (3) A

（1）大腰围。大腰围也被称为腹型肥胖或"苹果身材"，与身体其他部位（如臀部）的多余脂肪相比，胃部多余脂肪更易引发心脏病。（2）甘油三酯偏高。甘油三酯是血液中的一种脂肪。（3）高密度脂蛋白胆固醇偏低。HDL 代表高密度脂蛋白。HDL 有时也被称为"好"的胆固醇，因为它

low HDL cholesterol level. HDL stands for high-density lipoproteins. HDL sometimes is called "good" cholesterol. This is because it helps remove cholesterol from your arteries. A low HDL cholesterol level raises your risk of heart disease.

（4）High blood pressure. Blood pressure is the force of blood pushing against the walls of your blood vessels as your heart pumps blood. If this pressure rises and stays high over time, it can damage your heart and lead to plaque buildup. (5) High fasting blood sugar. Mildly high blood sugar may be an early sign of diabetes.

Metabolic syndrome is becoming more common due to a rise in obesity rates among adults. In the future, metabolic syndrome may overtake smoking as the leading risk factor for heart disease. It is possible to prevent or delay metabolic syndrome, mainly with lifestyle changes. A healthy lifestyle is a lifelong commitment. Heart-healthy lifestyle changes are the first line of treatment for metabolic syndrome.

Heart-healthy lifestyle changes

有助于清除动脉中的胆固醇。HDL 胆固醇水平偏低会增加心脏病风险。

（4）高血压。血压是心脏泵血时，血液作用于血管壁的压力。如果压力上升，长时间血压较高，就会损害心脏，并导致斑块堆积。（5）空腹血糖偏高。轻度高血糖可能是糖尿病的早期征兆。

由于成年人肥胖率的上升，代谢综合征正变得越来越普遍。未来，代谢综合征可能会取代吸烟成为心脏病的主要风险因素。改变生活方式可预防或延缓代谢综合征。健康的生活方式需要一生的努力。有益心脏健康的生活方式是治疗代谢综合征的第一步。

有益心脏健康的生活方式包括有

include heart-healthy eating, aiming for a healthy weight, managing stress, physical activity, and quitting smoking. If heart-healthy lifestyle changes aren't enough, your doctor may prescribe medicines. Medicines are used to treat and control risk factors, such as high blood pressure, high triglycerides, low HDL or good cholesterol, and high blood sugar.

益心脏健康的饮食、保持健康体重、压力管理、体育锻炼和戒烟。如果改变生活方式还不够，那么医生可能会给你开药。这些药物用于应对和控制风险因素，如高血压、高甘油三酯、高密度脂蛋白胆固醇或者说"好"的胆固醇偏低以及高血糖等。

4.2 汉译英

（一）低血糖 Hypoglycemia[5]

低血糖是指血液葡萄糖水平低于正常水平。葡萄糖是身体的主要能量来源。低血糖常与糖尿病治疗有关。但其他药物和情况也会导致没有糖尿病的人出现低血糖。低血糖患者在出现低血糖症状时需要立即治疗。对许多人来说，空腹血糖在每分升 70 毫克（mg/dL）或每升 3.9 毫摩尔（mmol/L）以下应该作为低血糖的预警。

Hypoglycemia is a condition in which your blood glucoselevel is lower than normal. Glucose is your body's main energy source. Hypoglycemia is often related to diabetes treatment. But other drugs and a variety of conditions can cause low blood sugar in people who don't have diabetes. Patients of hypoglycemia needs immediate treatment when blood sugar levels are low. For many people, a fasting blood sugar of 70 milligrams per deciliter (mg/dL), or 3.9 millimoles per liter (mmol/L), or below should serve as an alert for hypoglycemia.

治疗方式包括食用高糖食物、饮

Treatment involves quickly getting

料或药物使血糖迅速恢复正常。长期治疗则需要确定导致低血糖的病因，对症治疗。胰岛素能使葡萄糖进入细胞并提供细胞所需的"燃料"。多余的葡萄糖以糖原的形式储存在肝脏和肌肉中。

如果你已经好几个小时没吃东西了，血糖水平下降，那么胰腺中的另一种激素会向你的肝脏发出信号，分解储存的糖原，并将葡萄糖释放到血液中，使血糖保持在正常范围内，直到你再次进食。你的身体也有制造葡萄糖的能力。这一过程主要发生在肝脏，但也发生在肾脏。

如果你有糖尿病，可能你分泌的胰岛素量不够或胰岛反应差。因此，葡萄糖往往在血液中积聚，并可能达到危险的高水平。要解决这个问题，你可以使用胰岛素或其他药物来降低血糖水平。但过多的胰岛素或其他糖尿病药物也会导致血糖水平过低，从而导致低血糖。如果服用糖尿病药物后饮食比平时少，或者运动量比平时

your blood sugar back to normal either with high-sugar foods or drinks or with medications. Long-term treatment requires identifying and treating the cause of hypoglycemia. Insulin enables the glucose to enter the cells and provide the "fuel" your cells need. Extra glucose is stored in your liver and muscles in the form of glycogen.

If you haven't eaten for several hours and your blood sugar level drops, another hormone from your pancreas signals your liver to break down the stored glycogen and release glucose into your bloodstream. This keeps your blood sugar within a normal range until you eat again. Your body also has the ability to make glucose. This process occurs mainly in your liver, but also in your kidneys.

If you have diabetes, you might not make enough insulin or you might be less responsive to it. As a result, glucose tends to build up in the bloodstream and can reach dangerously high levels. To solve this problem, you might take insulin or other drugs to lower blood sugar levels. But too much insulin or other diabetes medications may cause your

大，也可能发生低血糖。

无糖尿病的人出现低血糖的情况要少得多。他们出现低血糖的原因如下：（1）药物。不小心服用别人的口服糖尿病药物可能会导致低血糖。其他药物也能引起低血糖，尤其是对儿童或肾衰竭患者而言，比如用来治疗疟疾的奎宁。（2）过量饮酒。大量空腹饮酒会阻碍肝脏将储存的葡萄糖释放到血液中，导致低血糖。（3）严重疾病。严重的肝病，如重型肝炎或肝硬化可导致低血糖。肾脏疾病会阻止身体正常排泄药物，导致药物堆积，从而影响血糖水平。（4）长期饥饿。神经性厌食症等会导致身体中产生葡萄糖所需的物质过少。（5）胰岛素过剩。一种罕见的胰腺肿瘤（胰岛素瘤）会使得胰岛素分泌过多，导致低血糖。其他肿瘤也会导致胰岛素样物质过度产生。胰腺细胞增大也可导致胰岛素释放过多，造成低血糖。（6）激素缺乏。某些肾上腺疾病和垂体瘤会导致调节葡萄糖生产的关键激素缺乏。如果生长激素太少，儿童也可能会出现低血糖。

blood sugar level to drop too low, causing hypoglycemia. Hypoglycemia can also occur if you eat less than usual after taking diabetes medication, or if you exercise more than you normally do.

Hypoglycemia in people without diabetes is much less common. Causes can include the following: (1) Medications. Taking someone else's oral diabetes medication accidentally is a possible cause of hypoglycemia. Other medications can cause hypoglycemia, especially in children or in people with kidney failure. One example is quinine, which is used to treat malaria. (2) Excessive alcohol drinking. Drinking heavily without eating can block your liver from releasing stored glucose into your bloodstream, causing hypoglycemia. (3) Some critical illnesses. Severe liver illnesses such as severe hepatitis or cirrhosis can cause hypoglycemia. Kidney disorders, which can keep your body from properly excreting medications, can affect glucose levels due to a buildup of those medications. (4) Long-term starvation. As can occur in the eating disorder anorexia nervosa, it can result in too little of substances your body needs to create glucose. (5) Insulin overproduction. A rare tumor of the pancreas (insulinoma) can cause you to produce too much insulin, resulting in hypoglycemia. Other tumors can also result in too much production of insulin-like substances. Enlargement of cells of the pancreas can result in excessive insulin release, causing hypoglycemia.

(6) Hormone deficiencies. Certain adrenal gland and pituitary tumor disorders can result in a deficiency of key hormones that regulate glucose production. Children can have hypoglycemia if they have too little growth hormone.

（二）人类生长激素与衰老 Human Growth Hormone and Aging[6]

人类生长激素真的能像那没人见过的青春之泉一样延缓衰老吗？1513年，西班牙探险家胡安·庞塞·德莱昂抵达佛罗里达州寻找青春之泉。如果说他得到了什么好处的话，那这些好处就是寻找过程中的身体锻炼带来的。今天很少有人再会相信这神奇的泉水，但似乎很多人却开始相信"青春注射器"：他们不是通过饮用生命之水，而是通过注射人类生长激素来减缓生物钟的滴答流逝。

Can human growth hormones really benefit aging, like the elusive fountain of youth? In 1513, the Spanish explorer Juan Ponce de Leon arrived in Florida to search for the fountain of youth. If he got any benefit from his quest, it was due to the exercise involved in the search. Few men today believe in miraculous waters, but many, it seems, believe in the syringe of youth. Instead of drinking rejuvenating waters, they inject human growth hormone to slow the tick of the clock.

一些人是受到了所谓的"抗衰老"言论的鼓动，另一些人则想效仿年轻运动员，寻求竞争优势。像庞

Some are motivated by the claims of the "anti-aging" movement, others by the examples of young athletes seeking a

塞·德莱昂一样，运动员仍然能从锻炼中获益，而老年人则可以用注射生长激素来代替锻炼。但生长激素会提高表现或延缓衰老吗？它安全吗？

Growth hormone（GH）is a small protein that is made by the pituitary gland and secreted into the bloodstream. GH production is controlled by a complex set of hormones produced in the hypothalamus of the brain and in the intestinal tract and pancreas. The pituitary puts out GH in bursts; levels rise following exercise, trauma, and sleep.

生长激素（GH）是由脑垂体分泌到血液中的小蛋白。生长激素的产生是由大脑的下丘脑、肠道和胰腺中产生的复杂激素体系控制。垂体一阵一阵地分泌生长激素；运动、创伤和睡眠后生长激素水平升高。

competitive edge. Like Ponce de Len, the athletes still benefit from exercise, while older men may use growth hormone shots as a substitute for working out. But will growth hormone boost performance or slow aging? And is it safe?

在正常情况下，夜间分泌的生长激素比白天多。这一生理过程很复杂，但至少它告诉我们，用一两次血液测试来衡量生长激素水平是没有意义的，因为一天当中激素水平是起伏变化的。但仔细测量生长激素总量的科学家发现，生长激素在儿童时期会上升，在青春期达到高峰，从中年开始下降。

Under normal conditions, more GH is produced at night than during the day. This physiology is complex, but at a minimum, it tells us that sporadic blood tests to measure GH levels are meaningless since high and low levels alternate throughout the day. But scientists who carefully measure overall GH production report that it rises during childhood, peaks during puberty, and declines from middle age onward.

生长激素是一种通过注射给药的

GH is available as a prescription

处方药，可用于帮助生长激素分泌不足的、身材矮小的儿童。它也被批准用于治疗成人生长激素缺乏症，这是一种罕见的情况，几乎总要涉及下丘脑、垂体或两者兼而有之的大问题。患有生长激素缺乏症的成年人可从注射生长激素中获益，可避免骨折，增加肌肉量，提高运动能力和能量，并减少未来患心脏病的风险。但这也要付出代价。高达30%的患者会出现副作用造成的液体潴留、关节和肌肉疼痛以及高血糖症状。

drug that is administered by injection. It is indicated for children with GH deficiency and others with very short stature. It is also approved to treat adult GH deficiency—an uncommon condition that almost always develops in conjunction with major problems afflicting the hypothalamus, pituitary gland, or both. Adults with GH deficiencies benefit from GH injections. They enjoy protection from fractures, increased muscle mass, improved exercise capacity and energy, and a reduced risk of future heart disease. But there is a price to pay. Up to 30% of patients experience side effects that include fluid retention, joint and muscle pain and high blood sugar levels.

（三）围绝经期、更年期和绝经后 Perimenopause, Menopause and Postmenopause[7]

自然更年期是经期的永久结束，不是由任何类型的医疗带来的。对于自然绝经的女性来说，这个过程是渐进的，分为三个阶段。

Natural menopause is the permanent ending of menstruation that is not brought on by any type of medical treatment. For women undergoing natural menopause, the process is gradual and is described in three stages.

（1）围绝经期或"绝经过渡期"。围绝经期可在绝经期前8至10年开始，此时卵巢产生的雌激素逐渐减少。

（1）Perimenopause or "menopause transition". Perimenopause can begin 8 to 10 years before menopause, when the

围绝经期通常在女性 40 多岁开始，但也可以从 30 多岁开始。在围绝经期的最后一到两年，雌激素的下降速度加快。在这个阶段，许多女性可能会出现更年期症状。女性在这段时间仍有月经，仍可能怀孕。（2）更年期。女性连续 12 个月不来月经，便可诊断为进入更年期。（3）绝经后。在这个阶段，很多女性的更年期症状如潮热可能会减轻。然而，有些女性在更年期之后仍会在长达十年或更长时间中出现更年期症状。由于雌激素水平较低，绝经后女性患骨质疏松症和心脏病等多种疾病的风险增加。

潮热是更年期最常见的症状之一。这是一种短暂的热感。潮热对每个人来说都不一样，也没有确切的原因。除了热，潮热还可能伴随着脸部潮红，出汗和热后发冷的感觉。不仅每个人对潮热有不同的感觉，潮热还会持续不同的时间。有些女性在更年期只有短暂的潮热，而另一些女性的余生都

ovaries gradually produce less estrogen. It usually starts in a woman's 40s, but can start in the 30s as well. In the last one to two years of perimenopause, the drop in estrogen accelerates. At this stage, many women may experience menopause symptoms. Women are still having menstrual cycles during this time, and can get pregnant. （2）Menopause. Menopause is diagnosed when a woman has gone without a menstrual period for 12 consecutive months. （3）Postmenopause. During this stage, menopausal symptoms, such as hot flashes, may ease for many women. However, some women continue to experience menopausal symptoms for a decade or longer after the menopause transition. As a result of a lower level of estrogen, postmenopausal women are at increased risk for a number of health conditions, such as osteoporosis and heart disease.

Hot flashes are one of the most frequent symptoms of menopause. It is a brief sensation of heat. Hot flashes aren't the same for everyone and there's no definitive reason that they happen. Aside from the heat, hot flashes can also come with a red, flushed face, sweating and a chilled feeling after the heat. Not only

可能会有潮热。一般来说，潮热会随着时间的推移而逐渐减弱。

在日常生活中，很多常见的东西都可能会引起潮热。需要注意的有咖啡因、吸烟、辛辣食物、酒精、紧身衣、压力和焦虑。某些日常行为也能引发潮热。注意晚上保持卧室凉爽，穿多层衣服，以及戒烟。减肥对缓解潮热也有帮助。如果你正在经历潮热，锻炼可能会很困难，但是锻炼还可以帮助缓解更年期的其他一些症状。锻炼可以助你彻夜安眠，如果你失眠，建议你加强锻炼。像瑜伽这样平静的运动也能帮助控制情绪，缓解你可能感觉到的恐惧或焦虑。

do different people feel different hot flashes, these hot flashes can also last for various amounts of time. Some women only have hot flashes for a short period of time during menopause. Others can have some kind of hot flash for the rest of their life. Typically, hot flashes are less severe as time goes on.

There are quite a few normal things in your daily life that could set off a hot flash. Some things to look out for include caffeine, smoking, spicy foods, alcohol, tight clothing, stress and anxiety. Certain things in your daily life could be triggers for hot flashes. Keep your bedroom cool at night, wear layers of clothing, and quit smoking. Weight loss can also help with hot flashes. Working out can be difficult if you are dealing with hot flashes, but exercising can help relieve several other symptoms of menopause. Exercise can help you sleep through the night and is recommended if you have insomnia. Calm, tranquil types of exercise like yoga can also help with your mood and relieve any fears or anxiety you may be feeling.

5 口译注释与学习资源

5.1 口译注释

"排尿"

排尿的正式和非正式的英文表达包括 urinate（*formal*），micturate（*formal*），wee（*informal*），piddle（*informal*），tinkle（*British*，*informal*），spend a penny（*British*，*informal*），wee-wee（*informal*），pass water（*euphemism*），make water（*euphemism*），pee（*slang*），take a leak（*slang*），take a whizz（*mainly US*，*slang*）等。

5.2 学习资源

登录中国大学 MOOC（慕课）平台，学习"医疗口译"课程"内分泌科"的口译实战示范视频。补充主题包括：（1）What is Type 1 diabetes? 什么是 1 型糖尿病？（2）What is Type 2 diabetes? 什么是 2 型糖尿病？（3）I Cured My Type 2 Diabetes 我治愈了我的 2 型糖尿病；（4）10 Food Tips for Diabetes 糖尿病饮食的 10 个小窍门；（5）How Does the Thyroid Manage Your Metabolism? 甲状腺如何管理你的新陈代谢？（6）The Endocrine System：An Overview 内分泌系统：概述；（7）How do your hormones work? 荷尔蒙如何发挥作用？另外，还可以参考中国疾病预防控制中心（CDC）、美国医师协会（AMA）、妙佑医疗国际、克利夫兰诊所、哈佛医学院、约翰斯·霍普金斯大学医学院等机构官网关于内分泌科及相关疾病的介绍。

参考文献

[1] FREIDA. (n. d.). *Endocrinology，diabetes，and metabolism(IM) residency and fellowship listing.* Retrieved November 12，2021，from https://freida. ama-assn. org/specialty/endocrinology-diabetes-and-metabolism-im.

[2] U. S. Department of Health and Human Services. National Institute of Diabetes and Digestive and Kidney Diseases. (n. d.). *What is diabetes?.* Retrieved November 13，2021，from https://www. niddk. nih. gov/health-information/diabetes/overview/what-is-diabetes.

[3] MediLexicon International. (n. d.). *Diabetic emergencies: Warning signs and what to do.* Medical News Today. Retrieved November 12，2021，from https://www. medicalnewstoday. com/

articles/317436#hyperglycemia.

[4] Mayo Foundation for Medical Education and Research. （2021，May 6）. *Metabolic syndrome.* Retrieved November 13, 2021, from https://www. mayoclinic. org/diseases-conditions/ metabolic-syndrome/symptoms-causes/syc － 20351916.

[5] Mayo Foundation for Medical Education and Research. （2020，March 13）. *Hypoglycemia.* Retrieved November 13, 2021, from https://www. mayoclinic. org/diseases-conditions/ hypoglycemia/symptoms-causes/syc － 20373685.

[6] *Growth hormone，athletic performance，and aging.* Harvard Health. （2021，August 13）. Retrieved November 13, 2021, from https://www. health. harvard. edu/diseases-and- conditions/growth-hormone-athletic-performance-and-aging.

第八章

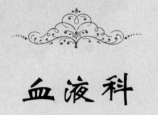

血液科

1　导读

本章的重点为交际技巧和血液科的 6 篇"口译实战"练习。口译实战练习中英译汉、汉译英各 3 篇，内容涵盖血液科/血液学，血型与输血，贫血的种类、病因和症状，白血病，淋巴瘤和多发性骨髓瘤。请结合本章口译技巧练习 6 篇口译实战文本。

2　口译技巧——交际技巧

当来自不同文化背景的交流双方在传递信息和交流思想时，作为语言服务提供者的译员必须是合格的跨文化交际者，并在双方由于政治制度、宗教信仰、价值标准、风俗习惯、历史传统等差异造成交流障碍时进行文化调解。只有适应文化环境的语言，才能促使交际双方的交际目的得以实现。

文化调解能力是区分机器翻译和人类译者的关键之处。因此，口译员除了要有良好的双语能力，还必须自觉提升跨文化交际意识，发挥桥梁作用，在不断丰富的口译实战经验中积累社会文化背景知识，避开不同文化背景的交际陷阱，准确传达双方真正的交际意图。以下是一些文化调解的小贴士。

中方在机场接机时，经常会说"您辛苦了"之类的话。如果译员直译为"You must be tired."，那么这个"忠实的翻译"事实上往往会让外宾介怀，因为西方文化崇尚个人主义，所以西方人喜欢自己看上去精力充沛、年轻、充满活力。因此，译员可以说"How was your flight?"。如果外宾自己抱怨长时间飞行令人沮丧，那么译员可以安慰一句"But you look great."。

送行时，中方可能会说"您慢走"之类的话，译员这时的恰当说法应是"Have a pleasant flight.""Have a safe journey home."。

假如中方很好奇外方同行的收入，忍不住询问，那译员一定不要不经大脑思考，直接译出"What's your salary?"，因为在跟西方人社交时"谈钱"会被认为是"恶俗"。译员可以礼貌地提醒中方这些西方文化禁忌，如果中方实在好奇，译员可以下来在劳工局之类的网站上帮忙查询。

由于有些西方国家移民较多，有时译员可能无法判断外宾姓名中的"姓"和"名"，例如对方是韩裔美国人，这时译员可以先礼貌地跟外宾确认称谓，"Do you prefer to be called Dr ... or Dr ... ?"。

西方文化对于社交着装有正式、商务、休闲等不同要求。如果是外方主办的活动，译员要提前确认着装要求，以便中方雇主和译员自己有时间准备妥当的着装；如果是中方主办的活动，译员也要将着装要求的相关信息提供给外宾，以便外宾做好准备。

3 口译词汇

3.1 英译汉

（一）Hematology 血液科/血液学

subspecialty of internal medicine or pathology 内科或病理科的亚专科

blood, bone marrow, vascular system, spleen, and lymph glands 血液、骨髓、血管系统、脾脏和淋巴腺

disorders of the hematopoietic, hemostatic, and lymphatic systems 造血、止血和淋巴系统的疾病

blood vessel wall 血管壁

hematologic malignancy 血液系统恶性肿瘤

leukemia and lymphoma 白血病和淋巴瘤

evaluation of tissue or cytological specimens 对组织或细胞学标本的评估

disorders of red and white blood cells, platelets, and the blood clotting system 红细胞和白细胞、血小板和凝血系统的疾病

benign and malignant 良性和恶性

blood products and blood derivatives 血液制品和血液衍生品

nutritional supplement 营养补充剂

immunosuppressant 免疫抑制剂

chemotherapy and other anti-tumor agents 化学疗法和其他抗肿瘤药物

stem cell therapy（bone marrow/hematopoietic stem cell transplantation）干细胞疗法（骨髓/造血干细胞移植）

hematological test 血液学检查

anemia, infection, hemophilia, blood-clotting disorders, and leukemia 贫血、感染、血友病、凝血紊乱和白血病

complete blood count（CBC）全血细胞计数

white blood cell count（WBC）白细胞计数

red blood cell count（RBC）红细胞计数

platelet count 血小板计数

hematocrit red blood cell volume（HCT）红细胞压积

hemoglobin concentration（Hb）血红蛋白浓度

differential white blood cell count 白细胞分类计数

（二）Blood Type and Blood Transfusions 血型与输血

blood type（group）血型

antigen 抗原

safe blood transfusion 安全输血

blood typing and cross-matching 血液分型和交叉配型

A（B）antigen A（B）抗原

A（B）antibody A（B）抗体

Rh factor Rh 因子

either present（＋）or absent（－）存在（＋阳性）或不存在（－阴性）

the 8 most common blood types（A＋，A－，B＋，B－，O＋，O－，AB＋，AB－）8 种最常见的血型（A＋，A－，B＋，B－，O＋，O－，AB＋，AB－）

compatible 相容的

rare blood type 稀有血型

sickle cell disease 镰状细胞病

African descent 非洲裔

emergency transfusion 紧急输血

immune deficient infant 免疫缺陷婴儿

（三）Anemia：Types，Causes and Symptoms 贫血的种类、病因和症状

hemoglobin 血红蛋白

hematocrit 红细胞压积

fatigue or shortness of breath 疲劳或呼吸急促

iron-deficiency anemia 缺铁性贫血

blood loss from period 经期失血

kidney disease 肾病

anemia caused by blood loss 失血性贫血

anemia caused by decreased or faulty red blood cell production 红细胞生成减少或缺陷性贫血

anemia caused by destruction of red blood cells 红细胞破坏性贫血

gastrointestinal conditions such as ulcers, hemorrhoids, gastritis and gastric cancer 胃肠道疾病，如溃疡、痔疮、胃炎和胃癌

non-steroidal anti-inflammatory drugs（NSAIDs）such as aspirin or ibuprofen 非甾体抗炎药（NSAIDs），如阿司匹林或布洛芬

heavy menstrual bleeding（menorrhagia） 月经过量

post-trauma or post-surgery blood loss 创伤后或手术后失血

vitamin-deficiency anemia 维生素缺乏性贫血

folate 叶酸

hemolytic anemia 溶血性贫血

lupus 狼疮

hemolytic disease of the newborn 新生儿溶血病

3.2 汉译英

（一）白血病 Leukemia

强大的感染卫士 potent infection fighters

过多的异常白细胞 excessive amount of abnormal white blood cells

淋巴结肿大 swollen lymph nodes

肝脏或脾脏肿大 enlarged liver or spleen

反复流鼻血 recurrent nosebleeds

皮肤上的小红点（瘀点）tiny red spots in your skin（petechiae）

压痛 tenderness

未成熟的血细胞（母/胚细胞）immature blood cells（blasts）

急性淋巴细胞白血病 acute lymphocytic leukemia（ALL）

急性骨髓细胞白血病 acute myelogenous leukemia（AML）

慢性淋巴细胞白血病 chronic lymphocytic leukemia（CLL）

慢性骨髓细胞白血病 chronic myelogenous leukemia（CML）

毛细胞白血病 hairy cell leukemia

骨髓增生异常综合征 myelodysplastic syndrome

骨髓增生性疾病 myeloproliferative disorders

（二）淋巴瘤 Lymphoma

淋巴系统 lymphatic system

抗菌网络 the germ-fighting network

淋巴结（淋巴腺）lymph nodes（lymph glands）

脾脏、胸腺 spleen，thymus gland

亚型 subtype

霍奇金淋巴瘤（旧称霍奇金病）Hodgkin's lymphoma（formerly called Hodgkin's disease）

非霍奇金淋巴瘤 non-Hodgkin's lymphoma

颈部、腋窝或腹股沟淋巴结的无痛肿胀 painless swelling of lymph nodes in your neck，armpits or groin

盗汗 night sweats

淋巴细胞 lymphocyte

EB 病毒 Epstein-Barr virus

幽门螺杆菌感染 Helicobacter pylori infection

（三）多发性骨髓瘤 Multiple Myeloma

浆细胞 plasma cell

并发症 complication

精神模糊或混乱 mental fogginess or confusion

双腿无力或麻木 weakness or numbness in your legs

极度口渴 excessive thirst

单克隆蛋白或 M 蛋白 monoclonal proteins or M proteins

4　口译实战

4.1　英译汉

（一）Hematology 血液科/血液学[1]

Hematology is a subspecialty of internal medicine or pathology concerned with the development, function, and diseases of the blood, bone marrow,

血液科是内科或病理科的亚专科，以血液、骨髓、血管系统、脾脏和淋巴腺的发育、功能和疾病为研究对象。血液科医生专门诊断、治疗、预防和

vascular system, spleen, and lymph glands. A hematologist specializes in the diagnosis, treatment, prevention, and investigation of disorders of the hematopoietic, hemostatic, and lymphatic systems as well as disorders of the interaction between blood cells and blood vessel walls.

研究造血、止血、淋巴系统的疾病以及血细胞和血管壁之间相互作用紊乱的疾病。

Through investigation and treatment of hematologic malignancies, for instance, leukemias and lymphomas, hematology also shares areas of interest and activity with medical oncology. Hematologists use the medical history, physical findings, specialized clinical laboratory tests, and evaluation of tissue or cytological specimens to diagnose and treat disorders of red and white blood cells, platelets, and the blood clotting system, as well as benign and malignant disorders of the bone marrow and lymph glands.

在研究和治疗白血病和淋巴瘤等血液系统恶性肿瘤时，血液科与肿瘤科有共同之处。血液科医生根据病史、体检结果、专业临床实验室检查以及对组织或细胞学标本的评估来诊断和治疗红细胞、白细胞、血小板和凝血系统的疾病，以及骨髓和淋巴腺的良性和恶性疾病。

They use a broad range of approaches to treat these diseases, including blood products and blood derivatives, nutritional supplements, immunosuppressants, chemotherapy and other anti-tumor agents, pain management, drugs that prevent or promote blood clotting, and stem cell therapies (bone marrow/hematopoietic

他们使用广泛的方法来治疗这些疾病，包括使用血液制品和血液衍生品、营养补充剂、免疫抑制剂、化疗和其他抗肿瘤药物、疼痛管理、预防或促进血液凝固的药物以及干细胞疗法（骨髓/造血干细胞移植）。血液科医生不仅必须具备普通内科医生的临床技能，还需要广博的细胞生物学、生物化学和实验室技术知识。

stem cell transplantation）. Not only must hematologists have the clinical skills of general internists, they also need a broad knowledge of cell biology, biochemistry, and laboratory techniques.

Hematological tests can help diagnose anemia, infection, hemophilia, blood-clotting disorders, and leukemia. One of the most common hematological tests is complete blood count（CBC）, which includes white blood cell count（WBC）, red blood cell count（RBC）, platelet count, hematocrit red blood cell volume（HCT）, hemoglobin concentration（Hb）, differential white blood count and red blood cell indices. CBC is used to aid in diagnosing anemia, certain cancers of the blood, inflammatory diseases, and to monitor blood loss and infection and to diagnose and/or to monitor certain types of bleeding and clotting disorders.

血液学检查可以帮助诊断贫血、感染、血友病、凝血紊乱和白血病。最常见的血液学检查之一是全血细胞计数（CBC），包括白细胞计数（WBC）、红细胞计数（RBC）、血小板计数、红细胞压积（HCT）、血红蛋白浓度（Hb），白细胞分类计数和红细胞指数。全血细胞计数用于帮助诊断贫血、特定血癌、炎症性疾病，监测失血和感染，以及诊断和/或监测特定类型的出血和凝血性疾病。

（二）Blood Type and Blood Transfusions 血型与输血[2]

Blood types are determined by the presence or absence of certain antigens — substances that can trigger an immune response if they are foreign to the body. Since some antigens can trigger a patient's immune system to attack the transfused blood, safe blood transfusions

血型由某些抗原的存在与否决定——抗原是能够触发免疫反应的异体物质。由于某些抗原会触发患者的免疫系统攻击输入的血液，因此安全输血建立在仔细的血液分型和交叉配型基础上。

depend on careful blood typing and cross-matching.

There are four major blood groups determined by the presence or absence of two antigens — A and B — on the surface of red blood cells. Group A has only the A antigen on red cells and B antibody in the plasma. Group B has only the B antigen on red cells and A antibody in the plasma. Group AB has both A and B antigens on red cells but neither A nor B antibody in the plasma. Group O has neither A nor B antigens on red cells but both A and B antibodies are in the plasma.

In addition to the A and B antigens, there is a protein called the Rh factor, which can be either present (＋) or absent (－), creating the 8 most common blood types (A＋, A－, B＋, B－, O＋, O－, AB＋, AB－). When a transfusion is given, it is preferable for patients to receive blood and plasma of the same ABO and RhD group. However, if the required blood type is unavailable, a patient may be given a product of an alternative but compatible group. The universal red cell donor has Type O negative blood. The universal

红细胞表面是否存在 A 和 B 两种抗原决定了四种主要血型。A 型血红细胞上只有 A 抗原，血浆中只有 B 抗体。B 型血红细胞上只有 B 抗原，血浆中只有 A 抗体。AB 型血的红细胞上有 A 抗原和 B 抗原，但在血浆中既没有 A 抗体也没有 B 抗体。O 型血在红细胞上既没有 A 抗原也没有 B 抗原，但 A 抗体和 B 抗体都存在其血浆中。

除了 A 抗原和 B 抗原之外，还有一种称为 Rh 因子的蛋白质，它可以存在（＋阳性）或不存在（－阴性），从而产生 8 种最常见的血型（A＋、A－、B＋、B－、O＋、O－、AB＋、AB－）。输血时，患者最好接受 ABO 和 RhD 同型的血液和血浆。但是，如果无法获得所需的血型，那也可为患者提供相容的替代血型。O 型阴性血是红细胞的万能供体。AB 型血则是血浆的万能供体。

plasma donor has Type AB blood.

There are more than 600 other known antigens, the presence or absence of which creates "rare blood types". Your blood type is considered rare if you lack antigens that 99% of the people are positive for. If you somehow lack an antigen that 99.99% are positive for, your blood type is extremely rare. Certain blood types are unique to specific ethnic or racial groups. That's why an African-American blood donation may be the best hope for the needs of patients with sickle cell disease, many of whom are of African descent.

有超过 600 种的其他已知抗原，它们的存在与否决定"稀有血型"。如果你缺乏 99% 的人均为阳性的抗原，则你的血型将是罕见型。如果你缺乏 99.99% 的人均为阳性的抗原，那么你的血型将是极为罕见型。某些血型是特定民族或种族所独有的。这就是为什么非裔美国人献的血最有可能满足镰状细胞病患者的需求，因为他们中许多人是非洲人后裔。

Each year 4.5 million lives are saved by blood transfusions. Every 2 seconds someone in the US needs a blood transfusion. Type O is routinely in short supply and in high demand by hospitals — both because it is the most common blood type and because type O negative blood is the universal blood type needed for emergency transfusions and for immune deficient infants.

每年有 450 万人因输血而被挽救了生命。在美国，每 2 秒就有一个人需要输血。O 型血通常供不应求，医院需求量很大，这既是因为它是最常见的血型，又因为 O 型阴性血是紧急输血和免疫缺陷婴儿所需的万能血型。

（三）Anemia: Types, Causes and Symptoms 贫血的种类、病因和症状[3]

Anemia is defined as a low number of red blood cells. In a routine blood

贫血是指红细胞数量很少。在血常规检查中，贫血表现为低血红蛋白

test, anemia is reported as low hemoglobin or hematocrit. Hemoglobin is the main protein in your red blood cells. It carries oxygen, and delivers it throughout your body. If you have anemia, your hemoglobin level will be low. If it is low enough, your tissues or organs may not get enough oxygen. Symptoms of anemia — like fatigue or shortness of breath — happen because your organs aren't getting what they need to work the way they should.

Anemia is the most common blood condition in the US. It affects almost 6% of the population. Women, young children, and people with long-term diseases are more likely to have anemia. Certain forms of anemia are passed down through your genes, and infants may have it from birth. Women are at risk of iron-deficiency anemia because of blood loss from their periods and higher blood supply demands during pregnancy. Older adults have a greater risk of anemia because they are more likely to have kidney disease or other chronic medical conditions.

There are many types of anemia. All have different causes and treatments. Some forms—like the mild anemia that

或红细胞压积。血红蛋白是红细胞中的主要蛋白质。它携带氧气，并将其输送到全身。如果患上贫血，那血红蛋白水平就会很低。如果太低，组织或器官就可能得不到足够的氧气。由于器官没有得到维持其正常运转所必需的氧气，疲劳或呼吸急促等贫血症状就会发生。

贫血是美国最常见的血液病，影响到差不多6%的人口。妇女、幼儿和长期患有疾病的人更容易贫血。某些形式的贫血来自基因遗传，婴儿可能从出生就有贫血。由于经期失血和孕期血液供应需求增加，女性有缺铁性贫血的风险。老年人贫血的风险更大，因为他们更可能患有肾病或其他慢性病。

贫血有很多种，有不同的病因和治疗方法。有些形式的贫血不是大问题，比如怀孕期间发生的轻度贫血。

happens during pregnancy—aren't a major concern. But some types of anemia may reflect a serious underlying medical condition. The signs of anemia can be so mild that you might not even notice them. As your blood cells decrease, symptoms often develop.

Depending on the cause of the anemia, symptoms may include dizziness, fast or unusual heartbeat, headache, pain (in your bones, chest, belly, and joints), problems with growth for children and teens, shortness of breath, skin that's pale or yellow, cold hands and feet, and tiredness or weakness. There are more than 400 types of anemia, and they're divided into three groups: anemia caused by blood loss, anemia caused by decreased or faulty red blood cell production and anemia caused by destruction of red blood cells.

You can lose red blood cells through bleeding. This can happen slowly over a long period of time, and you might not notice. Causes can include gastrointestinal conditions such as ulcers, hemorrhoids, gastritis and gastric cancer, the use of non-steroidal anti-inflammatory drugs (NSAIDs) such as

但某些类型的贫血可能反映出存在严重的潜在疾病。贫血的症状可能很轻微，你甚至都不会注意到。但随着血细胞的减少，症状往往会发展。

根据不同的贫血病因，可能出现的症状有头晕、心跳加快或不正常、头痛、其他部位疼痛（骨骼、胸部、腹部和关节疼痛）、儿童和青少年的生长问题、呼吸短促、皮肤苍白或发黄、手脚冰冷、疲倦或虚弱。贫血有400多种，可分为三类：失血性贫血、红细胞生成减少或缺陷性贫血、红细胞破坏性贫血。

患者可能会由于出血而损失红细胞。这种情况可能会在很长一段时间内缓慢发生，甚至难以察觉。病因可能包括胃肠道疾病，如溃疡、痔疮、胃炎和胃癌，非甾体抗炎药（NSAIDs）如阿司匹林或布洛芬的使用，女性经期，尤其是月经过量，以及创伤后或手术后失血。

aspirin or ibuprofen, a woman's period especially if she has a heavy menstruation, and post-trauma or post-surgery blood loss.

Anemia caused by decreased or faulty red blood cell production can happen because there's something wrong with your red blood cells or because you don't have enough minerals and vitamins for your red blood cells to form normally. Conditions include bone marrow and stem cell problems, iron-deficiency anemia, sickle cell anemia and vitamin-deficiency anemia, specifically B_{12} or folate.

When red blood cells are fragile and can't handle the stress of traveling through your body, they may burst, causing what's called hemolytic anemia. The causes of hemolytic anemia can include an attack by your immune system, as with lupus. This can happen to anyone, even a baby still in the womb or a newborn. That's called hemolytic disease of the newborn. Enlarged spleen can, in rare cases, trap red blood cells and destroy them too early.

如果红细胞有问题，或者因为缺乏足够的矿物质和维生素使红细胞正常生成，就可能会出现由红细胞生成减少或缺陷引起的贫血。病情包括骨髓和干细胞问题，缺铁性贫血，镰状细胞贫血和维生素缺乏性贫血，如维生素 B_{12} 或叶酸缺乏导致的贫血。

当红细胞很脆弱，且不能承受在身体中穿行的压力时，它们可能会破裂，导致所谓的溶血性贫血。溶血性贫血的病因可能包括免疫系统攻击，比如狼疮。溶血性贫血可能发生在任何人身上，即使是还在子宫里的婴儿或新生儿，这种情况被称为新生儿溶血病。在极少数情况下，脾脏肿大会捕获红细胞并过早破坏它们。

4.2　汉译英

（一）白血病 Leukemia[4]

　　白血病是身体造血组织的癌症，涉及骨髓和淋巴系统。白血病通常涉及白细胞。白细胞是强大的感染卫士，它们通常会在你的身体需要时有序地生长和分裂。但在白血病患者体内，骨髓会产生过多的异常白细胞，这些细胞不能正常工作。

Leukemia is cancer of the body's blood-forming tissues, including the bone marrow and the lymphatic system. Leukemia usually involves the white blood cells. Your white blood cells are potent infection fighters. They normally grow and divide in an orderly way as your body needs them. But in the bodies of people with leukemia, the bone marrow produces an excessive amount of abnormal white blood cells, which can't function properly.

　　白血病的症状因白血病的类型而异。常见的白血病体征和症状包括发烧或寒战、持续疲劳、虚弱、频繁或严重感染、体重易轻、淋巴结肿大、肝脏或脾脏肿大、容易出血或瘀伤、反复流鼻血、皮肤上长小红点（瘀点）、出汗过多（尤其是在夜间），以及骨痛或压痛。

Leukemia symptoms vary, depending on the type of leukemia. Common leukemia signs and symptoms include fever or chills, persistent fatigue, weakness, frequent or severe infections, losing weight without trying, swollen lymph nodes, enlarged liver or spleen, easy bleeding or bruising, recurrent nosebleeds, tiny red spots in your skin (petechiae), excessive sweating (especially at night), and bone pain or tenderness.

　　一般而言，当某些血细胞的遗传物质或 DNA 发生变化（突变）时，就会发生白血病。细胞 DNA 中含有告诉细胞该做什么的指令。通常，DNA

In general, leukemia is thought to occur when some blood cells acquire changes (mutations) in their genetic material or DNA. A cell's DNA contains

会告诉细胞以设定的速度增殖并在设定的时间死亡。在白血病中，突变导致血细胞持续生长和分裂。当这种情况发生时，血细胞的生产就会失控。随着时间的推移，这些异常细胞会排挤骨髓中的健康血细胞，导致健康的白细胞、红细胞和血小板减少，从而导致白血病的症状和体征出现。

医生根据白血病的进展速度和所涉的细胞类型对白血病进行分类。在急性白血病中，异常血细胞是未成熟的血细胞（母/胚细胞）。它们不能发挥正常的功能，而且繁殖速度很快，所以病情会迅速恶化。急性白血病需要积极、及时的治疗。

慢性白血病波及更成熟的血细胞。这些血细胞复制或积累的速度更慢，并且可以在一段时间内正常发挥作用。某些形式的慢性白血病最初不会产生早期症状，并且可能多年不被发现或不被诊断。淋巴细胞白血病会影响淋巴细胞，淋巴细胞会形成构成免疫系

the instructions that tell a cell what to do. Normally, the DNA tells the cell to proliferate at a set rate and to die at a set time. In leukemia, the mutations tell the blood cells to continue growing and dividing. When this happens, blood cell production becomes out of control. Over time, these abnormal cells can crowd out healthy blood cells in the bone marrow, reduce healthy white blood cells, red blood cells and platelets, and cause the signs and symptoms of leukemia.

Doctors classify leukemia based on its speed of progression and the type of cells involved. In acute leukemia, the abnormal blood cells are immature blood cells (blasts). They can't carry out their normal functions, and they multiply rapidly, so the disease worsens quickly. Acute leukemia requires aggressive, timely treatment.

Chronic leukemia involves more-mature blood cells. These blood cells replicate or accumulate more slowly and can function normally for a period of time. Some forms of chronic leukemia initially display no early symptoms and can go unnoticed or undiagnosed for

统的淋巴组织。骨髓细胞白血病影响产生红细胞、白细胞和血小板的髓细胞。

急性淋巴细胞白血病（ALL）是幼儿中最常见的白血病类型。成人也可能患上这一疾病。儿童和成人都可能患急性骨髓细胞白血病（AML）。它是成人中最常见的急性白血病类型。慢性淋巴细胞白血病（CLL）是最常见的慢性成人白血病。

慢性骨髓细胞白血病（CML）主要影响成人。在白血病细胞加速生长阶段到来之前，患有慢性骨髓细胞白血病的人可能在几个月或几年内几乎没有症状。也有其他罕见类型的白血病，包括毛细胞白血病、成人 T 细胞白血病、浆细胞白血病和肥大细胞白血病。

years. Lymphocytic leukemia affects the lymphocytes, which form lymphatic tissue that makes up your immune system. Myelogenous leukemia affects the myeloid cells which give rise to red blood cells, white blood cells and platelet-producing cells.

Acute lymphocytic leukemia （ALL） is the most common type of leukemia in young children. ALL can also occur in adults. Acute myelogenous leukemia （AML） occurs in children and adults. AML is the most common type of acute leukemia in adults. Chronic lymphocytic leukemia （CLL） is the most common chronic adult leukemia.

Chronic myelogenous leukemia （CML） mainly affects adults. A person with CML may have few or no symptoms for months or years before entering a phase in which the leukemia cells grow more quickly. Other, rarer types of leukemia exist, including hairy cell leukemia, adult T-cell leukemia, plasma cell leukemia, and mast cell leukemia.

（二）淋巴瘤 Lymphoma[5]

淋巴瘤是淋巴系统的癌症，淋巴系统是人体抗菌网络的一部分，包括淋巴结（淋巴腺）、脾脏、胸腺和骨髓。淋巴瘤可以影响所有这些区域以及全身其他器官。淋巴瘤有多种类型，主要的亚型是霍奇金淋巴瘤（旧称霍奇金病）和非霍奇金淋巴瘤。

采取哪种淋巴瘤治疗方式最合适取决于淋巴瘤类型和严重程度。淋巴瘤治疗方法包括化疗、免疫疗法、放疗、骨髓移植或这些的组合疗法。淋巴瘤的体征和症状可能包括颈部、腋窝或腹股沟淋巴结的无痛性肿胀，持续性疲劳、发烧、盗汗、呼吸急促，无法解释的体重减轻和皮肤瘙痒。

淋巴瘤始于淋巴细胞的基因突变，但具体病因不明。突变令细胞快速复制，导致许多病变的淋巴细胞持续繁殖。当其他正常细胞死亡时，突变却能使这些细胞继续存活。这会使淋巴

Lymphoma is a cancer of the lymphatic system, which is part of the body's germ-fighting network. The lymphatic system includes the lymph nodes (lymph glands), spleen, thymus gland and bone marrow. Lymphoma can affect all those areas as well as other organs throughout the body. Many types of lymphoma exist. The main subtypes are Hodgkin's lymphoma (formerly called Hodgkin's disease) and Non-Hodgkin's lymphoma.

Which lymphoma treatment is best for you depends on your lymphoma type and its severity. Lymphoma treatment may involve chemotherapy, immunotherapy medications, radiation therapy, bone marrow transplant or a combination of these. Signs and symptoms of lymphoma may include painless swelling of lymph nodes in your neck, armpits or groin, persistent fatigue, fever, night sweats, shortness of breath, unexplained weight loss and itchy skin.

Lymphoma begins when a lymphocyte develops a genetic mutation, but the causes remain unclear. The mutation tells the cell to multiply rapidly, causing many diseased lymphocytes to

结中病变和无效的淋巴细胞过多，并导致淋巴结、脾脏和肝脏肿大。

continue multiplying. The mutation also allows the cells to go on living when other normal cells would die. This causes too many diseased and ineffective lymphocytes in your lymph nodes and causes the lymph nodes, spleen and liver to swell.

淋巴瘤的危险因素包括年龄、男性、免疫系统受损和特定感染。有些类型的淋巴瘤在年轻人中更为常见，而另外类型的淋巴瘤却在 55 岁以上的人群中最为常见。男性患淋巴瘤的概率略高于女性。淋巴瘤在免疫系统疾病患者或服用免疫系统抑制药物的人群中更为常见。有些感染与淋巴瘤的风险增大有关，比如 EB 病毒和幽门螺杆菌感染。

Risk factors of lymphoma include your age, male, impaired immune system, and certain infections. Some types of lymphoma are more common in young adults, while others are most often diagnosed in people over 55. Males are slightly more likely to develop lymphoma than females. Lymphoma is more common in people with immune system diseases or in people who take drugs that suppress their immune system. Some infections are associated with an increased risk of lymphoma, e. g. the Epstein-Barr virus and Helicobacter pylori infection.

（三）多发性骨髓瘤 Multiple Myeloma[6-7]

多发性骨髓瘤是一种癌变的浆细胞在骨髓中产生、繁殖和积聚的罕见病。多发性骨髓瘤是一种浆细胞癌。健康的浆细胞通过制造识别和攻击细菌的抗体来帮助你抵抗感染。在多发性骨髓瘤中，癌变的浆细胞在骨髓中

Multiple myeloma is a rare condition that causes cancerous plasma cells to be produced, multiply and build up in the bone marrow. Multiple myeloma is a cancer of plasma cells. Healthy plasma cells help you fight infections by making

积聚并排挤健康的血细胞。癌细胞不会产生有益的抗体，而是产生异常的蛋白质，从而导致并发症。

多发性骨髓瘤不一定需要马上治疗。如果多发性骨髓瘤生长缓慢，且没有引起症状和体征，那么医生可能建议密切监测而不是立即治疗。多发性骨髓瘤的症状和体征包括脊柱或胸部骨痛、恶心、便秘、食欲不振、精神模糊或混乱、疲劳、频繁感染、体重减轻、双腿无力或麻木以及极度口渴。

骨髓是处于大部分骨骼中心的柔软造血组织。骨髓瘤始于骨髓的某个异常浆细胞。该异常细胞繁殖迅速。因为癌细胞不像正常细胞那样成熟，然后死亡，所以它们会积聚起来，最终压制健康细胞的生长。在骨髓中，骨髓瘤细胞排挤健康的血细胞，会导致身体疲劳，无法抵抗感染。

antibodies that recognize and attack germs. In multiple myeloma, cancerous plasma cells accumulate in the bone marrow and crowd out healthy blood cells. Rather than produce helpful antibodies, the cancer cells produce abnormal proteins that can cause complications.

Treatment for multiple myeloma isn't always necessary right away. If the multiple myeloma is slow growing and isn't causing signs and symptoms, your doctor may recommend close monitoring instead of immediate treatment. Signs and symptoms of multiple myeloma consist of bone pain in your spine or chest, nausea, constipation, loss of appetite, mental fogginess or confusion, fatigue, frequent infections, weight loss, weakness or numbness in your legs, and excessive thirst.

Bone marrow is the soft, blood-producing tissue that fills in the center of most of your bones. Myeloma begins with one abnormal plasma cell in your bone marrow. The abnormal cell multiplies rapidly. Because cancer cells don't mature and then die as normal cells do, they accumulate, eventually overwhelming the production of healthy cells. In the bone marrow, myeloma cells crowd out healthy blood cells, leading to fatigue and an inability to fight infections.

骨髓瘤细胞继续试图产生抗体，就像健康的浆细胞一样，但是身体无法使用骨髓瘤细胞产生的异常抗体。相反，异常抗体（单克隆蛋白或 M 蛋白）的体内积聚，又会导致肾脏受损等问题。癌细胞还会对骨骼造成损伤，从而增加骨折的风险。由于骨髓瘤细胞排挤正常的血细胞，所以多发性骨髓瘤也可引起贫血和其他血液问题。

The myeloma cells continue trying to produce antibodies, as healthy plasma cells do, but the myeloma cells produce abnormal antibodies that the body can't use. Instead, the abnormal antibodies (monoclonal proteins, or M proteins) build up in the body and cause problems such as damage to the kidneys. Cancer cells can also cause damage to the bones, which increases the risk of broken bones. As myeloma cells crowd out normal blood cells, multiple myeloma can also cause anemia and other blood problems.

5　口译注释与学习资源

5.1　口译注释

（一）白细胞分类计数

"白细胞分类计数"有三种表达：differential white blood cell count（最常见），white blood cell differential count，differential white blood count。

（二）凝血紊乱（凝血病，凝血功能障碍）

Blood clotting (coagulation) disorders are dysfunctions in the body's ability to control the formation of blood clots. These dysfunctions may result in too little clotting, leading to abnormal bleeding (hemorrhage), or too much clotting, leading to the development of blood clots (thrombosis). 凝血紊乱是身体控制血凝块形成的功能出现的障碍。这一功能障碍可能导致凝血过少，出现异常出血，或导致凝血过

多，形成血栓。

（三）细菌国际命名法

生物名称一般分两类：俗名（vernacular name）和学名（scientific name）。细菌的学名是国际通用的名称。林奈氏（Linnaeus）创立的"双名法"由两个拉丁（化）词或希腊词组成，一般用斜体，且第一个词的首字母大写，如：

幽门螺杆菌 *Helicobacter pylori*（*H. pylori*）

结核分枝杆菌 *Mycobacterium tuberculosis*（*Mtb*）

铜绿假单胞菌 *Pseudomonas aeruginosa*（*P. aeruginosa*）

金黄色葡萄球菌 *Staphylococcus aureus*（*S. aureus*）

5.2 学习资源

登录中国大学 MOOC（慕课），学习"医疗口译"课程中"血液科"的口译实战示范视频。补充主题包括：（1）什么是白血病？What Is Leukemia？（2）白血病：病因、体征和症状以及诊断和治疗 Leukemia：Causes，Signs and Symptoms，Diagnosis and Treatment；（3）什么是血友病？What Is Hemophilia？（4）血友病与基因疗法 Hemophilia and Gene Therapy；（5）镰状细胞病：这种疾病如何改变你的细胞形状 Sickle-Cell Disease：How Does This Disease Change the Shape of Your Cells；（6）输血的工作原理是什么？How Do Blood Transfusions Work？（7）骨头如何造血？How Do Bones Make Blood？

参考文献

[1] Careers in Medicine.（n. d.）. *Hematology*. Retrieved November 11，2021，from https://www. aamc. org/cim/explore-options/specialty-profiles/hematology.

[2] Red Cross Blood Services.（n. d.）. *Blood types*. Retrieved November 11，2021，from https://www. redcrossblood. org/donate-blood/blood-types. html.

[3] WebMD.（n. d.）. *Anemia: Causes，symptoms，diagnosis，treatments*. Retrieved November 11，2021，from https://www. webmd. com/a-to-z－guides/understanding-anemia-basics.

[4] Mayo Foundation for Medical Education and Research.（2021，January 13）. *Leukemia*. Retrieved November 12，2021，from https://www. mayoclinic. org/diseases-conditions/leukemia/symptoms-causes/syc－20374373.

[5] Mayo Foundation for Medical Education and Research.（2021，October 30）. *Lymphoma*. Retrieved November 12，2021，from https://www. mayoclinic. org/diseases-conditions/

lymphoma/symptoms-causes/syc－20352638.

［6］ Cleveland Clinic. *Multiple myeloma: Symptoms & treatment.* （n. d. ）. Retrieved November 12,
　　 2021, from https://my. clevelandclinic. org/health/articles/6178－multiple-myeloma.

［7］ Mayo Foundation for Medical Education and Research. （2021, June 16）. *Multiple myeloma.*
　　 Retrieved November 12, 2021, from https://www. mayoclinic. org/diseases-conditions/multiple-
　　 myeloma/symptoms-causes/syc－20353378.

第九章

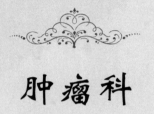

肿瘤科

1　导读

本章重点为口译技巧之公众演讲和肿瘤科的6篇"口译实战"练习。口译实战练习中英译汉、汉译英各3篇，内容涵盖肿瘤科介绍、癌症的病因与预防、皮肤癌、甲状腺腺瘤、癌症的治疗方案和肝癌。请结合本章口译技巧练习6篇口译实战文本。

2　口译技巧——公众演讲

无论是在一对一的谈话中，还是在会议、参观、展示等一对多的交际环境中，无论是所有交际方处于同一交际空间，还是交际方依靠远程连线的方式，口译员作为连接讲话者和听众的重要渠道，承担着向交际活动参与者发布信息与传达信息的责任。工作中的口译员可以看作某种意义上的公众演讲者，虽然其发布的信息内容大多来自交际方且听众人数可以是一人或多人。因此，公众演讲技巧可迁移至口译员的信息发布技巧中，帮助口译员高效、清晰地发布信息、传递信息。了解并运用下列两方面的公众演讲技巧有益于口译员开展工作。

2.1　语言输出

口译员的首要目标是准确、完整地翻译讲话者的信息，在此基础上需要注意以下与语言输出相关的演讲技巧。

（1）**保持清晰流利**。口译员需要发音清晰、吐字准确，避免吞音和错误的读音。口译员需有意识地避免重复词句或无意义的填补词及口头禅，也要避免不必要的停顿。

（2）**理清信息逻辑**。语言文化差异、信息差和个人讲话风格等因素都会使讲话者信息发布的逻辑和容易被听众接受的逻辑有差异，口译员需要对信息逻辑差异有一定的敏感度，使得信息的发布符合听众的逻辑。

（3）**调节声音质量**。悦耳的讲话声音一般音色清澈、音高音量适中。口译初学者在练习中，可根据自身的声音特色进行调整，避免声音过于低沉或尖锐、太大或者太小。

（4）**维持适当语速**。避免语速太快或者太慢，根据讲话者的语速和口译活动的时间安排适当调整语速，做到不快不慢，张弛有度。在口译开始时，由于内容偏向于程式化，也相对简单，切忌使用较快语速，以免与口译任务中段与后段差别太大。

2.2 形象仪态

（1）**着装简洁大方**。口译员在工作中须着装正式（根据具体的口译任务，正式程度可稍作调整），可参照我国外交部工作人员的着装风格，避免前卫、暴露、颜色过于鲜亮的着装和浓艳夸张的妆发。在医疗场合（如医院）工作的口译员，着装也需考虑场合，参照医护人员着装规范。

（2）**仪态端庄得体**。口译员应举止得体，坐、立、言、行都宜内敛、沉着和自信，应身姿挺拔，避免弯腰驼背。

（3）**肢体语言恰当**。口译员应避免过多的肢体语言或表情语言，动作幅度不宜过大，同时也应注意不同文化中的肢体语言禁忌。

因此，口译员在平时的训练中可以模拟口译信息发布场景，结合演讲技巧来训练良好的信息发布习惯。在练习时可以采取站姿和坐姿记笔记后发布信息，并对练习过程录像。通过回看，总结自身信息发布中的优点与不足。

3 口译词汇

3.1 英译汉

（一）Oncology 肿瘤科（肿瘤学）

epithelial cell 上皮细胞

breast duct 乳腺导管

airways 气道

connective tissue 结缔组织

lymphoma 淋巴瘤

benign 良性的

malignant 恶性的

mutation 突变

apoptosis 细胞凋亡

histological type 组织学类型

carcinoma 癌

sarcoma 肉瘤

myeloma 骨髓瘤

prostate 前列腺

colon 结肠

rectum 直肠

cervix 宫颈，颈部

uterus 子宫

non-small cell lung cancer 非小细胞肺癌

small cell lung cancer 小细胞肺癌

squamous cell carcinoma 鳞状细胞癌

adenocarcinoma 腺癌

large cell carcinoma 大细胞癌

chemotherapy 化疗

targeted therapy 靶向治疗

hormonal therapy 激素治疗

immunotherapy 免疫疗法

hematologist 血液学家，血液科医生

（二）Cancer：Causes and Prevention 癌症：病因与预防

neoplasm 肿瘤、赘生物

metastasis 转移

proto-oncogene 原癌基因

tumor suppressor gene 肿瘤抑制基因

DNA repair gene DNA 修复基因

ionizing radiation 电离辐射

radon 氡

radioactive 放射性的

natural decay 自然衰变

uranium 铀

HPV test 人乳头状瘤病毒检测

PAP cytology test 巴氏抹片细胞学检查（用于检测宫颈癌等疾病）

visual inspection with acetic acid（VIA）醋酸目视检查

mammography screening 乳房 X 光影像筛查

hepatitis B 乙型肝炎（乙肝）

（三）Skin Cancer 皮肤癌

lump 隆起、肿块

Actinic Keratosis 光化性角化病

pre-cancerous 癌前的

basal cell 基底细胞

melanoma 黑色素瘤

nodule 结节

scaly 鳞状的

pigmented area 色素沉淀区域

birthmark 胎记

texture 质地

3.2 汉译英

（一）甲状腺腺瘤 Thyroid Adenoma

甲状腺 thyroid

腺瘤 adenoma

腺体 gland

激素 hormone

新陈代谢 metabolism

囊肿 cyst

（非）癌性的（non）cancerous

病变 lesion

甲状腺功能正常的 euthyroid

甲状腺功能亢进 hyperthyroidism

毒性甲状腺腺瘤 toxic thyroid adenoma

易怒 irritability

情绪波动 mood swings

多汗 excessive sweating

燥热 sensitive to heat

声音嘶哑 hoarseness

喉管 larynx

气管 trachea/windpipe

超声波成像 ultrasound imaging

促甲状腺激素 thyroid-stimulating hormone（TSH）

活检 biopsy

放射碘－131 疗法 Iodine-131 therapy

同位素 isotope

甲状腺全切除术 thyroidectomy

甲状腺叶切除术 thyroid lobectomy

甲状腺峡部切除术 thyroid isthmusectomy

（二）癌症治疗 Cancer Treatment

免疫疗法 immunotherapy

免疫检查点抑制剂 immune checkpoint inhibitor

T 细胞转移疗法 T-cell transfer therapy

过继细胞疗法 adoptive cell therapy

单克隆抗体 monoclonal antibody

免疫系统调节剂 immune system modulator

（三）肝癌 Liver Cancer

膈膜 diaphragm

肝细胞癌 hepatocellular carcinoma

肝内胆管癌 intrahepatic cholangiocarcinoma

肝母细胞瘤 hepatoblastoma

转移性癌症 metastatic cancer

肝硬化 cirrhosis

血色素沉着病 hemochromatosis

黄曲霉素 aflatoxin

4 口译实战

4.1 英译汉

（一）Oncology 肿瘤科[1-3]

Oncology is the field of medicine that deals with the diagnosis, treatment,

肿瘤科（Oncology）是有关癌症的诊断、治疗、预防和早期发现的医

prevention, and early detection of cancer. While the term "onco" means mass, and "logy" means study, not all cancers cause a mass. There are hundreds of types of cancer that may arise from epithelial cells (such as breast ducts and airways in the lungs), connective tissue (such as sarcomas), or blood cells (such as leukemias and lymphomas).

A tumor is an abnormal growth of cells that serves no purpose. A benign tumor differs from a malignant tumor, which is cancer. It does not invade nearby tissues or spread to other parts of the body the way cancer can. In most cases, the outlook with benign tumors is very good. However, benign tumors can be serious if they press on vital structures such as blood vessels or nerves. Therefore, sometimes they require treatment and other times they do not.

Cancer is caused by the uncontrolled growth and reproduction of a cell that is initiated by a series of mutations in a normal cell. Cancer cells differ from normal cells in many ways. (1) Cancer cells grow in the absence of signals telling them to grow. Normal cells only grow

学领域。虽然"onco"的意思是"结块","logy"的意思是"研究",但并不是所有癌症都会引起"结块"。有数百种癌症起源于上皮细胞(如乳腺导管和肺部气道)、结缔组织(如肉瘤)或血细胞(如白血病和淋巴瘤)。

肿瘤是细胞出现的无意义的异常增生。良性肿瘤不同于恶性肿瘤,后者又称癌症。良性肿瘤不会入侵肿瘤部位附近的组织,也不会像恶性肿瘤一样扩散到身体的其他部位。在大多数情况下,良性肿瘤的预后较好。但是,即使是良性肿瘤,当其压迫血管或神经等重要结构时则会导致严重后果。因此,肿瘤是否需要治疗需视具体情况而定。

癌症是由正常细胞中的一系列突变引起的细胞不受控制的生长和增殖。癌细胞在很多方面区别于正常细胞。(1)癌细胞在没有接收到生长信号的情况下仍然生长,而正常细胞只有在收到此类信号时才会生长。(2)癌细胞会忽略让其停止分裂或死亡的信号

when they receive such signals. (2) Cancer cells ignore signals that normally tell cells to stop dividing or to die (a process known as programmed cell death, or apoptosis).

(3) Cancer cells invade into nearby areas and spread to other areas of the body. Normal cells stop growing when they encounter other cells, and most normal cells do not move around the body. (4) Cancer cells tell blood vessels to grow toward tumors. These blood vessels supply tumors with oxygen and nutrients and remove waste products from tumors. (5) Cancer cells hide from the immune system. Cancer cells trick the immune system into helping cancer cells stay alive and grow. For instance, some cancer cells convince immune cells to protect the tumor instead of attacking it.

(6) Cancer cells accumulate multiple changes in their chromosomes, such as duplications and deletions of chromosome parts. Some cancer cells have twice the normal number of chromosomes. (7) Cancer cells rely on different kinds of nutrients than normal cells. In addition, some cancer cells make energy from nutrients in a different

（此过程被称为细胞程序性死亡或细胞凋亡）。

（3）癌细胞侵入其附近区域并扩散到身体的其他部位，而正常细胞在遇到其他细胞时停止生长，大多数正常细胞不会在体内游走。（4）癌细胞让血管向肿瘤方向生长。这些血管为肿瘤提供氧气和营养物质，并将肿瘤中的废物排出。（5）癌细胞能躲避机体的免疫系统。癌细胞诱使免疫系统帮助其存活和生长。例如，一些癌细胞能使免疫细胞保护肿瘤，而不是攻击肿瘤。

（6）癌细胞会造成染色体产生多种改变，如复制或者删除染色体的一部分。有些癌细胞的染色体数量是正常数目的两倍。（7）与正常细胞相比，癌细胞依赖于不同种类的营养物质。此外，一些癌细胞利用营养物质产生能量的方式与正常细胞有所差异，这可以使癌细胞生长得更快。

way than most normal cells. This lets cancer cells grow more quickly.

Cancers are classified in two ways: by the type of tissue in which the cancer originates (histological type) and by primary site, or the location in the body where the cancer first developed. From a histological standpoint there are hundreds of different cancers, which are grouped into six major categories: carcinoma, sarcoma, myeloma, leukemia, lymphoma, Mixed Types.

Medical professionals usually refer to cancers based on their histological type. However, the general public is more familiar with cancer names based on their primary sites. The most common sites in which cancer develops include skin, lungs, female breasts, prostate, colon and rectum, cervix and uterus.

Compared with those based on histological type, cancers named after the primary site may not be as accurate. Take lung cancer for example, the name does not specify the type of tissue involved. It simply indicates where the cancer is located. In fact, depending on how the cells look under a microscope,

癌症可通过以下两种方式分类：癌症原发组织的类型（组织学类型）和癌症原发部位，也就是癌症最初在体内生长的部位。从组织学的角度来看，有数百种不同的癌症，可分为六大类：癌、肉瘤、骨髓瘤、白血病、淋巴瘤、混合型肿瘤。

医学专家经常以组织学类型来指称不同癌症。但是，公众更加熟悉的是基于其主要发病部位而命名的癌症名称。癌症发生的最常见部位包括皮肤、肺、女性乳房、前列腺、结肠和直肠、宫颈和子宫。

与基于组织学类型命名相比，以原发部位命名癌症可能不那么准确。以肺癌为例，该名称未明确癌症的组织学类型，它只表明癌症所在的位置。实际上，根据显微镜下观察到的细胞外观，肺癌主要分为非小细胞肺癌和

there are two major types of lung cancer: non-small cell lung cancer and small cell lung cancer. Non-small cell lung cancer can be further divided into various types for the type of cells in which the cancer develops, typically: squamous cell carcinoma, adenocarcinoma, and large cell carcinoma.

There are three primary types of oncologists or physicians who treat people with cancer. Medical oncologists treat people with medications such as chemotherapy, targeted therapy, hormonal therapy, and immunotherapy. Surgical oncologists perform surgeries to remove malignant tumors. Radiation oncologists use radiation to treat cancer. Oncologists and hematologists treat not only people who have cancer but also people who are coping with benign blood-based diseases such as anemia.

小细胞肺癌。非小细胞肺癌可以进一步分为多种类型，这些类型以发生癌症的细胞类型命名，典型的有鳞状细胞癌、腺癌和大细胞癌。

肿瘤科医生主要有三种类型：肿瘤内科医生，用化疗、靶向治疗、激素治疗和免疫疗法等药物手段治疗患者；肿瘤外科医生，使用手术的方式切除恶性肿瘤；放射肿瘤科医生，使用放射的方式来治疗癌症。肿瘤科医生和血液科医生不仅治疗癌症患者，还治疗良性血液疾病患者，如贫血症患者。

（二）Cancer: Causes and Prevention 癌症：病因与预防[2,4-5]

Cancer is a genetic disease—it is caused by changes to genes that control the way our cells function, especially those that control how they grow and divide. Other terms used are malignant tumours and neoplasms. One defining feature of cancer is the rapid creation of

癌症是一种基因性疾病，由控制细胞功能的基因发生变化引起，尤其是控制细胞生长和分裂的基因。癌症还可以称为恶性肿瘤或恶性赘生物。癌症的一个典型特征是异常细胞的快速增生，这些细胞的生长超出了正常生长界限，然后入侵相邻身体部位，

abnormal cells that grow beyond their usual boundaries and can then invade adjoining parts of the body and spread to other organs; the latter process is referred to as metastasis. Metastases are the primary cause of death from cancer.

并扩散到其他器官，后面的过程称为癌细胞转移。癌细胞转移是癌症患者死亡的主要原因。

Each person's cancer has a unique combination of genetic changes. As the cancer continues to grow, additional changes will occur. Even within the same tumor, different cells may have different genetic changes. The genetic changes that contribute to cancer tend to affect three main types of genes—proto-oncogenes, tumor suppressor genes, and DNA repair genes. These changes are sometimes called "drivers" of cancer.

每个癌症患者的癌症都有其独特的基因变化组合。随着癌症发展，这些变化还将持续发生。即使在同一个肿瘤中，不同的细胞也可能有不同的基因变化。导致癌症的基因变化往往主要会影响三种类型的基因——原癌基因、肿瘤抑制基因和 DNA 修复基因。这些变化有时被称为癌症的"驱动因素"。

Proto-oncogenes are involved in normal cell growth and division. However, when these genes are altered in certain ways or are more active than normal, they may become cancer-causing genes (or oncogenes), allowing cells to grow and survive when they should not. Tumor suppressor genes are also involved in controlling cell growth and division. Cells with certain alterations in tumor suppressor genes may divide in an uncontrolled manner. DNA repair genes

原癌基因参与正常的细胞生长和分裂。然而，当这些基因以某种方式被改变或比正常更活跃时，它们可能成为致癌基因（又称癌基因），使细胞在不该生长和存活时生长和存活。肿瘤抑制基因也参与控制细胞生长和分裂。肿瘤抑制基因发生了某些变化的细胞可能会以不受控制的方式分裂。DNA 修复基因参与修复受损的 DNA。

are involved in fixing damaged DNA.

Cells with mutations in these genes tend to develop additional mutations in other genes and changes in their chromosomes, such as duplications and deletions of chromosome parts. Together, these mutations may cause the cells to become cancerous. Doctors have identified several ways to reduce your risk of cancer, such as not using tobacco, maintaining a healthy body weight, having a healthy diet, exercising regularly, and avoiding harmful use of alcohol. These are some common advices for staying healthy. Additional measures are as follows:

First, avoid unnecessary exposure to radiation and pollution. Harmful ultraviolet（UV）rays from the sun and artificial tanning devices can increase your risk of skin cancer. Limit your sun exposure by staying in the shade, wearing protective clothing or applying sunscreen. Ensure safe and appropriate use of radiation in health care for diagnostic and therapeutic purposes. Minimize occupational exposure to ionizing radiation. Pollution can also trigger certain types of cancers; therefore,

这些基因发生突变的细胞，其他基因往往也会出现突变，并改变其染色体，如改变染色体的复制和删除。在所有这些突变共同作用下，细胞可能发生癌变。医生已经确定了降低患癌风险的几种方法，比如不吸烟、保持健康的体重、健康饮食、经常锻炼、避免过度饮酒。这些都是保持健康的一些常见建议。其他措施还包括：

首先，避免暴露于不必要的辐射和污染中。来自太阳和人工晒黑装置的有害紫外线（UV）会增加罹患皮肤癌的风险。待在遮阴处、穿防护服或涂防晒霜，以避免直接暴露在阳光照射之下。在医疗过程中出于诊疗目的需要接触辐射时，要确保安全和适量地使用辐射。尽量减少电离辐射的职业性暴露。污染也会引发某些类型的癌症，因此需要减少暴露于受污染的室内外空气中，包括氡污染。氡是一种由铀的自然衰变产生的放射性气体，它可以积聚在建筑物中，如住宅、学

reduce exposure to outdoor and indoor air pollution, including radon. Radon is a radioactive gas produced from the natural decay of uranium, which can accumulate in buildings—homes, schools and workplaces.

校和工作场所。

Second, schedule cancer screening exams. Screening aims to identify individuals with findings suggestive of a specific cancer or pre-cancer before they have developed symptoms. Talk to your doctor about what types of cancer screening exams are best for you based on your risk factors. Examples of screening methods are HPV testing for cervical cancer, PAP cytology test for cervical cancer, visual inspection with acetic acid (VIA) for cervical cancer, mammography screening for breast cancer, etc.

其次，安排癌症筛查。癌症筛查的目的是在出现症状之前，识别出有特定癌症或癌前病变的个人。可根据自身的风险因素，与医生讨论哪些类型的癌症筛查最为适合。例如筛查宫颈癌的方法有 HPV 检测、PAP 细胞学检测、醋酸（VIA）目视检查，筛查乳腺癌的方法有乳房 X 光检查等。

Lastly, ask your doctor about immunizations. Certain viruses increase your risk of cancer. Immunizations may help prevent those viruses, including hepatitis B, which increases the risk of liver cancer, and human papillomavirus (HPV), which increases the risk of cervical cancer and other cancer. Ask your doctor whether immunization against these viruses is appropriate for you.

最后，询问医生有关预防接种的问题。某些病毒感染会增加患癌风险。预防接种有助于预防这些病毒，包括增加肝癌风险的乙型肝炎病毒、增加宫颈癌和其他癌症风险的人乳头状瘤病毒（HPV）。询问医生接种这些病毒疫苗是否适合你个人。

（三）Skin Cancer 皮肤癌[6-7]

Skin cancer—the abnormal growth of skin cells—develops most often on skin long exposed to the sun. But this common form of cancer can also occur on areas of your skin not ordinarily exposed to sunlight. The beginning signs of skin cancer involve a change in the skin. This may mean that a new lump or sore has formed on the skin, that a new mole has popped up, or that an existing mole has begun to grow or change in shape.

Actini Keratosis（AK）is a pre-cancerous growth that may become skin cancer over time. AKs may show up as small patches on the skin that are pink, rough, dry, and/or scaly. The patches may be painful, burning, or itchy, particularly when pressure is applied. An AK isn't skin cancer, but it can turn into a common type of skin cancer, squamous cell carcinoma.

The type of skin cancer a person gets is determined by where the cancer begins. If the cancer begins in skin cells called basal cells, the person has basal cell skin cancer. When cells that give our skin its color become cancerous, melanoma develops. There are three

皮肤癌，也就是皮肤细胞的异常生长，发病部位通常为长期暴露在阳光下的皮肤。但是这种常见的癌症也可能发生在不常暴露在阳光下的皮肤部位。皮肤癌的早期症状通常与皮肤的变化相关，可能是皮肤上出现新的隆起或疼痛，也有可能是皮肤上长出新的痣，或者是皮肤上现有的痣开始生长或其形状产生变化。

光化性角化病（AK）是一种癌前病变，随着时间推移可变成皮肤癌。光化性角化病表现为皮肤粉红、粗糙、干燥和/或出现鳞片状小斑块。按压这些斑块时可能有疼痛感、灼烧感或发痒。光化性角化病不是皮肤癌，但它可以发展为一种常见的皮肤癌，即鳞状细胞癌。

一个人患皮肤癌的类型取决于癌症的起源部位。如果癌症起源于基底细胞，则此人患有基底细胞皮肤癌。当决定肤色的细胞发生癌变时，则形成黑色素瘤。皮肤癌主要有三种类型——基底细胞癌、鳞状细胞癌和黑色素瘤。

major types of skin cancer—basal cell carcinoma, squamous cell carcinoma and melanoma.

Basal cell carcinoma (BCC) is the most common type of skin cancer that usually occurs in sun-exposed areas of your body, such as your neck or face. It is likely to develop in people who have fair skin. But it doesn't mean that people who have skin of color are immune to this skin cancer. BCCs are common on the head, neck, and arms; however, they can form anywhere on the body, including the chest, abdomen, and legs.

Squamous cell carcinoma (SCC) is the second most common type of skin cancer, which can develop from a precancerous skin growth. Squamous cell carcinoma may appear as a firm, red nodule or a flat lesion with a scaly, crusted surface. The most common places for SCC to form are arms, legs, face, ears, and lips.

While it is very uncommon that basal or squamous cell carcinomas will cause death, melanoma may be fatal if the disease spreads to other organ systems

基底细胞癌（BCC）是最常见的皮肤癌类型，通常发生在人身体的阳光照射区域，如脖子或脸部。皮肤白皙的人更易患此病。但这并不意味着有色人种对这种皮肤癌天然免疫。基底细胞癌多发于头部、颈部和手臂，但也可以在身体的任何部位出现，包括胸部、腹部和腿部。

鳞状细胞癌（SCC）是第二常见的皮肤癌类型，这种皮肤癌可以由癌前皮肤生长发展而来。鳞状细胞癌可能表现为红色硬结，也可能表现为扁平的鳞状结壳。鳞状细胞癌最常见的部位是手臂、腿部、面部、耳朵和嘴唇。

基底细胞癌或鳞状细胞癌导致死亡的情况非常罕见，但黑色素瘤可能是致命的，尤其蔓延到身体的其他器官或部位时。黑色素瘤通常被称为

or places in the body. Melanoma is often called "the most serious skin cancer". It can develop from a mole that you already have on your skin, or appear suddenly as a dark spot on the skin that looks different from the rest.

Common early symptoms of melanoma include a new mole or freckle that pops up suddenly and grows quickly, or any change to a mole or other pigmented area such as birthmarks and large freckles. Any moles or blemishes that change texture, shape, or color, any spots that are black, or any pigmented areas that itch or bleed may also indicate the early stages of melanoma. In many instances, a self-exam will help reveal a melanoma in the beginning signs of skin cancer. If the melanoma has spread, it can be cured by removing the affected area through surgery.

"最严重的皮肤癌"。它可能从皮肤上已有的痣中发展而来，也可能以深色斑点的形式突然出现在皮肤上，这种深色斑点看起来有别于其他斑点。

黑色素瘤的常见早期症状为皮肤上突然出现的快速生长的痣或者斑点，或者皮肤上的痣或其他皮肤色素沉着区域（如胎记、大的雀斑）突然发生变化。任何改变质地、形状、颜色的痣或皮肤瑕疵，任何黑色斑点，任何发痒或出血的皮肤色素沉着区域，也都有可能是黑色素瘤的早期形态。在许多情况下，自我检查将有助于早日发现开始发生癌变的黑色素瘤。如果黑色素瘤已经扩散，可以通过手术切除受影响的区域来治疗。

4.2　汉译英

（一）甲状腺腺瘤 Thyroid Adenoma[8]

甲状腺是在喉部前方的一个小蝴蝶形的腺体，它分泌激素，影响新陈代谢、心率等诸多生理过程。甲状腺疾病是比较常见的疾病，如甲状腺腺瘤这一良性肿瘤。甲状腺腺瘤是甲状

The thyroid is a small, butterfly-shaped gland in the front of your throat that produces hormones. It affects a number of bodily processes, from metabolism to heart rate. Thyroid disease

腺上的非癌性病变。虽不是癌症，但仍会影响人的整体健康。

甲状腺腺瘤若不活跃则不产生甲状腺激素；若活跃，则产生激素。在极少数情况下，也就是对于大约1%的人而言，活跃的甲状腺腺瘤可导致甲状腺功能亢进，也就是甲状腺激素的过度分泌。然而，大多数甲状腺腺瘤患者没有任何症状。

在某些情况下，活跃的甲状腺腺瘤——毒性甲状腺腺瘤，可能导致甲状腺分泌过多的激素。这可能导致甲状腺功能亢进的症状，包括疲劳、体重减轻、易怒、情绪波动、多汗或燥热。除了甲状腺功能亢进，当甲状腺腺瘤压迫喉管、气管和喉部其他部位时，甲状腺腺瘤患者还可能会出现声音变化、声音嘶哑、吞咽困难或呼吸困难的症状。

is relatively common, such as thyroid adenoma, which is a benign tumor. A thyroid adenoma is a noncancerous lesion on the thyroid. Although they're not cancer, they can still affect your overall health.

Thyroid adenomas can be inactive, meaning that they don't produce thyroid hormones, or they can be active, meaning that they produce hormones. In rare cases, for about 1% of people, an active thyroid adenoma can cause hyperthyroidism, or an overproduction of thyroid hormones. However, most patients with a thyroid adenoma do not have any symptoms.

In some cases, having an active adenoma—also known as a toxic thyroid adenoma—can cause the thyroid to produce too many hormones. This can lead to symptoms of hyperthyroidism, including fatigue, weight loss, irritability, mood swings, excessive sweating or sensitivity to heat. In addition to hyperthyroidism, people with a thyroid adenoma might experience vocal changes, hoarseness, or might have trouble swallowing or breathing. These symptoms occur when the thyroid adenoma is pushing against the larynx, trachea (windpipe), and other structures in the throat.

在发现甲状腺生长异常后，医生需要确定这种异常生长是否影响激素水平，以及是否发生癌变。为了诊断甲状腺腺瘤，医生必须排除有类似症状的其他甲状腺疾病。因此，医生会要求做以下检查：超声波成像、血液测试——以测量促甲状腺激素（TSH）水平，以及活检。

After spotting an unusual growth on the thyroid, doctors need to determine whether the growth is affecting hormone levels, and whether or not it is cancerous. In order to diagnose a thyroid adenoma, doctors have to rule out other thyroid conditions that present in a similar way. To do this, doctors will order ultrasound imaging, a blood test to measure your thyroid-stimulating hormone (TSH) levels, and a biopsy.

如果患者促甲状腺激素水平受到了甲状腺腺瘤影响，则必须接受治疗以恢复正常的甲状腺功能。放射碘－131疗法通常用于抑制甲状腺的异常生长以使甲状腺恢复正常的功能。碘－131是一种由口腔吸收的放射性同位素。

People whose TSH levels are impacted by a thyroid adenoma must be treated in order to restore normal thyroid function. Iodine-131 therapy is often used to kill off abnormal growths on the thyroid and restore normal thyroid function. Iodine-131 is a radioactive isotope taken by mouth.

当甲状腺腺瘤引起严重症状时，医生可能会建议手术。手术可以立即缓解包括甲状腺功能亢进和压迫气管在内的症状。有三种手术可用于治疗甲状腺腺瘤患者。甲状腺切除术，也

In some cases, where the symptoms of a thyroid adenoma are severe, your doctor might recommend surgery. This is usually used for an immediate resolution of symptoms, including hyperthyroidism

就是切除整个甲状腺，或者有腺瘤的一部分甲状腺。甲状腺叶切除术，也就是切除腺瘤所在的一半甲状腺。甲状腺峡部切除术，只切除甲状腺的峡部。医生将综合考虑患者腺瘤的位置、大小、症状，以及患者的其他健康因素以确定最佳治疗方案。

or compression on the windpipe. There are three types of surgery used in patients with thyroid adenomas. Thyroidectomy removes all of the thyroid, or just a part, like the adenoma. Thyroid lobectomy removes the half of the thyroid that the adenoma is on. Isthmusectomy removes just the isthmus. Doctors will consider the position and size of your adenoma, your symptoms, and any other health considerations you have in order to determine the best treatment for you.

（二）癌症治疗 Cancer Treatment[9]

免疫疗法是一种癌症治疗方法，可帮助免疫系统抵抗癌症。免疫疗法是一种生物疗法，也就是使用由活体制成的物质来治疗癌症。以下简单介绍几种免疫疗法。

Immunotherapy is a type of cancer treatment that helps your immune system fight cancer. Immunotherapy is a type of biological therapy that uses substances made from living organisms to treat cancer. Here is a brief introduction to several types of immunotherapies.

免疫检查点抑制剂是阻断免疫检查点的药物。这些检查点是免疫系统的正常组成部分，可以防止免疫反应过强。通过阻断它们，这些药物使免疫细胞对癌症的响应更加强烈。

Immune checkpoint inhibitors are drugs that block immune checkpoints. These checkpoints are a normal part of the immune system and keep immune responses from being too strong. By blocking them, these drugs allow immune cells to respond more strongly to cancer.

T 细胞转移疗法，是一种通过增强 T 细胞能力来抗癌的疗法。在这一治疗过程中，免疫细胞取自患者的肿瘤。那些对患者自身癌症抵抗最活跃的细胞被筛选出来，并在实验室中修改变得更为强大，而后大批量培养这些细胞，最后通过静脉注射的方式放回患者体内。T 细胞转移疗法也可以称为过继细胞疗法、过继免疫疗法或免疫细胞疗法。

单克隆抗体，是实验室制作出的免疫系统蛋白，旨在与癌细胞上的特定靶标结合。一些单克隆抗体会标记癌细胞，使得后者能更容易被免疫系统发现并杀死。使用这样的单克隆抗体是一种免疫疗法。

治疗性疫苗，可通过增强免疫系统对癌细胞的应答来对抗癌症。癌症治疗性疫苗不同于疾病预防性疫苗。癌症治疗性疫苗的受众是已经患有癌症的患者。癌症治疗性疫苗针对的是癌细胞，而不是针对导致癌症的因素。

T-cell transfer therapy is a treatment that boosts the natural ability of your T cells to fight cancer. In this treatment, immune cells are taken from the patient's tumor. Those that are most active against your cancer are selected or changed in the lab to better attack your cancer cells. Then such cells are grown in large batches and put back into your body through a needle in a vein. T-cell transfer therapy may also be called adoptive cell therapy, adoptive immunotherapy, or immune cell therapy.

Monoclonal antibodies are immune system proteins created in the lab that are designed to bind to specific targets on cancer cells. Some monoclonal antibodies mark cancer cells so that they will be better seen and destroyed by the immune system. Using such monoclonal antibodies is a type of immunotherapy.

Treatment vaccines work against cancer by boosting your immune system's response to cancer cells. Treatment vaccines are different from the ones that help prevent disease. Cancer treatment vaccines are designed to be used in people who already have cance. They work against cancer cells, not against something that causes cancer.

免疫系统调节剂，可增强人体对癌症的免疫反应。有的试剂作用于免疫系统的特定部分，而另一些则以更全面的方式作用于免疫系统。

Immune system modulators enhance the body's immune response against cancer. Some of these agents affect specific parts of the immune system, whereas others affect the immune system in a more general way.

（三）肝癌 Liver Cancer[10-11]

人的肝脏位于腹部的右上方，横膈膜之下，胃部之上。肝癌是肝脏细胞癌变的结果。有几种类型的癌症是在肝脏中形成的。最常见的一种肝癌是肝细胞癌，始发于肝细胞。

Your liver sits in the upper right portion of your abdomen, beneath your diaphragm and above your stomach. Liver cancer is the cancer that begins in the cells of your liver. Several types of cancer can form in the liver. The most common type of liver cancer is hepatocellular carcinoma, which begins in hepatocytes.

其他类型的肝癌，如肝内胆管癌和肝母细胞瘤，更为少见。扩散到肝脏的癌症比原发性肝癌更为常见。身体其他部位的癌症，如结肠癌、肺癌或乳腺癌可能会扩散至肝脏，被称为转移癌，而不是肝癌。这种类型的癌症是以其初始癌变器官命名的，比如转移性结肠癌指的是由结肠扩散到肝脏的癌症。

Other types of liver cancer, such as intrahepatic cholangiocarcinoma and hepatoblastoma, are much less common. Cancer that spreads to the liver is more common than cancer that begins in the liver cells. Cancer that begins in another area of the body—such as the colon, lung or breast—and then spreads to the liver is called metastatic cancer rather than liver cancer. This type of cancer is named after the organ in which it begins—such as metastatic colon cancer—to describe cancer that begins in the colon and spreads to the liver.

大多数人在原发性肝癌的早期阶段没有症状。当出现症状时，症状可能包括不明原因的体重减轻、食欲不振、上腹疼痛、恶心、呕吐、全身虚弱和疲劳、腹部肿胀、黄疸、大便发白等。

Most people don't have signs or symptoms in the early stages of primary liver cancer. When signs and symptoms do appear, they may include weight lost without trying, loss of appetite, upper abdominal pain, nausea and vomiting, general weakness and fatigue, abdominal swelling, jaundice, white and chalky stools, etc.

以下行为或者情况可能增加患肝癌的风险：超重、长期感染乙型或丙型肝炎病毒、吸烟、饮酒、肝硬化、非酒精性脂肪肝、糖尿病、血色素沉着病、食用含有黄曲霉素的食物等。

Behaviors and conditions that increase risks for getting liver cancer include being overweight, having a long-term hepatitis B or C virus infection, smoking, drinking alcohol, having cirrhosis, having nonalcoholic fatty liver disease, having diabetes, having hemochromatosis, eating foods that have aflatoxin, etc.

预防肝癌，减少危险因素是关键。饮酒需适量，保持健康体重可以降低肝硬化的风险。接种乙肝疫苗可降低患乙型肝炎的风险。虽没有丙型肝炎疫苗，但可通过了解性伴侣的健康状况，在身体穿孔或文身时选择安全、

To prevent liver cancer, reducing the risk factors is the key. You can reduce the risk of cirrhosis if you drink alcohol in moderation and maintain a healthy weight. You can reduce the risk of hepatitis B by receiving the hepatitis B

干净的地方等措施降低感染丙型肝炎的风险。

vaccine. There is no vaccine for hepatitis C, but you can reduce the risk of hepatitis C infection by knowing the health status of your sexual partner, going to safe and clean shops when getting a piercing or tattoo.

5 口译注释与学习资源

5.1 口译注释

"produce"一词在医学英语中，多翻译为"分泌""生殖""合成""产生""制造"等，具体选择需视语境和其后的名词搭配而定。例如：

（1）英译汉第一篇中"Cancer is caused by the uncontrolled growth and **reproduction of a cell** that is initiated by a series of mutations in a normal cell." 这句中的加粗部分应翻译为"细胞的增殖"。

（2）汉译英第一篇中"The thyroid is a small, butterfly-shaped gland in the front of your throat that **produces hormones**." 这句中的加粗部分应翻译为"分泌激素"。

5.2 学习资源

登录中国大学 MOOC（慕课），学习"医疗口译"课程中"肿瘤科"的口译实战示范视频。

参考文献

［1］Lynne Eldridge, M. D.（2020, September 26）. *What is oncology?*. Verywell Health. Retrieved November 13, 2021, from https://www.verywellhealth.com/what-is-oncology-5074859.

［2］National Cancer Institute.（n. d.）. *What is cancer?*. Retrieved November 13, 2021, from https://www.cancer.gov/about-cancer/understanding/what-is-cancer.

［3］Stuart, A.（n. d.）. *Benign tumors: Types, causes, and treatments*. WebMD. Retrieved November 13, 2021, from https://www.webmd.com/a-to-z-guides/benign-tumors-causes-treatments.

［4］World Health Organization.（n. d.）. *Cancer*. World Health Organization. Retrieved November 13,

2021, from https://www. who. int/news-room/fact-sheets/detail/cancer.

[5] Mayo Foundation for Medical Education and Research. (2021, April 27). *Cancer.* Retrieved November 13, 2021, from https://www. mayoclinic. org/diseases-conditions/cancer/symptoms-causes/syc – 20370588.

[6] Illnessee. com. (n. d.). *Early signs of Skin cancer pictures.* Retrieved November 13, 2021, from https://illnessee. com/early-signs-of-skin-cancer-pictures/.

[7] American Academy of Dermatology. (n. d.). *Types of skin cancer.* Retrieved November 13, 2021, from https://www. aad. org/public/diseases/skin-cancer/types/common.

[8] Burch, K. (2021, June 8). *What is a thyroid adenoma?.* Verywell Health. Retrieved November 13, 2021, from https://www. verywellhealth. com/thyroid-adenoma – 5101465.

[9] National Cancer Institute. (n. d.). *Radiation therapy for cancer.* Retrieved November 13, 2021, from https://www. cancer. gov/about-cancer/treatment/types/radiation-therapy.

[10] Mayo Foundation for Medical Education and Research. (2021, May 18). *Liver cancer.* Retrieved November 13, 2021, from https://www. mayoclinic. org/diseases-conditions/liver-cancer/symptoms-causes/syc – 20353659.

[11] Centers for Disease Control and Prevention. (2021, January 19). *Liver cancer.* Centers for Disease Control and Prevention. Retrieved November 13, 2021, from https://www. cdc. gov/cancer/liver/index. htm.

第十章

心血管内科/外科

1　导读

本章重点为口译技巧之精力分配和心血管内科/外科的 6 篇"口译实战"练习。口译实战练习中英译汉、汉译英各 3 篇，内容涵盖心血管内科/外科介绍、心律失常、心肌病、风湿性心脏病、动脉粥样硬化和高血压。请结合本章口译技巧练习 6 篇口译实战文本。

2　口译技巧——精力分配

20 世纪 70 年代，Daniel Gile 提出了"认知负荷模型"（Effort Model，也称"精力分配模型"）。在交替传译中，"认知负荷模型"的公式为 Interpretation = L + M + N + C，即口译 = 听力和分析（L）＋短期记忆（M）＋笔记（N）＋协调（C）。口译活动过程中，可供使用的脑容量需要大于听力和分析、短期记忆、笔记和协调所需脑容量之和。

口译活动中，译员需要全程集中注意力，通常译员的注意力在翻译时都在饱和状态。但是在医疗口译中，由于专有名词多、信息密度大，"漏译"或者"错译"会造成重大后果，在某些场合下，译员的精力甚至会出现超负荷状态。医疗口译与法律口译等专业领域的口译一样，对于译员的相关专业知识要求较高，但相比其他领域，医疗口译对词汇、背景知识的要求更高。

对于听力和分析、短期记忆和笔记等口译技巧，本书已有专门的章节进行了阐述。译员需要提升应用技巧的能力，减少在每个技巧上分配的精力。需要强调的是，译员在不同的环节中的精力分配比例因人而异，同一位译员在不同的场合、不同的翻译领域中需要分配的精力也是有差异的。如果口译主题是译员非常熟悉的领域，那么译员可将大部分的精力用在语言表达上，在听力和分析上分配的精力就相应减少。

精力分配能力可以通过"影子练习"（shadowing）提升。"影子练习"即原语跟读复述。音频播放开始后，译员滞后 2～3 个单词开口跟读，边听边跟读完整个篇章。"影子练习"可以采取以下步骤：

（1）跟读一段 10 分钟之内的原语，可选取语速适中的篇章，同时对自己的跟读进行录音，便于跟读后检查准确率。

（2）跟读同一段原语，概括出该段的主要内容，可用原语和译语概括。

（3）在熟练掌握"影子练习"技巧后，在跟读过程中加入干扰因素，如尝试记下该段关键词。可能刚开始只能记下寥寥几个关键词，但是随着练习量的加大，译员找到"影子练习"的舒适区后，便能更好地分配精力。

3 口译词汇

3.1 英译汉

（一）Cardiovascular Medicine/Surgery 心血管内科/外科

cardiovascular disease（CVD）心血管疾病

cholesterol 胆固醇

obesity 肥胖

coronary 冠状位的，冠的

transient ischaemic attack（TIA）短暂性脑缺血发作

mini-stroke 微卒中

peripheral arterial disease 外周动脉疾病

aortic disease 主动脉疾病

aortic aneurysm 主动脉瘤

congestive heart failure 充血性心力衰竭

heart rhythm 心律

congenital 先天性

endocarditis 心内膜炎

surgeon 外科医生

heart valve 心脏瓣膜

repair and replacement 修复和置换

coronary artery bypass 冠状动脉搭桥术

transmyocardial laser revascularization 经心肌激光血运重建

heart transplantation 心脏移植

ventricular assist devices（VAD）心室辅助装置

（二）Heart Arrhythmia 心律失常

electrical impulse 电脉冲

atria 心房（单数为 atrium，复数为 atria 或者 atriums）

tachycardia 心动过速

bradycardia 心动过缓

atrial fibrillation 心房颤动（简称为颤）

quiver/fibrillate 颤动

ventricle 心室

heart block 心脏传导阻滞

ventricular fibrillation 心室颤动（简称室颤）

irregular rhythm 心律不规则

（三）Cardiomyopathy 心肌病

myocardium 心肌

heart failure 心力衰竭

shortness of breath 呼吸急促

swelling of lower limb 下肢肿胀

progression of the disease 疾病进展

viral infection 病毒感染

dilated cardiomyopathy（DCM）扩张型心肌病

heart chamber 心腔

genetic defect 遗传缺陷

hypertrophic cardiomyopathy 肥厚型心肌病

restrictive cardiomyopathy 限制型心肌病

main pumping chamber 心脏主泵室

3.2 汉译英

（一）风湿性心脏病 Rheumatic Heart Disease

急性风湿热 acute rheumatic fever（ARF）

心脏内膜 heart lining

肿胀 swell

心肌炎 carditis

风湿热 rheumatic fever

心力衰竭 heart failure

超声心动图 echocardiogram

心脏杂音 heart murmur

听诊器 stethoscope

胸痛 chest pain

呼吸困难 breathlessness

首次发作 initial episode

心律异常 abnormal heart rhythm

脑卒中，卒中，中风 stroke

心内膜炎 endocarditis

并发症 complication

进展性残疾 progressive disability

过早死亡 premature death

（二）动脉粥样硬化 Atherosclerosis

脂肪物质 fatty material

斑块 plaque

动脉壁 wall of artery/arterial wall

细胞代谢废物 cellular waste product

钙 calcium

纤维蛋白 fibrin

凝血物质 clotting material

骨盆 pelvis

心绞痛 angina

颈动脉疾病 carotid artery disease

内皮 inner lining

甘油三酯 triglyceride

（三）高血压 Hypertension

血压 blood pressure

血管壁 wall of blood vessel

动脉压 arterial pressure

体循环 systemic circulation

收缩 contract

主动脉 aorta

主动脉压 aortic pressure

体动脉压 systemic arterial pressure

心脏射血 ejection

收缩压 systolic pressure

心室 ventricle

舒张压 diastolic pressure

血压读数 blood pressure reading

心血管疾病 cardiovascular disease

动脉瘤 aneurysm

心脏病发作/心肌梗死 heart attack

终末器官 end organ

肾衰竭 renal failure

视力丧失 vision loss

4　口译实战

4.1　英译汉

（一）Cardiovascular Medicine/Surgery 心血管内科/外科[2-4]

Cardiovascular disease（CVD）is a type of disease that affects the heart or blood vessels. The risk of certain cardiovascular diseases may be increased by smoking, high blood pressure, high cholesterol, unhealthy diet, lack of exercise, and obesity. There are many different types of CVD. Four of the main types are described below.

心血管疾病（CVD）是一种影响心脏或血管的疾病。吸烟、高血压、高胆固醇、不健康饮食、缺乏运动和肥胖可能会增加患某些心血管疾病的风险。有许多不同类型的心血管疾病。下面介绍四种主要类型。

Coronary heart disease. Coronary heart disease occurs when the flow of oxygen-rich blood to the heart muscle is blocked or reduced. Strokes and

冠状动脉心脏疾病（冠心病）。当流向心肌的富含氧气的血液受阻或减少时，就会发生冠心病。脑卒中（中风）和短暂性脑缺血发作（TIA）。

transient ischaemic attack （TIA）. A stroke is where the blood supply to part of the brain is cut off, which can cause brain damage and even death. A transient ischaemic attack （also called a TIA or "mini-stroke"）is similar, but the blood flow to the brain is only temporarily disrupted.

脑卒中是指部分大脑的血液供应被切断，这会导致脑损伤甚至死亡。短暂性脑缺血发作（也称为 TIA 或 "微卒中"）与此类似，但流向大脑的血流只是暂时中断。

Peripheral arterial disease. Peripheral arterial disease occurs when there's a blockage in the arteries to the limbs, usually the legs. Aortic disease. Aortic diseases are a group of conditions affecting the aorta. This is the largest blood vessel in the body, which carries blood from the heart to the rest of the body. One of most common aortic diseases is an aortic aneurysm, where the aorta becomes weakened and bulges outwards.

外周动脉疾病。当通向四肢（通常是腿部）的动脉出现阻塞时，就会发生外周动脉疾病。主动脉疾病。主动脉疾病是一组影响主动脉的疾病。主动脉是体内最大的血管，它将血液从心脏输送到身体的其他部位。最常见的主动脉疾病之一是主动脉瘤，主动脉壁变薄并向外凸出。

The most common cardiovascular disease is coronary artery disease （narrow or blocked coronary arteries）, which can lead to chest pain, heart attacks, or stroke. Other cardiovascular diseases include congestive heart failure, heart rhythm problems, congenital heart disease （heart disease at birth）, and endocarditis （inflamed inner layer of the heart）.

最常见的心血管疾病是冠状动脉疾病（冠状动脉狭窄或阻塞），可导致胸痛、心脏病发作或脑卒中。其他心血管疾病包括充血性心力衰竭、心律问题、先天性心脏病（出生时即存在的心脏病）和心内膜炎（心脏内层发炎）。

Cardiovascular surgeons operate on your heart and blood vessels to repair damage caused by diseases or disorders of the cardiovascular system. Cardiovascular surgeons perform many different types of operations, including heart valve repair and replacement, heart defect repair, coronary artery bypass, aneurysm repair, transmyocardial laser revascularization, and heart transplantation.

心血管外科医生对病人的心脏和血管进行手术，以修复由心血管系统疾病或紊乱引起的损伤。心血管外科医生可做许多不同类型的手术，包括心脏瓣膜修复和置换、心脏缺损修复、冠状动脉搭桥术、动脉瘤修复、经心肌激光血运重建和心脏移植。

They also perform operations on the blood vessels in your body, including the aorta—the body's main blood supplier. Heart surgery today may also include the use or implantation of ventricular assist device (VAD), a mechanical device that "assists" the failing heart by helping it pump blood throughout the body.

他们还对病人的血管进行手术，包括主动脉——身体的主要血液供应渠道。如今的心脏手术还可能包括使用或植入心室辅助装置（VAD），这是一种通过帮助心脏将血液泵送到全身来"辅助"衰竭心脏工作的机械装置。

（二）Heart Arrhythmia 心律失常[5-6]

Heart is a muscular organ which lies in the center of your chest. Your heartbeat is controlled by electrical impulses which travel across the heart, making it contract. The atria contract first, sending blood into the ventricles. The ventricles then contract, sending blood to the lungs and around the body. Nerves supplying the heart change the rate at which impulses are sent across the

心脏是位于胸部中央的一个肌性器官。心跳受到电脉冲的控制，电脉冲在心脏中传导，使心脏收缩。心房首先收缩，将血液送入心室。然后，心室收缩，将血液输送到肺部和身体其他部位。支配心脏的神经改变了穿过心肌的电脉冲的速率，从而满足了身体的需求。

heart muscle to meet the needs of the body.

A heart arrhythmia is an irregular heartbeat. Heart rhythm problems (heart arrhythmias) occur when the electrical signals that coordinate the heart's beats don't work properly. The faulty signaling causes the heart to beat too fast (tachycardia), too slow (bradycardia) or irregularly.

In atrial fibrillation, the electrical impulses in the atria become disorganized, overriding the heart's normal rate and rhythm. The irregular impulses can be transmitted to the ventricles causing the heart to pump irregularly and too fast in supraventricular tachycardia or SVT. The irregular electrical impulses pass across the ventricles and back up into the atria in a circle rather than traveling from the atria to the ventricles in one direction as they should. This makes the heart beat faster.

In ventricular tachycardia abnormal electrical impulses are produced in the lower chambers of the heart. This causes the heart to pump faster than normal. The ventricles may not have enough time to fill up with blood properly. So less

心律失常是一种不规律的心脏搏动。当协调心脏跳动的电信号不能正常工作时，就会出现心律问题（心律失常）。错误的信号会导致心脏跳动过快（心动过速）、过慢（心动过缓）或节律异常。

心房颤动时，心房中的电脉冲变得混乱，打乱了心脏的正常搏动和节律。不规律的电脉冲可能会传递到心室，导致室上性心动过速（SVT），心脏不规律地、过快地跳动。不规律的电脉冲穿过心室，然后以一个回路的形式返回心房，而不是按照应有的方向从心房向心室传导。这使得心脏跳动更快。

室性心动过速时，在心脏的下腔室中会产生异常的电脉冲。这会导致心脏跳动快于正常速度。心室可能没有足够的时间来充满血液。因此，被泵送到身体其他部位的血液减少。心律失常的治疗手段有药物、导管、植

blood is pumped around your body. Heart arrhythmia treatment may include medications, catheter procedures, implanted devices or surgery to control or eliminate fast, slow or irregular heartbeats. A heart-healthy lifestyle can help prevent heart damage that can trigger certain heart arrhythmias.

入装置或手术,以控制或消除快速、缓慢或不规则的心跳。有益心脏健康的生活方式有助于预防可引发某些心律失常的心脏损伤。

(三) Cardiomyopathy 心肌病[7-9]

Cardiomyopathy is a group of diseases that weaken the heart muscle—the myocardium, making it harder for the heart to pump blood. Cardiomyopathy reduces blood output, and may lead to heart failure. The condition may be inherited from a parent, or develop as a consequence of another disease or factor.

心肌病是一系列削弱心脏肌肉——心肌的疾病总称,心肌病使心脏泵血更为困难。心肌病会减少血液输出,并可能导致心力衰竭。该疾病可能是从父母那里遗传的,也可能由另一种疾病或因素导致。

When present, symptoms may include shortness of breath, fatigue, rapid heartbeats, chest pain, swelling of lower limbs, dizziness and fainting. Progression of the disease varies greatly from person to person. In some people, symptoms may appear suddenly, and worsen quickly; while others see a gradual development over a long period of time.

患心肌病时,可能出现以下症状:呼吸急促,疲劳,心跳加快,胸痛,下肢肿胀,头晕和昏厥。病情的进展因人而异。在某些人身上,症状可能突然出现并迅速恶化,而其他人则可能经历很长一段时间的逐步发展。

There are many causes of cardiomyopathy, including alcohol

心肌病的病因很多,包括酗酒、高血压、冠状动脉疾病、病毒感染,

abuse, high blood pressure, coronary artery disease, viral infections and certain medicines. Often, the exact cause of the muscle disease is never found. Treatment varies depending on the type of cardiomyopathy, the underlying cause and severity of symptoms, and can range from life style changes, to medications and surgeries.

There are generally three types of cardiomyopathy. (1) Dilated cardiomyopathy. In this type of cardiomyopathy, your heart's main pumping chamber—the left ventricle—enlarges (dilates) and can't effectively pump blood out of the heart. Although this type can affect people of all ages, it occurs most often in middle-aged people and is more likely to affect men. The most common cause is coronary artery disease or heart attack. However, it can also be caused by genetic defects.

(2) Hypertrophic cardiomyopathy. This type involves abnormal thickening of your heart muscle, which makes it harder for the heart to work. It mostly affects the muscle of your heart's main pumping chamber (left ventricle). (3) Restrictive cardiomyopathy. In this type, the heart muscle becomes stiff and less flexible, so it can't expand and fill

以及某些药物的影响。肌肉疾病通常很难找到确切病因。治疗方法视心肌病的类型、根本原因和症状的严重程度而异,心肌病可通过改变生活方式、服药和手术进行治疗。

心肌病一般分为三种类型。(1)扩张型心肌病。在这种类型的心肌病中,心脏主泵室(左心室)变大(扩张)并且不能有效地将血液泵出心脏。虽然各年龄段的人都有可能患这种类型的心肌病,但它最常发生在中年人身上,并且男性更易患病。冠状动脉疾病或心脏病发作是心肌病的最常见原因。然而,它也可能由遗传缺陷引起。

(2)肥厚型心肌病。这种类型涉及心肌异常增厚,使心脏更难工作。它主要影响心脏主泵室(左心室)的肌肉。(3)限制型心肌病。在这种类型中,心肌变得僵硬、不那么灵活,因此它不能在两次心跳之间扩张并使血液充满心脏。任何年龄的人都有可能患上这种最不常见的心肌病,但老年人患此病的最多。

with blood between heartbeats. This least common type of cardiomyopathy can occur at any age, but it most often affects older people.

4.2 汉译英

（一）风湿性心脏病 Rheumatic Heart Disease[10-11]

风湿性心脏病（RHD）是一种严重的心脏疾病，涉及四个心脏瓣膜中的一个或多个受损。患急性风湿热（ARF）后，会出现瓣膜损伤。患急性风湿热期间，心脏瓣膜组织，以及有时心脏的其他部位（心脏内膜或肌肉）会肿胀，这被称为心肌炎。

Rheumatic heart disease (RHD) is a serious disease of the heart, involving damage to one or more of the four heart valves. The valve damage remains after an illness called acute rheumatic fever (ARF). During ARF the heart valve tissue, and sometimes other parts of the heart (the heart lining or muscle) can become swollen, and this is called carditis.

风湿性心脏病是由风湿热引起的，风湿热是一种炎症性疾病，可影响许多结缔组织，尤其是心脏、关节、皮肤或大脑中的结缔组织。随着时间的推移，心脏瓣膜可能会发炎并留下瘢痕。这会导致心脏瓣膜变窄或关闭不全，使心脏难以正常运作。进展到这一步可能需要数年时间，且可能导致心力衰竭。

Rheumatic heart disease is caused by rheumatic fever, an inflammatory disease that can affect many connective tissues, especially in the heart, joints, skin, or brain. The heart valves can be inflamed and become scarred over time. This can result in narrowing or leaking of the heart valve, making it harder for the heart to function normally. This may take years to develop and can result in heart failure.

风湿热可发生于任何年龄，但在

Rheumatic fever can occur at any

5 至 15 岁的儿童中较常见。这种疾病在美国这样的发达国家很少见。风湿性心脏病可通过超声心动图（超声波）诊断。轻度风湿性心脏病可能很多年都无明显症状。

当症状出现时，症状因具体受损心脏瓣膜、受损类型和严重程度而异。许多风湿性心脏病患者都有心脏杂音，可通过听诊器听到。更严重的症状有胸痛、体力活动或躺下时呼吸困难、虚弱和疲倦以及腿部肿胀。

半数以上的急性风湿热患者在首次发病后的 10 年内会进展成风湿性心脏病，其中超过三分之一的人会进展成严重风湿性心脏病。严重的风湿性心脏病患者可能出现心律失常、脑卒中、心内膜炎，孕期可能出现并发症。这些并发症会逐渐导致残疾，降低生活质量，并可能导致年轻人过早死亡。

age, but usually occurs in children ages 5 to 15 years old. It's rare in developed countries like the United States. RHD is diagnosed by echocardiogram (ultrasound). Symptoms of mild RHD may not be noticed for many years.

When they do develop, symptoms usually depend on which heart valves are affected, and the type and severity of the damage. Many people with RHD have a heart murmur, which can be heard through a stethoscope. Symptoms of more severe disease can include chest pain, breathlessness during physical activity or when lying down, weakness and tiredness, and swelling of the legs.

More than half of those with ARF progress to RHD within 10 years of their initial ARF episode, and more than one-third of these people develop severe RHD. With severe RHD there is a risk of abnormal heart rhythms, stroke, endocarditis, and complications during pregnancy. These complications cause progressive disability, reduce quality of life, and can lead to premature death in young adults.

（二）动脉粥样硬化 Atherosclerosis[12]

动脉粥样硬化是一种可能在儿童时期就开始进展的可危及生命的疾病。在动脉粥样硬化过程中，脂肪物质沉积物，即斑块，在动脉壁内积聚，从而减少或完全阻塞血流。动脉中积聚斑块称为动脉粥样硬化。这些沉积物由胆固醇、脂肪物质、细胞代谢废物、钙和纤维蛋白（血液中的凝血物质）组成。

Atherosclerosis is a life-threatening disease that may have begun to develop during childhood. This condition is a process in which deposits of fatty material called plaque build up inside the walls of arteries reducing or completely blocking blood flow. Plaque build up in your arteries is called atherosclerosis. These deposits are made up of cholesterol, fatty substances, cellular waste products, calcium and fibrin (a clotting material in the blood).

随着斑块积聚，血管壁变厚。这会使动脉内的通道变窄，减少血流量，减少输送给身体的氧气和其他营养物质。斑块形成的位置和受影响的动脉类型因人而异。斑块可能会部分阻止或完全阻止血液流经心脏、大脑、骨盆、腿部、手臂或肾脏的大动脉或中动脉。

As plaque builds up, the wall of the blood vessel thickens. This narrows the channel within the artery, reducing blood flow, which lessens the amount of oxygen and other nutrients reaching the body. Where plaque develops, and the type of artery affected, vary with each person. Plaque may partially or totally block blood flow through large- or medium-sized arteries in the heart, brain, pelvis, legs, arms or kidneys.

这可能导致以下情况：冠心病（心脏内或通向心脏的动脉斑块）、心绞痛（流向心肌的血流量减少导致的胸痛）、颈动脉疾病（向大脑供血的颈部动脉斑块）、外周动脉疾病或四

This can lead to the following conditions: coronary heart disease (plaque in arteries in or leading to the heart), angina (chest pain from reduced blood flow to the heart muscle),

肢动脉斑块（尤其是腿部）及慢性肾病。

动脉粥样硬化是一个缓慢的、持续终生的血管变化过程，可能从儿童时期开始，随着年龄的增长而恶化得更快。动脉粥样硬化的病因尚不完全清楚。许多科学家认为，当动脉内层（内皮）受损时，斑块就开始形成。

造成此类损坏的四种可能原因是血液中胆固醇和甘油三酯水平升高、高血压、吸烟，以及糖尿病。其中，吸烟在主动脉（身体的主要动脉）、冠状动脉和腿部动脉粥样硬化的进展中起着重要作用。吸烟使脂肪沉积更容易形成，并加速斑块的生长。

（三）高血压 Hypertension[13-14]

血压是指循环的血液对血管壁施加的力。在不同类型的血管中血压的叫法是不同的。但除非有特别的说明，

carotid artery disease (plaque in neck arteries supplying blood to the brain), peripheral artery disease, or PAD (plaque in arteries of the extremities, especially the legs), and chronic kidney disease.

Atherosclerosis is a slow, lifelong progression of changes in the blood vessels that may start in childhood and get worse faster as you age. The cause of atherosclerosis isn't completely known. Many scientists believe plaque begins when an artery's inner lining (the endothelium) becomes damaged.

Four possible causes of such damage are elevated levels of cholesterol and triglycerides in the blood, high blood pressure, cigarette smoking and diabetes. Smoking plays a big role in the progression of atherosclerosis in the aorta (the body's main artery), coronary arteries and arteries in the legs. Smoking makes fatty deposits more likely to form, and it accelerates the growth of plaque.

Blood pressure is the force the circulating blood exerts on the walls of blood vessels. It is different in different

"血压"这个术语是指体循环中的动脉压。当心脏收缩并将血液泵入主动脉时，主动脉压升高，体动脉压也升高。心脏射血后的最大压力称为收缩压。在两次心跳之间，当心室再充盈时，血压降至最低值，称为舒张压。这是血压读数上的两个数值。

血压通常在夜间较低。白天，它会随着身体活动和情绪状态而波动。高血压是指持续的血压偏高。在美国，高血压的定义曾为血压读数大于140/90 mmHg，但为了更好地预防和治疗高血压，最新的指南已将数值更改为130/80 mmHg。正常血压应低于120/80 mmHg。

实际上，只有在产生症状时我们才认为血压过低。高血压本身不会引起症状，但会缓慢损害血管，从长远

types of vessels, but the term "blood pressure", when not specified otherwise, refers to arterial pressure in the systemic circulation. When the heart contracts and pumps blood into the aorta, the aortic pressure rises, and so does the systemic arterial pressure. The maximum pressure following an ejection is called the systolic pressure. In between heart beats, when the ventricles refill, blood pressure falling to its lowest value is called the diastolic pressure. These are the 2 numbers on a blood pressure reading.

Blood pressure is usually lower at night. During day-time, it fluctuates with physical activities and emotional states. Hypertension refers to a persistent high blood pressure. In the US, high blood pressure used to be defined as greater than 140/90 mmHg on a blood pressure reading, but recent guidelines have changed these values to 130/80 mmHg to better prevent and treat the condition. Normal blood pressure is below 120/80 mmHg.

In practice, blood pressure is considered too low only if it produces symptoms. Hypertension does not cause

来看，是脑卒中、动脉瘤和心脏病发作等多种心血管疾病的主要致病因素；它还可能造成终末器官损害，如肾衰竭或视力丧失。因此，高血压被称为"沉默的杀手"。

symptoms on its own, but it slowly damages blood vessels. In the long-term, it is a major risk factor for a variety of cardiovascular diseases such as stroke, aneurysm and heart attack. It way cause end organ damage such as renal failure or vision loss. For these reasons, hypertension is known as the "silent killer".

全世界估计共有 11.3 亿人患有高血压，大多数（约三分之二）患者生活在低收入和中等收入国家。2015年，四分之一的男性和五分之一的女性患有高血压。

An estimated 1.13 billion people worldwide suffer from hypertension, and most (about two-thirds) of these patients live in low-and middle-income countries. In 2015, one in four men and one in five women had high blood pressure.

不到五分之一的高血压患者的病情得到控制。高血压是世界各地人口过早死亡的一个主要原因。非传染性疾病领域的一项全球目标是，2010年至 2025 年期间将高血压患病率降低 25%。

Fewer than one-fifth of patients with hypertension have their problems under control. High blood pressure is a leading cause of premature death worldwide. A global goal in the field of noncommunicable diseases is to reduce the prevalence of hypertension by 25% between 2010 and 2025.

5 口译注释与学习资源

5.1 口译注释

梳理心血管疾病相关的词根有助于提高词汇学习和记忆的效率，"配对"的词根尤为常见，如动脉和静脉、高血压和低血压、心室和心房、收缩压和舒张压等。现梳理部分词根及其衍生词和表达方式，以供读者参考。

（一）动脉（**artery**）vs 静脉（**vein**）

这两个词的衍生词和表达方式在本章中比较常见，以 artery 和 vein 的形容词或者词根形式出现，如动脉压（**arterial** pressure）和静脉压（**venous** pressure）、动脉粥样硬化（**ather**osclerosis）、动脉壁（**arterial** wall）和静脉壁（**venous** wall）、动脉瘤（**aneur**ysm）等。

（二）心房（**atrium**）vs 心室（**ventricle**）

本章口译词汇中出现的房颤（**atrial** fibrillation）和室颤（**ventricular** fibrillation），英文缩写为 AF 和 VF。只需牢牢记住心房和心室的首字母分别为 a 和 v，即可"省力"记忆。英译汉第一篇中出现了室上性心动过速（supra**ventricular** tachycardia）。

（三）高血压（**hyper**tension）vs 低血压（**hypo**tension）

hyper 和 hypo 分别是指高和低。虽然本章未涉及更多的与 hyper 和 hypo 相关的词汇，但其应用非常广泛，如胃酸过多导致的呕吐（**hyper**acid vomiting）、轻狂躁的（**hypo**manic）、张力减退（**hyp**otonic）等。

（四）扩张（**dilate**）vs 收缩（**contract**）

本章中出现的与扩张和收缩相关的词汇有扩张型心肌病（**dilated** cardiomyopathy）、血管扩张剂（vaso**dilator**）、舒张压（**diastolic** pressure）、收缩力（**contract**ility）等。但是值得注意的是收缩压的表述为 systolic pressure。

5.2　学习资源

登陆中国大学 MOOC（慕课），学习"医疗口译"课程中"心血管内科/外科"的口译实战示范视频。此外还可登录美国心脏协会、世界卫生组织、美国妙佑医疗国际、约翰斯·霍普金斯大学医学院等机构官网学习相关知识。

参考文献

［1］Gile，D.（2009）. *Basic concepts and models for interpreter and translator training*. Rev. edn. Amsterdam: John Benjamins.

［2］NHS.（n. d.）. *Cardiovascular disease*. Retrieved November 14，2021，from https://www. nhs. uk/conditions/cardiovascular-disease/.

［3］National Cancer Institute.（n. d.）. *NCI dictionary of cancer terms*. Retrieved November 14，2021，from https://www. cancer. gov/publications/dictionaries/cancer-terms/def/cardiovascular-disease.

[4] Texas Heart Institute. (2020, September 30). *What is a cardiovascular surgeon?*. Retrieved November 14, 2021, from https://www. texasheart. org/heart-health/heart-information-center/topics/what-is-a – cardiovascular-surgeon/.

[5] Bupa, inc. (n. d.). *Arrhythmia (palpitations)*. Retrieved November 14, 2021, from https://contenidos. bupasalud. com/en/health-and-wellness/bupa-life/arrhythmia-palpitations.

[6] Mayo Foundation for Medical Education and Research. (2021, October 1). *Heart arrhythmia*. Retrieved November 14, 2021, from https://www. mayoclinic. org/diseases-conditions/heart-arrhythmia/symptoms-causes/syc – 20350668.

[7] Alila Medical Media (n. d.). *Cardiomyopathy*. Retrieved November 14, 2021, from https://www. alilamedicalmedia. com/?search = Cardiomyopathy&orientation = &media_ type = .

[8] Johns Hopkins Medicine. (n. d.). *Cardiomyopathy*. Retrieved November 14, 2021, from https://www. hopkinsmedicine. org/health/conditions-and-diseases/cardiomyopathy.

[9] Mayo Foundation for Medical Education and Research. (2021, April 9). *Cardiomyopathy*. Retrieved November 14, 2021, from https://www. mayoclinic. org/diseases-conditions/cardiomyopathy/symptoms-causes/syc – 20370709.

[10] Noonan, S. (2021, February 26). *What is rheumatic heart disease?*. Rheumatic Heart Disease Australia. Retrieved November 14, 2021, from https://www. rhdaustralia. org. au/what-rheumatic-heart-disease.

[11] Johns Hopkins Medicine. (n. d.). *Rheumatic heart disease*. Retrieved November 14, 2021, from https://www. hopkinsmedicine. org/health/conditions-and-diseases/rheumatic-heart-disease.

[12] Heart org. (n. d.). *Atherosclerosis*. Retrieved November 14, 2021, from https://www. heart. org/en/health-topics/cholesterol/about-cholesterol/atherosclerosis.

[13] Alila Medical Media (n. d.). *Hypertension*. Retrieved November 14, 2021, from https://www. alilamedicalmedia. com/?search = hypertension&orientation = &media_ type = .

[14] World Health Organization. (n. d.). *Hypertension*. Retrieved November 14, 2021, from https://www. who. int/news-room/fact-sheets/detail/hypertension.

第十一章

神经内科/外科

1 导读

本章重点为口译技巧之数字转换（1）和神经内科/外科的 6 篇"口译实战"练习。口译实战练习中英译汉、汉译英各 3 篇，内容涵盖神经内科/外科介绍、癫痫、帕金森病、渐冻症、脑卒中和三叉神经痛。请结合本章口译技巧练习 6 篇口译实战文本。

2 口译技巧——数字转换（1）

数字转换是口译中的难点。由于中文和英文的计数规则存在差别，单纯的数字转换需要一定的时间才能熟练习得。英文中，三位一个计数节，如：123, 345, 789；中文中，四位一个计数节，如：1234, 5678。数字转换中容易出错的有中文数字中的"十万"（100, 000）和"亿"（100 million）。由于中文"十万"中"十"的出现，"十万"容易被错误翻译为 ten thousand（10, 000，即一万）；"亿"容易错误翻译为 one billion。

在口译环境中，数字转换的难度成倍增加，主要源于以下因素：原语中，数字所附带的信息，包括单位，如人民币、美元等，以及数字所代表的意思，如进出口值、血小板计数等，与数字同时出现，容易造成顾此失彼的情况。单纯大数字的转换在口译过程中准确率已是较低，再加之译员精力在数字上分配较多，导致翻译数字附带信息时也容易出错。口译的即时性容易给译员带来较大的心理压力，特别是当数字连续出现，并且所指代意义不属于同一个类型时，如基数词、序数词和百分比等交替出现。英文为原语的文本中，可能出现译员不熟悉的读法，如 2, 300，我们熟悉的读法是 two thousand and three hundred，但 2, 300 可以读成 twenty three hundred。

本章着重介绍分数、小数、不确定数目的转换技巧。

（一）分数

分数（fraction）由分子（numerator）和分母（denominator）构成，其中分子用基数词（cardinal number）表示，分母用序数词（ordinal number）表示，如 $\frac{1}{5}$ 读作 one fifth。当分子为 1 时，分母用序数词单数；当分子大于 1 时，分母用序数词复数，如 $\frac{2}{3}$ 读作 two thirds。分子和分母数值较大的情况下，如 $\frac{123}{456}$ 可以读作 one hundred and twenty-three over four hundred and fifty-six。更多示例如下：

$\frac{1}{2}$：a/one half

$\frac{1}{3}$：a/one third

$\frac{1}{4}$：a/one quarter

$\frac{2}{3}$：two thirds

$\frac{7}{8}$：seven eighths

$\frac{20}{75}$：twenty over seventy-five

$\frac{4}{123}$：four over one hundred and twenty-three；four over one two three

（二）小数

英文中的小数点（.）读作 point。小数点前的数字按照数字规则读出，小数点后的数字逐一读出，如 123.45 读作 one hundred and twenty-three point four five。请注意 123.45 中小数点后面的 .45 一般读作 point four five，但在表示钱的数量时，如 $123.45，可读作 one hundred and twenty-three dollars and forty-five cents，日常简略拼读可以是 one hundred and twenty-three forty-five，即钱里面的小数点可以不读出来。小数点前面如果是零，可读作 zero 或者 nought，如 0.23 读作 zero/nought point two three。小数点后面的零，通常读作 o（/əʊ/），如 0.0034 读作 zero/nought point o o three four。

（三）不确定数目

英文表示"大约/大概"的词或短语有 about，around，some，approximately，roughly，more or less，in the neighborhood of，or so 等。更多示例如下：

几个：some，a few，several，a number of

两三个：two or three

五六个：five or six

十几个：more than ten，over a dozen，less/no more than twenty

三十来个：about/around thirty

几十个：dozens of

几十年：decades

十几岁：in one's teens

四十出头：a little/a bit over forty

五十岁左右：more or less fifty（years old），about fifty（years old）

近八十岁：nearly/almost eighty（years old）

九十好几：well over ninety（years old）

五点左右：around five o'clock

三天左右：three days or so

大约 150 米处：somewhere about 150 meters

好几百：hundreds of

成千上万，千千万万：thousands of

几十万：hundreds of thousands of

几百万：millions of

亿万：hundreds of millions of

以下段落为《2021 年国务院政府工作报告》中涉及数字的部分内容，可先通过段落练习熟悉数字的转换。

例 1：全年为市场主体减负超过 2.6 万亿元，其中减免社保费 1.7 万亿元。

We reduced the burden on market entities by more than 2.6 trillion yuan for the year, including 1.7 trillion yuan in social insurance premium cuts and exemptions.

例 2：城镇新增就业 1186 万人，年末全国城镇调查失业率降到 5.2%。作为最大发展中国家，在巨大冲击下能够保持就业大局稳定，尤为难能可贵。加强生活必需品保供稳价，居民消费价格上涨 2.5%。

A total of 11.86 million urban jobs were added, and the year-end surveyed urban unemployment rate dropped to 5.2 percent. It is truly remarkable that China, the largest developing country in the world, has kept overall employment stable in the face of such an enormous shock. The supply and price stability of daily necessities was ensured; the consumer price index（CPI）posted a 2.5 percent growth.

例 3：年初剩余的 551 万农村贫困人口全部脱贫、52 个贫困县全部摘帽。

All remaining poor rural residents, totaling 5.51 million in early 2020, were lifted from poverty, as were all of China's remaining 52 poor counties.

例 4：今年发展主要预期目标是：国内生产总值增长 6% 以上；城镇新增就

业 1100 万人以上，城镇调查失业率 5.5% 左右；居民消费价格涨幅 3% 左右……单位国内生产总值能耗降低 3% 左右……粮食产量保持在 1.3 万亿斤以上。

The main projected targets for development this year include a GDP growth of over 6 percent, over 11 million new urban jobs, a surveyed urban unemployment rate of around 5.5 percent, CPI increase of around 3 percent... a drop of around 3 percent in energy consumption per unit of GDP... grain output of over 650 million metric tons.

3　口译词汇

3.1　英译汉

（一）Neurology／Neurological Surgery 神经内科／外科

central nervous system 中枢神经系统

spinal cord 脊髓

peripheral nervous system 周围神经系统

sensory receptor 感觉受体

neurologist 神经病学家

cerebrovascular 脑血管的

demyelinating disease 脱髓鞘疾病

multiple sclerosis 多发性硬化症

Parkinson's disease 帕金森病

neurodegenerative disorder 神经退行性疾病

Alzheimer's disease 阿尔茨海默病

Amyotrophic Lateral Sclerosis（ALS）肌萎缩侧索硬化症（渐冻症）

seizure disorder 痉挛性疾病

epilepsy 癫痫

autonomic nervous system 自主神经系统

pathological process 病理过程

hypophysis 垂体

meninges 脑膜

extracranial carotid 颅外颈动脉

vertebral artery 椎动脉

skull 颅骨

pituitary gland 垂体

vertebral column 脊柱

spinal fusion 脊柱融合术

instrumentation 器械治疗

（二）Epilepsy 癫痫

muscle tone 肌肉张力

stiffness 僵硬

twitching 抽搐

limpness 跛行

sensation 感觉

state of awareness 意识状态

focal seizure 局灶性癫痫发作

electrical discharge 放电

generalized seizure 全身性癫痫发作

trauma 外伤

vascular malformation 血管畸形

arteriovenous malformations （AVM）动静脉畸形

cavernous malformation 海绵状血管畸形

viral encephalitis 病毒性脑炎

parasitic infection 寄生虫感染

prenatal injury 产前损伤

oxygen deficiency 缺氧

cerebral palsy 脑瘫

developmental disorder 发育异常

autism 自闭症

（三）Parkinson's Disease 帕金森病

progressive 进行性

tremor 震颤

pill-rolling tremor 捻丸样震颤

bradykinesia 运动迟缓

3.2 汉译英

（一）渐冻症（肌萎缩侧索硬化症）Amyotrophic Lateral Sclerosis （ALS）

神经系统疾病 neurological disease

神经元 neuron

自主肌肉运动 voluntary muscle movement

肌肉无力 muscle weakness

呼吸衰竭 respiratory failure

遗传病史 genetic history

迟发 late onset

常染色体显性遗传 autosomal dominant

超氧化物歧化酶 superoxide dismutase

（二）脑卒中 Cerebral Stroke

脑血管意外 cerebrovascular accident

缺血性卒中 ischemic stroke

出血性卒中 hemorrhagic stroke

短暂性脑缺血发作 transient ischemic attack （TIA）

破坏血栓 clot-busting

溶栓剂 thrombolytics

心房颤动 atrial fibrillation

胆固醇 cholesterol

（三）三叉神经痛 Trigeminal Neuralgia

三叉神经 trigeminal nerve

剧烈疼痛 excruciating pain

灼痛 searing pain

颅神经 cranial nerve

眼神经 ophthalmic nerve

上颌神经 maxillary nerve

眼睑 eyelid

鼻孔 nostril

牙龈 gum

下颌神经 mandibular nerve

高分辨率核磁共振 high-resolution Magnetic Resonance Imaging（MRI）

血管异常 blood vessel abnormality

4　口译实战

4.1　英译汉

（一）Neurology/Neurological Surgery[1-2] 神经内科/外科

Neurology is the branch of medicine concerned with the study and treatment of disorders of the nervous system. The nervous system is a complex, sophisticated system that regulates and coordinates body activities. It has two major divisions, central nervous system, which includes the brain and spinal cord, and peripheral nervous system, which covers all other neural elements, such as eyes, ears, skin, and other "sensory receptors".

神经病学是与神经系统疾病的研究和治疗有关的医学分支。神经系统是一个复杂、精密的系统，可以调节和协调身体活动，包含两个主要部分：中枢神经系统和周围神经系统。前者包括脑和脊髓，后者包括所有其他神经结构，如眼睛、耳朵、皮肤和其他"感觉受体"。

A doctor who specializes in neurology is called a neurologist. The neurologist treats disorders that affect the brain, spinal cord, and nerves. These conditions include cerebrovascular disease, such as stroke, demyelinating diseases of the central nervous system, such as multiple sclerosis, headache disorders, and infections of the brain and peripheral nervous system, movement disorders, such as Parkinson's disease,

研究神经病学的专家被称为神经病学家。神经科医生治疗影响大脑、脊髓和神经的疾病，包括脑血管疾病，如脑卒中；中枢神经系统脱髓鞘疾病，如多发性硬化症、头痛病、脑部和周围神经系统感染；运动功能障碍，如帕金森病；神经退行性疾病，如阿尔茨海默病、帕金森病和肌萎缩侧索硬化症；痉挛性疾病，如癫痫、脊髓疾病和言语及语言障碍。

neurodegenerative disorders, such as Alzheimer's disease, Parkinson's disease, and Amyotrophic Lateral Sclerosis, seizure disorders, such as epilepsy, spinal cord disorders, and speech and language disorders.

Neurological Surgery is a discipline of medicine and specialty of surgery that provides the operative and nonoperative management (including critical care, prevention, diagnosis, evaluation, treatment, and rehabilitation) of disorders of the central, peripheral, and autonomic nervous systems. It also provides the evaluation and treatment of pathological processes which modify the function or activity of the nervous system, including the hypophysis, and the operative and nonoperative management of pain.

神经外科是一个涉及内科和外科的专业，提供中枢、周围和自主神经系统疾病的手术和非手术治疗（包括重症监护、预防、诊断、评估、治疗和康复）；评估和治疗改变神经系统功能或活动的病理过程，包括垂体；并提供缓解疼痛的手术和非手术治疗。

As such, neurological surgery encompasses treatment of adult and pediatric patients with disorders of the nervous system: disorders of the brain, meninges, and skull, and their blood supply, including the extracranial carotid and vertebral arteries; disorders of the pituitary gland, the spinal cord, and vertebral column, including those which may require treatment by spinal fusion or

因此，神经外科治疗患有神经系统疾病的成人和儿童患者，治疗大脑、脑膜和颅骨及其血液供应问题，包括颅外颈动脉和椎动脉问题，治疗垂体疾病、脊髓疾病和脊柱疾病，包括可能需要通过脊柱融合或固定治疗的疾病，以及治疗颅神经和脊神经功能紊乱。

instrumentation; and disorders of the cranial and spinal nerves throughout their distribution.

（二）Epilepsy 癫痫 [3-5]

A seizure is a burst of uncontrolled electrical activity between brain cells (also called neurons or nerve cells) that causes temporary abnormalities in muscle tone or movements (stiffness, twitching or limpness), behaviors, sensations or states of awareness.

Sometimes it is hard to tell when a person is having a seizure. A person having a seizure may seem confused or look like they are staring at something that isn't there. Other seizures can cause a person to fall, shake, and become unaware of what's going on around them.

There are two main types of seizures—focal, which are also called partial seizures, and generalized. (1) Focal Seizures. Focal seizures begin with an abnormal electrical discharge restricted to one small region of the brain. (2) Generalized Seizures. Generalized seizures begin with a widespread, excessive electrical discharge involving both hemispheres, or sides, of the brain.

癫痫发作是脑细胞（也称为神经元或神经细胞）之间爆发的不受控制的电活动，导致肌肉张力或运动（僵硬、抽搐或跛行）、行为、感觉或意识状态的暂时异常。

有时很难判断一个人何时癫痫发作。癫痫发作的人可能看起来很困惑，或者看起来像是在盯着不存在的东西。有些癫痫发作会导致跌倒、颤抖，或对周围发生的事情失去意识。

癫痫发作有两种主要类型——局灶性（也称为部分性）癫痫发作和全身性癫痫发作。（1）局灶性癫痫发作。局灶性癫痫发作始于仅限于大脑一个小区域的异常放电。（2）全身性癫痫发作。全身性癫痫发作始于大脑的两个半球或两侧的大面积过度放电。症状包括凝视和眨眼、抽搐、肌肉张力丧失和四肢僵硬。当整个大脑受到影响时，症状包括有节奏的全身抽搐。

Symptoms include staring and blinking, jerking movements, loss of muscle tone, and stiffening of limbs. When the entire brain is involved, symptoms include rhythmic, full-body jerking.

Epilepsy has no identifiable cause in about half the people with the condition. In the other half, the condition may be traced to various factors. (1) Genetic influence. Some types of epilepsy, which are categorized by the type of seizure you experience or the part of the brain that is affected, run in families. In these cases, it's likely that there's a genetic influence. (2) Head trauma. Head trauma as a result of a car accident or other traumatic injury can cause epilepsy.

大约一半的患者癫痫发作没有确切病因。另一半患者的癫痫发作可以追溯到各种因素。（1）遗传影响。某些类型的癫痫（根据癫痫发作类型或受影响的大脑部分进行分类）是家族性的。在这些情况下，很可能存在遗传影响。（2）颅脑外伤。车祸或其他外伤导致的颅脑外伤可导致癫痫。

(3) Brain abnormalities. Abnormalities in the brain, including brain tumors or vascular malformations such as arteriovenous malformations (AVM) and cavernous malformations, can cause epilepsy. Stroke is a leading cause of epilepsy in adults older than age 35. (4) Infections. Meningitis, HIV, viral encephalitis and some parasitic infections can cause epilepsy.

（3）大脑异常。脑部异常包括脑肿瘤或血管畸形，如动静脉畸形（AVM）和海绵状血管畸形可导致癫痫。脑卒中是 35 岁以上成年人患癫痫的主要原因。（4）感染。脑膜炎、艾滋病、病毒性脑炎和一些寄生虫感染可引起癫痫。

(5) Prenatal injury. Before birth,

（5）产前损伤。在出生之前，由

babies are sensitive to brain damage that could be caused by several factors, such as an infection in the mother, poor nutrition or oxygen deficiencies. This brain damage can result in epilepsy or cerebral palsy. （6） Developmental disorders. Epilepsy can sometimes be associated with developmental disorders, such as autism.

于母亲感染、营养不良或缺氧等多种因素，胎儿易出现脑损伤。这种脑损伤可导致癫痫或脑瘫。（6）发育障碍。癫痫有时与发育障碍如自闭症等有关。

（三） Parkinson's Disease 帕金森病[6-7]

Parkinson's disease is a progressive nervous system disorder that affects movement. Symptoms start gradually, sometimes starting with a barely noticeable tremor in just one hand. Tremors are common, but the disorder also commonly causes stiffness or slowing of movement. Signs and symptoms of Parkinson's disease can be different for everyone. Early signs may be mild and go unnoticed. Symptoms often begin on one side of your body and usually remain worse on that side.

帕金森病是一种影响运动的进行性神经系统疾病。症状逐渐产生，初期症状有时候是一只手的轻微震颤。震颤很常见，但这种疾病也常导致僵硬或行动迟缓。帕金森病的体征和症状可能因人而异。早期迹象可能是轻微的，不会引起注意。症状通常从身体的一侧开始，并在该侧症状较重。

Signs and symptoms of Parkinson's disease may include the following: (1) Tremor. A tremor, or shaking, usually begins in a limb, often your hand or fingers. You may rub your thumb and forefinger back and forth, known as a pill-

帕金森病的体征和症状可能包括：（1）震颤。震颤或颤抖通常始于四肢，常见于手或手指。可能出现来回摩擦拇指和食指的现象，这称为捻丸样震颤。（2）行动迟缓。随着时间的推移，帕金森病可能会使行动速度减

rolling tremor. (2) Slowed movement (bradykinesia). Over time, Parkinson's disease may slow your movement, making simple tasks difficult and time-consuming. (3) Rigid muscles. Muscle stiffness may occur in any part of your body. (4) Impaired posture and balance.

As the condition progresses, the symptoms of Parkinson's disease can get worse and it can become increasingly difficult to carry out everyday activities without help. Many people respond well to treatment and only experience mild to moderate disability, whereas the minority may not respond as well and can, in time, become more severely disabled.

Parkinson's disease does not directly cause people to die, but the condition can place great strain on the body, and can make some people more vulnerable to serious and life-threatening infections. But with advances in treatment, most people with Parkinson's disease now have a normal or near-normal life expectancy.

慢，使简单的任务变得困难且耗时。（3）肌肉僵硬。肌肉僵硬可能发生在身体的任何部位。（4）姿势和平衡受损。

随着病情的发展，帕金森病的症状会变得更糟，在无人帮助的情况下进行日常活动会变得越来越困难。许多人对治疗反应良好，只会出现轻度至中度残疾，而少数人可能反应不佳，其病情随着时间的推移可能会变得更严重。

帕金森病不会直接导致人死亡，但会给身体带来巨大影响。如果发生感染，更容易恶化，威胁生命。但随着治疗手段的进步，现在大多数帕金森病患者的预期寿命正常或接近正常。

4.2 汉译英

（一）渐冻症 Amyotrophic Lateral Sclerosis[8-9]

"渐冻症"医学名称叫肌萎缩侧索硬化症（ALS）。肌萎缩侧索硬化症

ALS stands for Amyotrophic Lateral Sclerosis. ALS is a rare neurological

是一种罕见的神经系统疾病，主要影响控制自主肌肉运动的神经细胞（神经元）。自主肌肉负责咀嚼、行走和说话等运动。"渐冻症"是进行性的，症状会随着时间的推移而恶化。目前，"渐冻症"无法治愈，也没有有效的治疗方法来阻止或逆转疾病的进展。

"渐冻症"的早期症状通常包括肌肉无力或僵硬。渐渐地，所有自主肌肉都受到影响，患者失去力量，失去说话、进食、移动甚至呼吸的能力。大多数"渐冻症"患者死于呼吸衰竭，通常在症状首次出现后的3至5年内死亡。然而，大约10%的"渐冻症"患者存活了10年或更长时间。

"渐冻症"是一种有些神秘的疾病。十分之九以上的确诊病例没有明确的病因，即患者没有明显的遗传病史及患"渐冻症"的家庭成员。此外，患者的生活方式也无法为科学家和临床医生提供关于"渐冻症"病因的线索。患者的饮食、居住地、生活方式或生活经历中没有任何信息可以

disease that primarily affects the nerve cells (neurons) responsible for controlling voluntary muscle movement. Voluntary muscles produce movements like chewing, walking, and talking. ALS is progressive, meaning the symptoms get worse over time. Currently, there is no cure for ALS and no effective treatment to halt or reverse the progression of the disease.

Early symptoms of ALS usually include muscle weakness or stiffness. Gradually all voluntary muscles are affected, and individuals lose their strength and the ability to speak, eat, move, and even breathe. Most people with ALS die from respiratory failure, usually within 3 to 5 years from when the symptoms first appear. However, about 10 percent of people with ALS survive for 10 or more years.

ALS is a somewhat mystifying disease. In more than 9 out of every 10 cases diagnosed, no clear identifying cause of the disease is apparent, that is, patients lack an obvious genetic history or affected family members. Also, nothing about the way patients live their lives gives scientists and

很容易地解释为什么他们会患上这种迟发和进行性的疾病。

然而，在大约5%的病例中存在明确的遗传病史。在此类患者中，该疾病被归类为常染色体显性遗传；也就是说，其几乎一半的家庭成员都有明确的"渐冻症"病史。在15%~20%的"渐冻症"家族性病例中发现了超氧化物歧化酶1（SOD1）或铜锌超氧化物歧化酶基因的突变。1%~2%的"渐冻症"病例涉及这种特定的基因突变。

（二）脑卒中 Cerebral Stroke[10-11]

当大脑的一部分失去血液供应并停止工作时，就会发生脑卒中。这会导致受伤的大脑控制的身体部位停止工作。脑卒中也称为脑血管意外、CVA或中风。从出现中风症状开始，只有3到4.5小时的窗口期可以使用破坏血栓的药物（溶栓剂）来尝试恢复大脑受影响部位的血液供应。

clinicians clues as to what causes ALS. Nothing in patients' diet, where they've lived, how they've lived or what they've done with their lives can easily explain why they've developed this late onset and progressive disease.

However, in about 5 percent of cases, a clear genetic history exists. The disease is classed as autosomal dominant in these patients; that is, almost half of their family members show a clear history of ALS. Mutations in the gene for the enzymes superoxide dismutase 1 (SOD1) or copper zinc superoxide dismutase have been found in 15 - 20 percent of the familial cases of ALS. Approximately 1 to 2 percent of all cases of ALS involve this particular gene mutation.

A stroke occurs when part of the brain loses its blood supply and stops working. This causes the part of the body that the injured brain controls to stop working. A stroke is also called a cerebrovascular accident, CVA, or brain attack. From onset of stroke symptoms, there is only a 3 to 4.5 hour window to use clot-busting drugs

脑卒中的分类如下：（1）缺血性卒中（大脑的一部分失去血供）；（2）出血性卒中（脑内发生出血）；（3）短暂性脑缺血发作或微卒中（卒中症状会在几分钟内消失，但在没有治疗的情况下也可能需要长达24小时。这是一个警告信号，表明在不久后可能会发生卒中）。

某些因素会增加脑卒中的风险。主要风险因素如下：（1）高血压。这是脑卒中的首要风险因素。（2）糖尿病。（3）心脏疾病。房颤和其他心脏病会导致血栓，从而导致脑卒中。（4）吸烟。吸烟会损害血管并使血压升高。（5）脑卒中或短暂性脑缺血发作的个人或家族史。（6）年龄。随着年龄的增长，患脑卒中的风险会增加。（7）种族和民族。非裔美国人患脑卒中的风险更高。

还有其他因素与较高的脑卒中风险有关，例如饮酒和使用非法药物、

(thrombolytics) to try to restore blood supply to the affected part of the brain.

The types of cerebral strokes are as follows：(1) Ischemic stroke (part of the brain loses blood flow)；(2) Hemorrhagic stroke (bleeding occurs within the brain)；(3) Transient ischemic attack (TIA), or mini-stroke (The stroke symptoms resolve within minutes, but may take up to 24 hours on their own without treatment. This is a warning sign that a stroke may occur in the near future).

Certain factors can raise your risk of a stroke. The major risk factors are as follows：(1) High blood pressure. This is the primary risk factor for a stroke. (2) Diabetes. (3) Heart diseases. Atrial fibrillation and other heart diseases can cause blood clots that lead to stroke. (4) Smoking. When you smoke, you damage your blood vessels and raise your blood pressure. (5) A personal or family history of stroke or TIA. (6) Age. Your risk of stroke increases as you get older. (7) Race and ethnicity. African Americans have a higher risk of stroke.

There are also other factors that are linked to a higher risk of stroke, such as

身体活动不足、高胆固醇、不健康的饮食和肥胖。脑卒中的症状往往出现得非常迅速，包括面部、手臂、腿部（尤其是身体的一侧）突然麻木或无力，突然混乱、说话困难或理解困难，一只或两只眼睛突然看不清，突然行走困难、头晕、失去平衡或协调，以及突然发生的不明原因的剧烈头痛。

alcohol and illegal drug use, not getting enough physical activity, high cholesterol, unhealthy diet and obesity. The symptoms of stroke often happen quickly. They include sudden numbness or weakness of the face, arm, or leg（especially on one side of the body）, sudden confusion, trouble speaking or understanding speech, sudden trouble seeing in one or both eyes, sudden difficulty walking, dizziness, loss of balance or coordination, and sudden severe headache with no known cause.

（三）三叉神经痛 Trigeminal Neuralgia [12-14]

三叉神经痛是一种影响三叉神经的慢性疼痛病症，三叉神经将感觉从面部传递到大脑。如果患有三叉神经痛，即使是轻微的面部刺激（例如刷牙或化妆）也可能引发剧烈疼痛。一开始，发作可能会短暂而轻微。但三叉神经痛会进展并导致更长时间、更频繁的灼痛。女性比男性更易受三叉神经痛影响，50岁以上的人群发病率更高。

Trigeminal neuralgia is a chronic pain condition that affects the trigeminal nerve, which carries sensation from your face to your brain. If you have trigeminal neuralgia, even mild stimulation of your face—such as from brushing your teeth or putting on makeup—may trigger a jolt of excruciating pain. You may initially experience short, mild attacks. But trigeminal neuralgia can progress and cause longer, more frequent bouts of searing pain. Trigeminal neuralgia affects women more often than men, and it's more likely to occur in people who are older than 50.

三叉神经是头部的一组颅神经。它是负责为面部提供感觉的神经。一根三叉神经连接头部右侧，而另一根连接头部左侧。这些神经中的每一根都有三个不同的分支。"Trigeminal"源自拉丁语"tria"，意思是三个，"geminus"意思是双胞胎。

三叉神经离开大脑并进入颅骨后，分成了控制整个面部感觉的三个分支：(1) 眼神经（V1）：第一分支控制人的眼睛、上眼睑和前额的感觉。(2) 上颌神经（V2）：第二分支控制下眼睑、脸颊、鼻孔、上唇和上牙龈的感觉。(3) 下颌神经（V3）：第三分支控制下颌、下唇、下牙龈和一些咀嚼肌的感觉。

三叉神经痛的诊断需进行体格检查，了解详细的病史，以排除面部疼痛的其他原因。医生会询问疼痛的频率和强度、引起疼痛的原因以及什么

The trigeminal nerve is one set of the cranial nerves in the head. It is the nerve responsible for providing sensation to the face. One trigeminal nerve runs to the right side of the head, while the other runs to the left. Each of these nerves has three distinct branches. "Trigeminal" derives from the Latin word "tria", which means three, and "geminus", which means twin.

After the trigeminal nerve leaves the brain and travels inside the skull, it divides into three smaller branches, controlling sensations throughout the face: (1) Ophthalmic Nerve (V1): The first branch controls sensation in a person's eye, upper eyelid and forehead. (2) Maxillary Nerve (V2): The second branch controls sensation in the lower eyelid, cheek, nostril, upper lip and upper gum. (3) Mandibular Nerve (V3): The third branch controls sensations in the jaw, lower lip, lower gum and some of the muscles used for chewing.

Diagnosing trigeminal neuralgia involves a physical exam and a detailed medical history to rule out other causes of facial pain. Your doctor will ask about

会加剧或者减轻疼痛。由于没有针对三叉神经痛的单一测试，了解疼痛的性质是诊断的关键。

the frequency and intensity of the pain, what seems to set it off and what makes it feel better or worse. Since there is no single test for trigeminal neuralgia, getting to the nature of the pain is key to the diagnosis.

医生也可能会推荐患者做影像学或实验室检查，例如对三叉神经和周围区域进行 CAT 扫描或做高分辨率核磁共振。这些检查可以帮助确定疼痛是由肿瘤或血管异常引起的，还是由未确诊的多发性硬化症引起的。某些先进的核磁共振技术可以帮助医生查看血管压在三叉神经分支的位置。

Your doctor may also recommend imaging or laboratory tests, such as a CAT scan or a high-resolution MRI of the trigeminal nerve and surrounding areas. These tests can help determine if the pain is caused by a tumor or blood vessel abnormality, or by undiagnosed multiple sclerosis. Certain advanced MRI techniques may help the doctor see where a blood vessel is pressing against a branch of the trigeminal nerve.

5 口译注释与学习资源

5.1 口译注释

（一）癫痫

Seizure disorders 和 epilepsy 都常用来指癫痫，seizure disorders 包含了 epilepsy，因此可将 seizure disorders 翻译成痉挛性疾病。

（二）卒中、中风

中风是卒中的通俗说法，包括缺血性卒中（脑梗死）和出血性卒中（脑实质出血、脑室出血、蛛网膜下腔出血）。

5.2 学习资源

登陆中国大学 MOOC（慕课），学习"医疗口译"课程中"神经内科/外科"的口译实战示范视频。此外，还可登录世界卫生组织、英国国民医疗服务体系、美国妙佑医疗国际、美国神经外科医生协会等组织机构官网学习相关知识。

参考文献

[1] University of Rochester Medical Center. (n. d.). Neurology at Highland Hospital. *What is a Neurologist?*. Retrieved November 14, 2021, from https://www.urmc.rochester.edu/highland/departments-centers/neurology/what-is-a－neurologist.aspx.

[2] American College of Surgeons. (n. d.). *Neurological surgery*. Retrieved November 14, 2021, from https://www.facs.org/education/resources/residency-search/specialties/neuro.

[3] Johns Hopkins Medicine. (n. d.). *Types of seizures*. Retrieved November 14, 2021, from https://www.hopkinsmedicine.org/health/conditions-and-diseases/epilepsy/types-of-seizures.

[4] NYU Langone Health. (n. d.). *Types of epilepsy & seizure disorders in adults*. Retrieved November 14, 2021, from https://nyulangone.org/conditions/epilepsy-seizure-disorders-in-adults/types.

[5] Mayo Foundation for Medical Education and Research. (2021, October 7). *Epilepsy*. Retrieved November 14, 2021, from https://www.mayoclinic.org/diseases-conditions/epilepsy/symptoms-causes/syc－20350093.

[6] UCLA Neurosurgery, Los Angeles, CA. (n. d.). *Parkinson's syndrome*. Retrieved November 14, 2021, from https://www.uclahealth.org/neurosurgery/parkinsons-syndrome.

[7] Mayo Foundation for Medical Education and Research. (2020, December 8). *Parkinson's disease*. Retrieved November 14, 2021, from https://www.mayoclinic.org/diseases-conditions/parkinsons-disease/symptoms-causes/syc－20376055.

[8] Heller, L. (2019, June 11). *Amyotrophic Lateral Sclerosis, Lou Gehrig's disease*. Retrieved November 14, 2021, from https://www.hopkinsmedicine.org/neurology_ neurosurgery/centers_ clinics/als/conditions/als_ amyotrophic_ lateral_ sclerosis. html.

[9] U. S. Department of Health and Human Services National Institute of Neurological Disorders and Stroke. (n. d.). *Amyotrophic lateral sclerosis (ALS) fact sheet*. Retrieved November 14, 2021, from https://www.ninds.nih.gov/Disorders/Patient-Caregiver-Education/Fact-Sheets/Amyotrophic-Lateral-Sclerosis-ALS-Fact-Sheet.

[10] Benjamin Wedro, M. D. (2021, November 12). *Stroke: Fast, symptoms, causes, types, treatment, prevention*. MedicineNet. Retrieved November 14, 2021, from https://www.medicinenet.com/stroke_ symptoms_ and_ treatment/article.htm.

[11] Centers for Disease Control and Prevention. (2021, August 2). *Types of stroke*. Retrieved November 14, 2021, from https://www.cdc.gov/stroke/types_ of_ stroke.htm.

[12] Mayo Foundation for Medical Education and Research. (2017, July 26). *Trigeminal neuralgia*.

Retrieved November 14，2021，from https：//www. mayoclinic. org/diseases-conditions/trigeminal-neuralgia/symptoms-causes/syc－20353344.

[13] Johns Hopkins Medicine. (n. d.). *Trigeminal neuralgia*. Retrieved November 14，2021，from https：//www. hopkinsmedicine. org/health/conditions-and-diseases/trigeminal-neuralgia.

[14] AANS. (n. d.). *Trigeminal neuralgia*. Retrieved November 14，2021，from https：//www. aans. org/Patients/Neurosurgical-Conditions-and-Treatments/Trigeminal-Neuralgia.

第十二章

骨科

1　导读

本章重点为口译技巧之数字转换（2）和骨科的 6 篇"口译实战"练习。口译实战练习中英译汉、汉译英各 3 篇，内容涵盖骨科介绍、腰椎间盘突出症、骨关节炎、半月板撕裂伤、骨癌和骨髓炎。请结合本章口译技巧练习 6 篇口译实战文本。

2　口译技巧——数字转换（2）

本章数字转换技巧着重介绍倍数的表达。中英文倍数转换的关键在于厘清容易混淆的倍数表达。首先仔细区分含义，然后选用恰当句型，最后灵活准确地表达。

中文的倍数表达归纳起来有两类：第一类表示 A 是 B（原来）的几倍；第二类表示 A 比 B（原来）大几倍。这两类说法含义不同：第一类表示包括基数在内的倍数；第二类表示净增倍数。

例如，下面三句中文表达的意思相同：（1）门诊人数增长了两倍。（2）门诊人数是原来的三倍。（3）门诊人数上升了 200%。英文对应翻译为：（1）The number of outpatients saw a three-fold increase.（2）The number of outpatients has tripled.（3）The number of outpatients increased by 200%. 也可以说（4）The outpatients were three times as many as before. 意思也和中文一样。

接下来，我们来看看更多倍数表达的中英转换。

例如，"A 是 B 的两倍"与"A 比 B 大 1 倍"意思相同，翻译为英语，至少有三种表达：（1）A is twice as big as B.（2）A is twice bigger than B.（3）A is twice the size of B.

再如，"A 是原来的 2 倍"与"A（比原来）增长了 1 倍"意思相同。翻译为英语，至少有四种表达：（1）A increases by 100%.（2）A is twice as much as the original amount.（3）A is 200% of the original amount.（4）A has doubled.

又如，"航运产生的二氧化碳是空运的两倍（航运产生的二氧化碳比空运多一倍）。"翻译为英语有两种表达：

（1）Carbon dioxide output from shipping is twice as much as that from airlines.

（2）Carbon dioxide output from shipping is twice more than that from airlines.

英文两倍、三倍、四倍表达如下：

两倍

twice as much/many/as ...

twice the amount/number/size/length ... of

double

to increase by 100%

三倍

three times as much/many/as ...

treble，triple

to increase by 200%

四倍

four times/fourfold as much/many/as ...

quadruple

to increase by 300%

以下例句中包含较多涉及倍数的表达，可先通过段落练习熟悉倍数的转换。

例 1：The earth is 49 times the size of the moon.

地球的大小是月球的 49 倍（地球比月球大 48 倍）。

例 2：Within 30 years there will be twice as many urban people as countryside people in the world.

30 年内，全世界的城市居民将是农村人口的两倍。

例 3：城镇居民人均居住面积由 1978 年的 3.6 平方米提高到 1997 年的 8.8 平方米，增长约 2.4 倍。

The per capita living space for urban residents expanded from 3.6 square meters in 1978 to 8.8 square meters in 1997，a rise of about 2.4 times.

例 4：1997 年，全国高等学校在校生总数为 608 万人，其中研究生 18 万人，分别是 1979 年的 2.2 倍和 9.6 倍。

In 1997，6.08 million students were studying in colleges and universities, including 180,000 postgraduates，2.2 times and 9.6 times the figures of 1979 respectively.

3 口译词汇

3.1 英译汉

（一）Orthopedics 骨科

correction 矫正

Anterior Cruciate Ligament（ACL）前交叉韧带

skeletal deformity 骨骼畸形

ligament 韧带

tendon 肌腱

musculoskeletal system 肌肉骨骼系统

limb deformity 四肢畸形

rehabilitative 康复的

fracture 骨折

dislocation 脱位

torn ligament 韧带撕裂

sprain 扭伤

strain 拉伤

pulled muscle 肌肉拉伤

bursitis ruptured disc 滑囊炎椎间盘破裂

sciatica 坐骨神经痛

scoliosis 脊柱侧弯

knock knee 膝外翻

bow leg 弓形腿

bunion 拇囊炎

hammer toe 锤状脚趾

arthritis 关节炎

osteoporosis 骨质疏松症

muscular dystrophy 肌肉萎缩症

cerebral palsy 脑瘫

club foot 足内翻，马蹄内翻足

growth abnormality 生长异常

（二）Lumbar Disc Herniation 腰椎间盘突出症

spinal/vertebral disc 椎间盘

nucleus 核

slipped disc 椎间盘滑脱

ruptured disc 椎间盘破裂

sciatic nerve 坐骨神经

tingling 刺痛

radiate 放射

buttock 臀部

acute sciatica 急性坐骨神经痛

laminotomy 椎板切开术

lamina 椎板

discectomy 椎间盘切除术

spinal fusion 脊柱融合术

physical therapy 物理治疗

back brace 背部支具

（三）Osteoarthritis 骨关节炎

arthritis 关节炎

protective cartilage 保护性软骨

cushion 缓冲

deteriorate 退化，恶化

wear and tear disease 磨损疾病

connective tissue 结缔组织

obesity 肥胖

metabolic effect 代谢效应

over-the-counter 非处方

pain reliever 止痛药

prescription drug 处方药

3.2 汉译英

（一）半月板撕裂伤 Meniscus Tear

膝关节 knee joint

楔形软骨 wedge-shaped cartilage

大腿骨 thigh bone

胫骨 shinbone

肿胀 swelling

僵硬 stiffness

并发症 complication

电磁能束 electromagnetic energy beam

射频 radiofrequency

韧带 ligament

膝关节镜检查 knee arthroscopy

微创手术 minimally invasive procedure

关节镜 arthroscope

修剪 trim out

（二）骨癌 Bone Cancer

骨盆 pelvis

非癌性骨肿瘤 noncancerous bone tumor

手术切除 surgical removal

化学疗法 chemotherapy

放射疗法 radiation therapy

骨肉瘤 osteosarcoma

尤文氏肉瘤 Ewing sarcoma

软骨肉瘤 chondrosarcoma

遗传性综合征 inherited syndromes

佩吉特骨病 Paget's disease of bone

阴性切缘 negative margin

新诊断 newly diagnosed

复发 recurrent

脊索瘤 chordoma

冷冻手术 cryosurgery

液氮 liquid nitrogen

靶向治疗 targeted therapy

（三）骨髓炎 Osteomyelitis

椎骨 vertebrae

脓液 pus

步态改变 changes in gait

抗生素 antibiotics

脓肿 abscess

脊髓 spinal cord

清创术 debridement

抗生素敷料 antibiotic dressing

4 口译实战

4.1 英译汉

（一）Orthopedics 骨科[1-2]

Orthopedics is a medical specialty that focuses on the diagnosis, correction, prevention, and treatment of skeletal diseases—disorders of the bones, joints, muscles, ligaments, tendons, nerves and skin. These elements make up the musculoskeletal system. Once devoted to the care of children with spine and limb deformities, orthopedics now cares for patients of all ages.

骨科专注于骨骼疾病的诊断、矫正、预防和治疗，涉及骨骼、关节、肌肉、韧带、肌腱、神经和皮肤，它们构成了肌肉骨骼系统。骨科曾经主要专注于治疗脊柱和四肢畸形的儿童，现在覆盖所有年龄段的患者。

Orthopedists use medical, physical and rehabilitative methods as well as surgery and are involved in all aspects of

骨科医生使用药物、物理、康复手段以及手术，来保护肌肉骨骼系统的健康。骨科医生治疗的疾病和创伤

heath care pertaining to the musculoskeletal system. Orthopedists treat a immense variety of diseases and conditions, including fractures and dislocations, torn ligaments, sprains and strains, tendon injuries, pulled muscles and bursitis ruptured discs, sciatica, low back pain, scoliosis, knock knees, bow legs, bunions and hammer toes, arthritis and osteoporosis, bone tumors, muscular dystrophy and cerebral palsy, club foot and unequal leg length, abnormalities of the fingers and toes, and growth abnormalities.

Top reasons you may need to see an orthopedic surgeon are as follows: (1) Sports medicine. Orthopedists often specialize in the prevention and treatment of sports related injuries. (2) Knee surgery. Knee arthroscopy is a procedure where the orthopedic surgeon creates small incisions in the knee and uses a very powerful camera to perform ACL (Anterior Cruciate Ligament) reconstruction, repair torn meniscus, remove damaged tissue (debridement), or realign the kneecap (lateral release).

(3) Shoulder surgery. Shoulder arthroscopy, much like knee surgery,

较为广泛，包括骨折和脱位、韧带撕裂、扭伤和拉伤、肌腱受伤、肌肉拉伤和滑囊炎椎间盘破裂、坐骨神经痛、腰痛、脊柱侧弯、弓形腿、拇囊炎和锤状脚趾、关节炎和骨质疏松症、骨肿瘤、肌肉萎缩症和脑瘫、畸形足、下肢不等长、手指和脚趾畸形，以及生长异常。

可能需要看骨外科医生的主要原因如下：（1）需要运动医疗。骨科医生通常专门从事运动相关损伤的预防和治疗。（2）需要做膝关节手术。骨科医生在膝关节上做小切口，使用高能镜头进行前交叉韧带重建，修复撕裂的半月板，去除受损组织（清创术）或重新调整膝盖骨（横向松解），这就是膝关节镜手术。

（3）肩部手术。肩部关节镜手术与膝部手术非常相似，它利用微型摄

employs the use of a tiny camera to repair rotator cuffs, labral tears, impingement syndromes, etc. (4) Joint replacements. If your knee, shoulder, or hip joint is damaged, an orthopedic surgeon can replace it with a new one.

像机辅助修复肩袖、盂唇撕裂，治疗撞击综合征等。（4）关节置换。如果膝关节、肩关节或髋关节受损，骨外科医生可以为患者更换一个新的关节。

(5) Fracture care. When a bone is broken it will heal itself, but an orthopedic surgeon provides the reduction, casting, and sometimes surgical intervention needed to make sure the bones line up properly and recover full strength and movement. (6) Arthritis. The inflammation of joints is a common condition, an orthopedist can help provide physical therapy and surgery that can reduce the pain and stiffness.

（5）骨折治疗。当骨头断裂时，它会自行愈合，但骨科医生会帮助复位，安装支具，有时还需要手术干预，以确保骨对线良好，并恢复全部力量和运动能力。（6）关节炎。关节炎是一种常见疾病，骨科医生可以提供物理治疗以及手术，以减轻疼痛，缓解关节僵硬。

（二）Lumbar Disc Herniation 腰椎间盘突出症[3-4]

A spinal disc has a soft, jellylike center (nucleus) encased in a tougher, rubbery exterior (annulus). Sometimes called a slipped disc or a ruptured disc, a herniated disc occurs when some of the nucleus pushes out through a tear in the annulus. A herniated disc, which can occur in any part of the spine, can irritate a nearby nerve. Depending on where the herniated disc is, it can result in pain, numbness or weakness in an

椎间盘有一个柔软的、果冻状的中心（核），外面包裹着一层坚韧的富有弹性的物质（纤维环）。椎间盘突出也称为椎间盘滑脱或椎间盘破裂，即内核撕裂外环突出。椎间盘突出可能发生在脊柱的任何部位，会刺激附近的神经。根据椎间盘突出的位置，它可能导致手臂或腿部疼痛、麻木或无力。

arm or leg.

Lumbar disc herniation （LDH） results from a herniated disc in the lower back. Pressure on one or several nerves that contribute to the sciatic nerve can cause pain, burning, tingling and numbness that radiates from the buttock into the leg and sometimes into the foot. Usually, one side （left or right） is affected. This pain is often described as sharp and electric shock-like. It may be more severe when standing, walking or sitting. Straightening the leg on the affected side can often make the pain worse. Along with leg pain, one may experience low back pain; however, for acute sciatica the pain in the leg is often worse than the pain in the low back.

Lumbar laminotomy is a procedure often utilized to relieve leg pain and sciatica caused by a herniated disc. During this procedure, a portion of the lamina may be removed. After the disc is removed through a discectomy, the spine may need to be stabilized. Spinal fusion is often performed in conjunction with a laminotomy. In more involved cases, a laminectomy may be performed.

腰椎间盘突出是由下背部的椎间盘突出引起。压迫坐骨神经的一根或几根神经会使人感到疼痛、灼热、刺痛和麻木，这些感觉会从臀部传到腿部，有时传到足部。通常，身体的一侧（左侧或右侧）会受到影响。这种疼痛通常被描述为剧烈的、电击般的疼痛。站立、行走或坐着时可能更严重。拉直患侧的腿通常会使疼痛加剧。除了腿部疼痛，患者还可能会感到腰痛；然而，对急性坐骨神经痛患者来说，腿部疼痛通常比腰部疼痛更严重。

腰椎椎板切开术是一种常用于缓解由椎间盘突出引起的腿部疼痛和坐骨神经痛的手术。在此手术过程中，部分椎板可能会被移除。通过椎间盘切除术移除椎间盘后，可能需要稳定脊柱。脊柱融合术通常与椎板切开术一起进行。在更复杂的情况下，可以进行椎板切除术。

Most times, the patient must have undergone at least three months of treatment, such as physical therapy, pain medication or wearing a back brace, without showing improvement. Then, surgical treatment of lumbar disc herniation should be considered.

大多数情况下，患者必须在接受至少 3 个月的治疗后，例如做理疗、服用止痛药或佩戴背部支具，但情况仍未改善，才能考虑手术治疗腰椎间盘突出症。

（三）Osteoarthritis 骨关节炎[5-6]

Osteoarthritis (OA) is the most common form of arthritis, affecting millions of people worldwide. It occurs when the protective cartilage that cushions the ends of the bones wears down over time. Although OA can damage any joint, the disorder most commonly affects joints in your hands, knees, hips and spine.

骨关节炎是最常见的关节炎，影响着全世界几百万人。当缓冲骨骼末端的保护性软骨随着时间的推移而磨损时，就会发生骨关节炎。虽然任何关节都有可能发生骨关节炎，但这种疾病最常影响手、膝盖、臀部和脊柱的关节。

OA symptoms can usually be managed, although the damage to joints can't be reversed. OA has often been referred to as a wear and tear disease. But besides the breakdown of cartilage, OA affects the entire joint. It causes changes in the bone and deterioration of the connective tissues that hold the joint together and attach the muscle to the bone. It also causes inflammation of the joint lining.

骨关节炎症状通常是可以控制的，尽管关节的损害无法逆转。骨关节炎通常被称为磨损性疾病。除了破坏软骨，骨关节炎还会影响整个关节。它会导致骨骼的变化，使得关节固定在一起，肌肉连接到骨骼的结缔组织退化。它还会导致关节内膜发炎。

Risk factors for OA are as follows:
(1) Joint injury or overuse—such as excessive knee bending and repetitive stress on a joint, can damage a joint and increase the risk of OA in that joint.
(2) Age—The risk of developing OA increases with age. (3) Gender—Women are more likely to develop OA than men, especially after age 50.

(4) Obesity—Extra weight puts more stress on joints, particularly weight-bearing joints like the hips and knees. This stress increases the risk of OA in that joint. Obesity may also have metabolic effects that increase the risk of OA. (5) Genetics—People who have family members with OA are more likely to develop this disease. People who have hand OA are more likely to develop knee OA. (6) Race—Some Asian populations have lower risk for OA.

There is no cure for OA, so doctors usually treat OA symptoms with a combination of therapies, including increasing physical activity, physical therapy with muscle strengthening exercises, weight loss, medications such as over-the-counter pain relievers and prescription drugs, supportive devices

骨关节炎的风险因素如下：
（1）关节损伤或过度使用——例如过度弯曲膝盖，对关节施加重复性压力，会损坏关节并增加该关节发生骨关节炎的风险。（2）年龄——发生骨关节炎的风险随着年龄的增长而增加。（3）性别——女性比男性更容易患骨关节炎，尤其是50岁以后。

（4）肥胖——额外的重量会给关节带来更大压力，尤其是髋关节和膝关节等承重关节。这种压力会增加该关节发生骨关节炎的风险。肥胖的代谢效应也可能增加骨关节炎风险。（5）遗传——家庭成员患有骨关节炎的人更有可能患上这种疾病。患有手部骨关节炎的人更容易患上膝部骨关节炎。（6）种族——一些亚洲人群患骨关节炎的风险较低。

骨关节炎无法治愈，医生通常采用联合疗法来缓解骨关节炎症状，包括增加体育活动，进行针对肌肉强化练习的物理治疗，减肥，服用药物（包括非处方止痛药和处方药），使用辅助设备（如拐杖或手杖），以及手术（当其他治疗方案无效时）。

such as crutches or canes, and surgery (if other treatment options have not been effective).

4.2 汉译英

（一）半月板撕裂伤 Meniscus Tear[7-8]

膝关节由三块骨头组成，通常是一个坚韧、强壮的关节。但在朝某些方向旋转时，膝关节不一定是最灵活的。在某些活动中，尤其是接触性运动中，扭转膝盖的力量和幅度过大会撕裂在大腿骨和胫骨之间起缓冲作用的楔形软骨，这个软骨就是半月板。每个膝关节都有两个半月板。

Formed by three bones, the knee joint is typically a tough, strong joint. But it is not necessarily the most flexible when it comes to rotating in certain directions. During some activities—especially contact sports—the force and degree of twisting your knee can tear some of the wedge-shaped cartilage that provides cushioning between your thigh bone and shinbone. This cartilage is your meniscus. Each of your knees has two meniscus wedges.

半月板撕裂伤在运动员中很常见，尤其是那些从事的运动需要做大量下蹲、扭转动作和变换姿势的运动员。半月板撕裂时，可能会有以下症状：膝关节反复疼痛，对关节施加压力时疼痛加重，肿胀和僵硬，或者弯曲膝盖时感觉膝盖错位、锁定或卡住。

Meniscus tears are common among athletes, especially those who play sports that require a lot of squatting, twisting, and changing positions. When your meniscus is torn, you may experience pain in the knee joint that comes and goes, and gets worse when putting pressure on the joint, swelling and stiffness, and the feeling that your knee is giving way, locking, or catching when you bend it.

如果不治疗，部分半月板可能会松动并滑入关节。可能需要手术来恢复膝关节的全部功能。如不治疗，半月板撕裂会扩大并导致并发症，例如关节炎。如果怀疑半月板撕裂，骨科医生会进行全面的病史询问和膝关节评估，也可能会让患者拍 X 光、做核磁共振成像（MRI）来确诊，并进一步评估膝关节情况。

X 光是一种诊断手段，它使用不可见的电磁能束在胶片上生成内部组织、骨骼和器官的图像。核磁共振成像是结合大磁铁、射频和计算机生成体内器官和结构详细图像的诊断手段，通常可以用来确定周围韧带或肌肉的损伤或疾病。

膝关节镜检查是一种微创手术，常用于治疗半月板撕裂伤。在关节镜检查中，会从关节上的一个小切口插入一个小的、发光的视管（关节镜）。然后将膝关节内的图像投影到屏幕上，

If not treated, part of the meniscus may come loose and slip into the joint. You may need surgery to restore full knee function. Untreated meniscus tears can increase in size and lead to complications, such as arthritis. If a meniscal tear is suspected, your orthopedist will conduct a thorough health history and evaluation of the knee, and may also order X-rays and magnetic resonance imaging（MRI）to confirm the diagnosis and further evaluate the knee joint.

An X-ray is a diagnostic test that uses invisible electromagnetic energy beams to produce images of internal tissues, bones, and organs onto film. An MRI is a diagnostic procedure that uses a combination of large magnets, radiofrequencies, and a computer to produce detailed images of organs and structures within the body. It can often determine damage or disease in a surrounding ligament or muscle.

Knee arthroscopy, a minimally invasive procedure, is often used to treat meniscal tears. During an arthroscopy, a small, lighted, optic tube （arthroscope）is inserted through a small

供医生修复或修剪半月板撕裂的部分。

incision in the joint. Images of the inside of the knee are then projected on a screen allowing the provider to repair or trim out the torn portion of the meniscus.

（二）骨癌 Bone Cancer[9-11]

骨癌可以发生在身体的任何骨骼，但最常影响的是骨盆以及手臂和腿部的长骨。骨癌是罕见病，占所有癌症的不到1%。事实上，非癌性骨肿瘤比癌性骨肿瘤更常见。某些类型的骨癌主要发生在儿童身上，而其他类型的骨癌主要影响成年人。手术切除是最常见的治疗方法，但也可以使用化学疗法和放射疗法。使用手术、化学疗法还是放射疗法，要根据所治疗的骨癌类型来决定。

Bone cancer can begin in any bone in the body, but it most commonly affects the pelvis and the long bones in the arms and legs. Bone cancer is rare, making up less than 1 percent of all cancers. In fact, noncancerous bone tumors are much more common than cancerous ones. Some types of bone cancer occur primarily in children, while others affect mostly adults. Surgical removal is the most common treatment, but chemotherapy and radiation therapy may also be utilized. The decision to use surgery, chemotherapy or radiation therapy is based on the type of bone cancer being treated.

骨癌的主要类型如下：（1）骨肉瘤——最常见的骨癌类型，主要影响儿童和 20 岁以下的年轻人。（2）尤文氏肉瘤——最常影响 10 至 20 岁的人。（3）软骨肉瘤——往往会影响 40 岁以上的成年人。

The main types of bone cancer are as follows：（1）Osteosarcoma— the most common type, which mostly affects children and young adults under 20. （2）Ewing sarcoma—which most commonly affects people aged between 10 and 20. （3）Chondrosarcoma—which tends to affect adults aged over 40.

目前尚不清楚骨癌的致病原因，但医生发现某些因素会增加患癌风险：（1）遗传综合征。某些通过家族遗传的罕见遗传综合征会增加患骨癌的风险，包括李－佛美尼综合征和遗传性视网膜母细胞瘤。（2）佩吉特骨病。佩吉特骨病最常见于老年人，会增加以后患骨癌的风险。（3）癌症放射治疗。暴露于大剂量辐射，例如在癌症放射治疗期间受到的辐射，会增加未来患骨癌的风险。

手术是骨癌的常用治疗方法。外科医生以阴性切缘切除整个肿瘤（即在手术过程中切除的组织边缘未发现癌细胞）。化疗则使用抗癌药物杀死癌细胞。尤文氏肉瘤患者（新诊断和复发患者）和新诊断骨肉瘤的患者通常在接受手术前联合使用抗癌药物。化疗通常不用于治疗软骨肉瘤或脊索瘤。

It's not clear what causes bone cancer, but doctors have found that certain factors are associated with an increased risk: （1）Inherited genetic syndromes. Certain rare genetic syndromes passed through families increase the risk of bone cancer, including Li-Fraumeni syndrome and hereditary retinoblastoma. （2）Paget's disease of bone. Most commonly occurring in older adults, Paget's disease of bone can increase the risk of bone cancer developing later. （3）Radiation therapy for cancer. Exposure to large doses of radiation, such as those given during radiation therapy for cancer, increases the risk of bone cancer in the future.

Surgery is the usual treatment for bone cancer. The surgeon removes the entire tumor with negative margins (that is, no cancer cells are found at the edge of the tissue removed during surgery). Chemotherapy is the use of anticancer drugs to kill cancer cells. Patients who have Ewing sarcoma (newly diagnosed and recurrent) or newly diagnosed osteosarcoma usually receive a combination of anticancer drugs before undergoing surgery. Chemotherapy is not typically used to treat chondrosarcoma or chordoma.

放射治疗,也称为放射疗法,使用高能 X 射线杀死癌细胞。这种治疗方式可以与手术结合使用。它通常用于治疗尤文氏肉瘤。冷冻手术是使用液氮冷冻和杀死癌细胞。有时可以使用这种技术代替传统手术来破坏骨骼中的肿瘤。靶向治疗则使用的是药物,该药物可与癌细胞生长和扩散相关的特定分子发生作用。

Radiation therapy, also called radiotherapy, involves the use of high-energy X-rays to kill cancer cells. This treatment may be used in combination with surgery. It is often used to treat Ewing sarcoma. Cryosurgery is the use of liquid nitrogen to freeze and kill cancer cells. This technique can sometimes be used instead of conventional surgery to destroy tumors in bone. Targeted therapy is the use of a drug that is designed to interact with a specific molecule involved in the growth and spread of cancer cells.

(三)骨髓炎 Osteomyelitis [12-13]

骨髓炎是一种感染,通常会导致腿部长骨疼痛。其他骨骼,例如背部或手臂的骨骼,也会受到影响。骨髓炎可影响成人和儿童。然而,导致不同年龄人群感染骨髓炎的细菌和真菌不同。对成人来说,骨髓炎通常会影响椎骨和骨盆。对儿童来说,骨髓炎通常影响长骨的相邻末端。

Osteomyelitis is an infection that usually causes pain in the long bones in the legs. Other bones, such as those in the back or arms, can also be affected. Osteomyelitis can affect both adults and children. The bacteria or fungus that can cause osteomyelitis, however, differs among age groups. In adults, osteomyelitis often affects the vertebrae and the pelvis. In children, osteomyelitis usually affects the adjacent ends of long bones.

骨髓炎的症状可能包括感染区域

The symptoms of osteomyelitis can

疼痛或一触就痛，感染区域肿胀、发红、发热，发烧，恶心，全身不适、不安，皮肤渗脓（浓稠的黄色液体）。

可能与这种疾病相关的其他症状包括出汗过多，发冷，下背部疼痛（如果涉及脊柱），脚踝、脚和腿肿胀，关节运动的丧失或减少，步态变化（行走痛苦，导致跛行），儿童不愿负重。

骨髓炎可用抗生素治疗。通常服用抗生素 4 到 6 周。如果感染严重，服药周期可能长达 12 周。如果感染得到迅速治疗（在感染开始后 3 到 5 天内），通常能彻底治愈。还可以服用止痛药来缓解疼痛。如果感染发生在长骨（例如手臂或腿）中，可能要安装夹板，以尽量保持不动。

骨髓炎手术。如果出现以下情况，

include pain or tenderness in the infected area; swelling, redness and warmth in the infected area; fever; nausea; general discomfort, uneasiness; and drainage of pus (thick yellow fluid) through the skin.

Additional symptoms that may be associated with this disease include excessive sweating; chills; lower back pain (if the spine is involved); swelling of the ankles, feet, and legs; loss or decrease of motion of a joint; and/or Changes in gait (walking pattern that is painful, yielding a limp) or unwillingness to bear weight in children.

Osteomyelitis is treated with antibiotics. You'll usually take antibiotics for 4 to 6 weeks. If you have a severe infection, the course may last up to 12 weeks. If the infection is treated quickly (within 3 to 5 days of it starting), it often clears up completely. You can take painkillers to ease the pain. If the infection is in a long bone (such as an arm or leg), you may be fitted with a splint so you do not move it as often.

Surgery for osteomyelitis. You'll

通常需要进行手术：（1）骨中形成脓液（脓肿），需要排出脓肿中的脓液；（2）感染压迫其他组织，如脊髓；（3）感染持续了很长时间并破坏了骨骼。

如果感染破坏了骨骼，则需要做手术（称为清创术）以去除损坏的部分。清创会在骨头上留下缺损，可在其中填充抗生素敷料。有时需要不止一次手术来治疗感染。身体其他部位的肌肉和皮肤可用于修复受影响骨骼附近的区域。

usually need an operation in the following conditions：（1）A build-up of pus（abscess）develops in the bone，and the pus in an abscess needs to be drained.（2）The infection presses against something else，for example，the spinal cord. （3）The infection has lasted a long time and damaged the bone.

If the infection has damaged the bone，you'll need surgery（known as debridement）to remove the damaged part. Debridement can leave an empty space in the bone，which may be packed with antibiotic dressing. Sometimes more than one operation is needed to treat the infection. Muscle and skin from another part of the body might be used to repair the area near the affected bone.

5　口译注释与学习资源

5.1　口译注释

（一）与骨骼、关节等相关的词根

oste/o 骨骼

myel/o 骨髓

chondr/o 软骨

arthr/o 关节

synov/i 滑膜液、关节

burs/o 滑囊

（二）中轴骨

中轴骨（axial skeleton）包括头骨（skull）、脊柱（spinal column）、胸廓（thorax）等。

5.2　学习资源

登陆中国大学 MOOC（慕课），学习"医疗口译"课程中"骨科"的口译实战示范视频。此外还可登录美国约翰斯·霍普金斯大学医学院、美国神经外科医生协会等组织机构官网学习相关知识。

参考文献

[1] Atlanta, GA: Perimeter Orthopaedics. (n. d.). *What is orthopaedics?*. Retrieved November 15, 2021, from https://www. perimeterortho. com/contents/patient-information/what-is-orthopaedics.

[2] Washington University Orthopedics. (n. d.). *Introduction to orthopaedic surgery*. Retrieved November 15, 2021, from https://www. ortho. wustl. edu/content/Education/2453/Training-Programs/Med-Student-Programs/WUMS-III-Surgery-Clerkship-Program/Introduction-to-Orthopaedic-Surgery. aspx.

[3] Mayo Foundation for Medical Education and Research. (2019, September 26). *Herniated disk*. Retrieved November 15, 2021, from https://www. mayoclinic. org/diseases-conditions/herniated-disk/symptoms-causes/syc－20354095.

[4] AANS. (n. d.). *Herniated disc*. Retrieved November 15, 2021, from https://www. aans. org/en/Patients/Neurosurgical-Conditions-and-Treatments/Herniated-Disc.

[5] Mayo Foundation for Medical Education and Research. (2021, June 16). *Osteoarthritis*. Retrieved November 15, 2021, from https://www. mayoclinic. org/diseases-conditions/osteoarthritis/symptoms-causes/syc－20351925.

[6] Centers for Disease Control and Prevention. (2020, July 27). *Osteoarthritis* (OA). Retrieved November 15, 2021, from https://www. cdc. gov/arthritis/basics/osteoarthritis. htm.

[7] Sheehan, M. (2020, April 6). *Meniscus tears: Why you should not let them go untreated*. Retrieved November 15, 2021, from https://www. pennmedicine. org/updates/blogs/musculoskeletal-and-rheumatology/2018/september/meniscus-tears-why-you-should-not-let-them-go-untreated.

[8] Johns Hopkins Medicine. (n. d.). *Torn meniscus*. Retrieved November 15, 2021, from https://www. hopkinsmedicine. org/health/conditions-and-diseases/torn-meniscus.

［9］ NHS. (n. d.). *Bone cancer.* Retrieved November 15, 2021, from https: // www. nhs. uk/ conditions/bone-cancer/.

［10］ Mayo Foundation for Medical Education and Research. (2020, March 10). *Bone cancer.* Retrieved November 15, 2021, from https: // www. mayoclinic. org/diseases-conditions/bone-cancer/symptoms-causes/syc－20350217.

［11］ National Cancer Institute. (n. d.). *Primary bone cancer.* Retrieved November 15, 2021, from https: // www. cancer. gov/types/bone/bone-fact-sheet.

［12］ Cleveland Clinic. (n. d.). *Osteomyelitis: Causes, symptoms, diagnosis & treatments.* Retrieved November 15, 2021, from https: // my. clevelandclinic. org/health/diseases/9495 － osteomyelitis.

［13］ NHS. (n. d.). *Osteomyelitis.* Retrieved November 15, 2021, from https: // www. nhs. uk/ conditions/osteomyelitis/.

第十三章

精神科

第十三章

林中作

1　导读

本章的重点为口译技巧之双语转换（1）和精神科的 6 篇"口译实战"练习。口译实战练习中英译汉、汉译英各 3 篇，内容涵盖精神科/精神病学、情绪障碍、焦虑症、精神分裂症、物质使用障碍和进食障碍。请结合本章口译技巧练习 6 篇口译实战文本。

2　口译技巧——双语转换（1）

双语转换的速度和质量是口译的关键。汉语和英语在词语、句式、语篇等层面存在较大差异：中文重归纳，逻辑重心在后，讲求"悟"，"四字格"多，句子蜿蜒冗长，语法呈"意合"；英文重演绎，逻辑重心在前，讲求"理"，主谓结构清晰，语法呈"形合"。

因此，中英双语转换需要运用增减、变换、调序等技巧，对译语进行适当调整，以符合目的语使用规范。本节以下面关于"糖尿病足"（diabetic foot）的双语文本为例，讨论中英转换中的增减。

If you have diabetes, your blood glucose levels are too high. Over time, this can damage your nerves or blood vessels. Nerve damage from diabetes can cause you to lose feeling in your feet. You may not feel a cut, a blister or a sore. Foot injuries such as these can cause ulcers and infections. Serious cases may even lead to amputation. Damage to the blood vessels can also mean that your feet do not get enough blood and oxygen. It is harder for your foot to heal, if you do get a sore or infection.

如果患有糖尿病，表示你的血糖水平过高。随着时间推移，会损害神经或血管。糖尿病引起的神经损伤会导致足部失去知觉，可能会感觉不到伤口、水疱或疼痛。诸如此类的足部损伤会导致溃疡和感染，严重的甚至可能导致截肢。血管受损也可能意味着足部无法获得足够的血液和氧气。足部一旦有疼痛或感染，就更难愈合。

第一，英译汉时多做"减法"，减掉主语、宾语或定语的人称（you）或指称（this）代词也不影响意义的传递理解；减少句子数量，越少越精炼。

第二，汉译英时多做"加法"，增补主语、宾语或定语中的人称或指称代词；增加句子数量，避免长句太多太长，单句语法完整，前后逻辑清晰。

第三，主谓结构和指代明确是英语的"必需品"，是汉语的"非必需品"。

在下一章中，我们会说明在双语转换时如何进行词性变换和结构调序。

3 口译词汇

3.1 英译汉

（一）Psychiatry 精神科/精神病学

mental, emotional and behavioral disorders 精神、情绪和行为异常/紊乱

mental health 精神健康，心理健康

psychiatrist 精神科医生

panic attack 惊恐发作，急性焦虑症

American Psychiatric Association（APA）美国精神病学协会

Diagnostic and Statistical Manual of Mental Disorders（DSM-5）《精神疾病诊断和统计手册（第 5 版）》

psychotherapy 心理治疗，心理疗法

talk therapy 谈话疗法

cognitive behavior therapy（CBT）认知行为治疗

psychoanalysis 精神分析

antidepressant 抗抑郁药

panic disorder 恐慌症

post-traumatic stress disorder（PTSD）创伤后应激障碍

obsessive-compulsive disorder 强迫症

borderline personality disorder 边缘型人格障碍

eating disorder 进食障碍

antipsychotic medication 抗精神病药物

psychotic symptom（delusion and hallucination）精神病性症状（妄想和幻觉）

schizophrenia 精神分裂症

bipolar disorder 双相情感障碍，躁郁症

sedative 镇静剂

anxiolytic 抗焦虑药

insomnia 失眠

hypnotic 催眠药

mood stabilizer 情绪稳定剂

stimulant 兴奋剂

attention deficit hyperactivity disorder（ADHD）多动症（注意力缺陷多动障碍）

electroconvulsive therapy（ECT）电休克疗法

deep brain stimulation（DBS）脑深部电刺激

vagus nerve stimulation（VNS）迷走神经刺激

transcranial magnetic stimulation（TMS）经颅磁刺激

light therapy 光疗法

severe depression 严重抑郁症

seasonal depression 季节性抑郁症

（二）Mood Disorder 情绪障碍

mania 躁狂症

major depressive disorder 重度抑郁症

manic depression 躁狂抑郁症，双相情感障碍

seasonal affective disorder（SAD）季节性情感障碍

cyclothymic disorder 循环性障碍

premenstrual dysphoric disorder 经前烦躁症

persistent depressive disorder（dysthymia）持续性抑郁症（恶劣心境）

disruptive mood dysregulation disorder 破坏性心境失调障碍

substance use 物质使用（如酗酒、吸毒、药品滥用）

（三）Anxiety Disorder 焦虑症

heart palpitations 心悸

Cognitive behavioural therapy（CBT）认知行为治疗

exercise-induced increase in blood circulation to the brain 运动引起的大脑血液循环增加

mindfulness 正念

the hypothalamic-pituitary-adrenal（HPA）axis 下丘脑－垂体－肾上腺（HPA）轴

physiologic reactivity to stress 对压力的生理反应

the limbic system 边缘系统

amygdala 杏仁核

hippocampus 海马体

distraction，self-efficacy，and social interaction 转移注意力、自我效能和社交互动

3.2 汉译英

（一）精神分裂症 Schizophrenia

精神病 psychosis，psychotic illness

人格分裂 split personality

教养不良或教养不好 poor parenting or a bad upbringing

错误信念或妄想 false beliefs or delusions

缺陷 defect

基因构成 genetic make-up

（二）物质使用障碍 Substance Use Disorder

非法药物（毒品）illicit（illegal）drug

成瘾 addiction

强烈渴望 intense craving

脑成像研究 brain imaging studies

中毒（陶醉）intoxication

极度兴奋 euphoria

耐受性 tolerance

美国药物滥用研究所 National Institute on Drug Abuse

（三）进食障碍 Eating Disorder

神经性厌食症 anorexia nervosa

限制性亚型和暴食/催吐亚型 restrictive subtype and binge-purge subtype

使用泻药和利尿剂 use of laxatives and diuretics

消瘦 emaciation

骨质减少或骨质疏松症 osteopenia or osteoporosis

肌肉萎缩无力 muscle wasting and weakness

呼吸和脉搏减慢 slowed breathing and pulse

全身细毛生长，毳毛，胎毛 growth of fine hair all over the body（lanugo）

严重便秘 severe constipation

嗜睡，呆滞 lethargy，sluggishness

不孕症，脑损伤和多器官功能衰竭 infertility，brain damage and multiorgan failure

4　口译实战

4.1　英译汉

（一）Psychiatry 精神科/精神病学[1-2]

Psychiatry is the branch of medicine focused on the diagnosis, treatment and prevention of mental, emotional and behavioral disorders. A psychiatrist is a medical doctor who specializes in mental health. Psychiatrists are qualified to assess both the mental and physical aspects of psychological problems. People seek psychiatric help for many reasons.

精神病学是专注于诊断、治疗和预防精神、情绪和行为障碍的医学分支。精神科医生是专门研究精神健康的医生。精神科医生具有评估心理问题的精神和身体两个层面的资质。人们出于多种原因寻求精神科帮助。

The problems can be sudden, such as a panic attack, frightening hallucinations, thoughts of suicide, or hearing "voices". Or they may be more long-term, such as feelings of sadness, hopelessness, or anxiousness that never seem to lift or problems functioning, causing everyday life to feel distorted or out of control.

心理问题可能是突发的，例如突然惊恐发作，出现可怕幻觉，产生自杀念头或听到"声音"。心理问题也可能是长时间存在的，例如产生似乎永远不会缓解的悲伤、绝望或焦虑的感觉，或是出现导致日常生活扭曲或失控的功能性问题。

Psychiatrists can order or perform a

精神科医生可以通过为患者做医

full range of medical laboratory and psychological tests which, combined with discussions with patients, help provide a picture of a patient's physical and mental state. Specific diagnoses are based on criteria established in APA's *Diagnostic and Statistical Manual of Mental Disorders* (*DSM* − *5*), which contains descriptions, symptoms and other criteria for diagnosing mental disorders.

学实验和心理测试，结合与患者的交谈，全面评估患者的身心状态。具体诊断是基于美国精神病学协会的《精神疾病诊断和统计手册（第 5 版）》中建立的标准，该手册包含了用于诊断精神障碍的描述、症状和其他标准。

Psychotherapy, sometimes called talk therapy, is a treatment that involves a talking relationship between a therapist and patient. It can be used to treat a broad variety of mental disorders and emotional difficulties. The goal of psychotherapy is to eliminate or control disabling or troubling symptoms so the patient can function better. Depending on the extent of the problem, treatment may take just a few sessions over a week or two, or may take many sessions over a period of years.

心理治疗，有时也称为谈话疗法，是一种通过使治疗师和患者建立谈话关系来进行治疗的方法。它可用于治疗各种精神障碍和情绪问题。心理治疗的目标是消除或控制使人丧失能力或者焦虑不安的症状，让患者趋于正常。根据问题的严重程度，可能只需要在一两个星期内进行几个疗程的治疗，也可能需要在几年内进行许多个疗程的治疗。

Psychotherapy can be done individually, as a couple, with a family, or in a group. There are many forms of psychotherapy. Cognitive behavior therapy is a goal-oriented therapy focusing on problem solving.

心理治疗可以单独进行，也可以以夫妻、家人或团体的方式进行。心理治疗有多种形式。认知行为治疗是以解决问题为核心的目标导向治疗。精神分析是个人心理治疗的强化形式，需要数年的频繁治疗。在完成全面评

Psychoanalysis is an intensive form of individual psychotherapy which requires frequent sessions over several years. After completing thorough evaluations, psychiatrists can prescribe medications to help treat mental disorders.

Class of medications include antidepressants—used to treat depression, panic disorder, PTSD, anxiety, obsessive-compulsive disorder, borderline personality disorder and eating disorders; antipsychotic medications—used to treat psychotic symptoms (delusions and hallucinations), schizophrenia, and bipolar disorder; sedatives and anxiolytics—used to treat anxiety and insomnia; hypnotics—used to induce and maintain sleep; mood stabilizers—used to treat bipolar disorder; and stimulants—used to treat ADHD. Psychiatrists often prescribe medications in combination with psychotherapy.

Other treatments are also sometimes used. Electroconvulsive therapy (ECT), a medical treatment that involves applying electrical currents to the brain, is used most often to treat severe depression that has not responded to other treatments. Deep brain stimulation (DBS), vagus

估后，精神科医生可以给患者开药以帮助治疗精神障碍。

这些药物包括：抗抑郁药——用于治疗抑郁症、恐慌症、创伤后应激障碍、焦虑症、强迫症、边缘型人格障碍和进食障碍；抗精神病药物——用于治疗精神病性症状（妄想和幻觉）、精神分裂症、双相情感障碍；镇静剂和抗焦虑药——用于治疗焦虑和失眠；催眠药——用于诱导和维持睡眠；情绪稳定剂——用于治疗双相情感障碍；中枢兴奋剂——用于治疗多动症。药物治疗通常会结合心理治疗来进行。

精神科医生有时也使用其他治疗方法。电休克疗法（ECT）是一种向大脑施加电流的医学疗法，最常用于治疗对其他疗法没有反应的严重抑郁症。脑深部电刺激（DBS）、迷走神经刺激（VNS）和经颅磁刺激（TMS）则是用于治疗某些精神障碍的新型疗

nerve stimulation (VNS), and transcranial magnetic stimulation (TMS) are a few of the newer therapies being used to treat some mental disorders. Light therapy is used to treat seasonal depression.

法。光疗法可用于治疗季节性抑郁症。

（二）Mood Disorder 情绪障碍[3]

If you have a mood disorder, your general emotional state or mood is distorted or inconsistent with your circumstances and interferes with your ability to function. You may be extremely sad, empty or irritable (depressed), or you may have periods of depression alternating with being excessively happy (mania). Anxiety disorders can also affect your mood and often occur along with depression. Mood disorders may increase your risk of suicide.

如果你有情绪障碍，那你的总体情绪状态或情感是扭曲的，或者说是与你所处环境不协调的，这会干扰你身体机能的正常运转。你可能感到极度悲伤、空虚或易怒（抑郁），可能会经历抑郁和过度快乐（躁狂）的交替出现。焦虑症也会影响你的情绪，并且经常与抑郁症一起出现。情绪障碍可能会增加你自杀的风险。

Some examples of mood disorders include major depressive disorder—prolonged and persistent periods of extreme sadness, bipolar disorder—also called manic depression that includes alternating times of depression and mania, and seasonal affective disorder (SAD) —a form of depression most often associated with fewer hours of

情绪障碍包括：重度抑郁症——长期和持续的极度悲伤；双相情感障碍——也称躁狂抑郁症，指抑郁症和躁狂症交替发生；季节性情感障碍（SAD）——常与深秋到早春的高纬度地区的日照时间变短有关的抑郁症。

daylight in the high latitudes from late fall to early spring.

Other examples include cyclothymic disorder—a disorder that causes emotional ups and downs that are less extreme than bipolar disorder, premenstrual dysphoric disorder—mood changes and irritability that occur during the premenstrual phase of a woman's cycle and go away with the onset of menses, persistent depressive disorder (dysthymia)—a long-term form of depression, and disruptive mood dysregulation disorder—a disorder of chronic, severe and persistent irritability in children that often includes frequent temper outbursts that are inconsistent with the child's developmental age.

Patients may also suffer from depression related to medical illness—a persistent depressed mood and a significant loss of pleasure in most or all activities that's directly related to the physical effects of another medical condition, and depression induced by substance use or medication—depression symptoms that develop during or soon after substance use or withdrawal or after exposure to a medication.

另外还有循环性障碍——导致情绪起伏但不如双相情感障碍严重的病症；经前烦躁症——发生在女性月经周期前的情绪变化和易怒，会随着月经开始而消失；持续性抑郁症（恶劣心境）——长期的抑郁症；破坏性心境失调障碍——慢性、严重和持续的儿童易怒症，患儿往往会频繁发脾气，表现得与其年龄不符。

患者还可能患上继发于疾病的抑郁症——与另一种身体疾病直接相关的抑郁情绪，对大多数或所有活动丧失乐趣，以及由物质使用或药物治疗引起的抑郁症——抑郁症症状在物质使用或戒断期间，在使用或戒断之后不久，以及在接触药物后出现。

For most people, mood disorders can be successfully treated with medications and talk therapy. If you're concerned that you may have a mood disorder, make an appointment to see your doctor or a mental health professional as soon as you can. If you're reluctant to seek treatment, talk to a friend or loved one or someone else you trust.

Talk to a health care professional if you feel like your emotions are interfering with your work, relationships, social activities or other parts of your life or if you have trouble with drinking or drugs. If you have suicidal thoughts or behaviors, seek emergency treatment immediately. Your mood disorder is unlikely to simply go away on its own, and it may get worse over time. Seek professional help before your mood disorder becomes severe.

（三）Anxiety Disorder 焦虑症[4-5]

Anxiety is a natural response to stressful life events. Most individuals will experience worry, nerves and apprehension during their lifetime. In fact, some degree of anxiety can be helpful, such as motivating you to

大多数人都可以通过药物和谈话疗法成功治疗情绪障碍。如果你担心自己可能患有情绪障碍，请尽快预约医生或心理健康专家进行咨询。如果你不愿意寻求治疗，请与朋友、亲人或其他信任的人交谈。

如果你觉得情绪干扰了你的工作、人际关系、社交活动或生活的其他方面，或者你有酗酒或吸毒问题，请咨询医疗保健专业人员。如果你有自杀念头或行为，请立即寻求紧急治疗。情绪障碍不太可能自行消失，而且随着时间的推移可能会变得更严重。在情绪障碍变得非常严重之前，应寻求专业帮助。

焦虑是对生活压力事件的自然反应。大多数人在一生中都会存在担忧、紧张和忧虑情绪。事实上，某种程度的焦虑可能是有益的，例如它会激励你为大型考试或演讲做好准备。然而，在某些时候，它会对机体的日常功能

prepare for a big exam or presentation. However, at a certain point it negatively interferes with daily functioning and physical health.

和身体健康产生负面影响。

Anxiety disorder looks different for everyone. You may get easily overwhelmed, feel on edge and avoid places, people or things. You may experience constant and uncontrollable worry about any aspect of your life including career, health, family and social life. You may experience panic attacks or sudden peaks of anxiety that cause intense physical sensations like heart palpitations and breathing trouble.

每个人的焦虑症看起来都不一样。你可能很容易不知所措，感到紧张，并避免前往某些地方，接触某些人或事物。你可能会对生活的任何方面（包括职业、健康、家庭和社交生活）感到持续和无法控制的担忧。你可能会经历惊恐发作或突然的焦虑高峰，出现强烈的躯体反应，如心悸和呼吸困难。

You may experience struggles in social situations or when you feel like attention is focused on you. And you may experience specific anxiety, like constantly worrying about your health or an extreme fear about a specific situation or object. There are also common physical symptoms associated with anxiety including feeling restless or on edge, sleeping trouble, nausea, sweating, trembling, feeling weak or tired, trouble concentrating or feeling irritable.

你可能会在社交场合中或被人关注时觉得为难。你可能会对特定情况或物体产生焦虑，比如不断担心自己的健康或对特定情况或物体极度恐惧。与焦虑相关的常见躯体症状还有感到不安或紧张、失眠、恶心、出汗、颤抖、感觉虚弱或疲倦、注意力不集中或感觉烦躁。

Research indicates that CBT is an

研究表明，认知行为治疗（CBT）

effective treatment for a range of anxiety disorders. Based on the idea that thoughts, feelings and behaviors constantly interact and influence us, CBT aims to alleviate anxiety by adjusting unhelpful thought patterns, beliefs and behavioral patterns of avoidance. CBT is an overarching type of therapy with many different types to help with different symptoms and needs. For example, individuals experiencing panic attacks might go through exposures to get used to certain physiological sensations. This helps patients relearn beliefs about what those sensations mean.

Exercise, sleep, mindfulness, nutrition and medication are also helpful in managing anxiety and everyday stressors. Aerobic exercises, including jogging, swimming, cycling, walking, gardening, and dancing, have been proved to reduce anxiety and depression. These improvements in mood are proposed to be caused by exercise-induced increase in blood circulation to the brain.

Exercise also influences the hypothalamic-pituitary-adrenal (HPA) axis and, thus, on the physiologic

是治疗一系列焦虑症的有效方法。认知行为治疗建立在这一理念基础上：思想、感觉和行为不断相互作用和影响我们。它旨在通过调整无益性思维模式、信念以及回避性行为模式来缓解焦虑。认知行为治疗是多种不同类型疗法的总称，可帮助缓解不同症状，满足不同需求。例如，经历惊恐发作的人可以通过多次暴露来习惯某些生理感觉。这有助于患者重新了解这些感觉意味着什么，重塑信念。

锻炼、睡眠、正念、营养和药物治疗也有助于控制焦虑和日常压力。有氧运动，包括慢跑、游泳、骑自行车、散步、园艺和跳舞，已被证明可以减少焦虑和抑郁。这些情绪改善被认为是源于运动引起的大脑血液循环增加。

运动也会影响下丘脑－垂体－肾上腺（HPA）轴，从而影响对压力的生理反应。这种生理影响可能由 HPA

reactivity to stress. This physiologic influence is probably mediated by the communication of the HPA axis with several regions of the brain, including the limbic system, which controls motivation and mood; the amygdala, which generates fear in response to stress; and the hippocampus, which plays an important part in memory formation as well as in mood and motivation. Other hypotheses that have been proposed to explain the beneficial effects of physical activity on mental health include distraction, self-efficacy, and social interaction.

轴与大脑多个区域的交流介导，包括：边缘系统，它控制动机和情绪；杏仁核，它使我们对压力产生恐惧；海马体，它在记忆形成以及情绪和动机方面起着重要作用。已提出的解释运动对心理健康有益影响的其他假设包括转移注意力、自我效能和社交互动。

4.2　汉译英

（一）精神分裂症 Schizophrenia[6]

精神分裂症是一种被称为"精神病"的精神疾病，这种精神疾病使人无法分辨真实与想象。有时，患有精神病的人会与现实脱节。世界可能看起来像是一堆混乱的想法、图像和声音。精神分裂症比大多数人想象的更常见。

在美国，大约每200人中就有1人会在他们的一生中患上精神分裂症。了解精神分裂症可以以不同的方式表

Schizophrenia is a type of mental illness known as a "psychosis", which is a mental illness in which a person cannot tell what is real from what is imagined. At times, people with psychotic illnesses lose touch with reality. The world may seem like a jumble of confusing thoughts, images, and sounds. Schizophrenia is more common than most people think.

About 1 in 200 of the people in the United States will develop schizophrenia over the course of their lives. It's also

现出许多不同的症状也很重要。精神分裂症与"人格分裂"不同，这是另一种精神疾病。人格分裂远不如精神分裂症常见。

精神分裂症没有单一病因。它不是因为教养不良或教养不好。尽管压力会引发或加重症状，但压力不会导致精神分裂症。精神分裂症是一种大脑疾病。它很可能由多种因素共同促成，这些因素可能包括某些大脑中控制思维和理解的化学物质的缺陷、个体的基因构成，或是大脑塑造人格的缺陷。

精神分裂症患者可能会突然出现严重的精神病性症状。这些症状可能会阶段性发生，时有时无，但也可能一生只发生一次或两次。在发病期，病人可能仍能理解部分现实。他可能过着还算正常的生活，能有一些基本活动，例如吃饭、工作和走动。在其他情况下，病人却可能无法正常生活。

important to know that schizophrenia has many different symptoms and can show up in many different ways. Schizophrenia is not the same as a "split personality". A split personality is another type of mental illness. It is much less common than schizophrenia.

There's no single cause for schizophrenia. It does not happen because of poor parenting or a bad upbringing. Although stress can trigger or worsen symptoms, it does not cause schizophrenia. Schizophrenia is a disorder of the brain. It most likely develops from a mix of factors that may include a defect in certain chemicals in the brain that control thinking and understanding, a person's genetic make-up, or a defect in how the brain forms a person's personality.

People with schizophrenia may have sudden and severe psychotic symptoms. These symptoms can come and go in phases, or they can happen only once or twice in a lifetime. During psychotic phases, the person may still understand parts of reality. He or she may lead a somewhat normal life, doing basic activities such as eating, working and

精神病发病期症状包括看到、听到、感觉到或闻到不存在的事物（幻觉）或具有与事实不符的奇怪信念（错误信念或妄想）。例如，病人可能坚信人们可以听到自己的想法，或者人们正在将想法放入自己脑中。病人可能存在思维障碍，无法从世界上整理出秩序，从一个想法迅速转移到另一个想法。并且此人可能有与发生的事件不符的情绪、想法和情感。

getting around. In other cases, the person may be unable to function.

Symptoms during psychotic phases include seeing, hearing, feeling or smelling things that are not real (hallucinations) or having strange beliefs that are not based on facts (false beliefs or delusions). For example, the person may believe that people can hear his or her thoughts, or that people are putting thoughts into his or her head. The person may think in a confused way, being unable to make order out of the world, shifting quickly from one thought to the next. And the person may have emotions, thoughts and moods that do not fit with events.

（二）物质使用障碍 Substance Use Disorder [7]

物质使用障碍（SUD）是一种复杂的病症，在这种情况下，尽管会产生有害后果，但患者仍会无法控制地使用该物质。患有物质使用障碍的人强烈地专注于使用某种物质，例如酒精、烟草或非法药物，以至其日常生活能力受损。他们即使知道该物质正在引起或将会引起问题，但仍会继续使用。最严重的物质使用障碍有时被称为成瘾。

Substance use disorder (SUD) is a complex condition in which there is uncontrolled use of a substance despite harmful consequence. People with SUD have an intense focus on using a certain substance(s) such as alcohol, tobacco, or illicit drugs, to the point where the person's ability to function in day to day life becomes impaired. People keep using the substance even when they know it is causing or will cause problems. The most severe SUDs are sometimes called addictions.

物质使用障碍患者的思维和行为可能发生扭曲。大脑的结构和功能变化是导致他们对物质产生强烈渴求，出现性格变化，做出异常动作和其他行为的原因。脑成像研究显示，患者与判断、决策、学习、记忆和行为控制相关的大脑区域发生了改变。重复使用物质也会导致大脑功能进一步发生变化。

People with a substance use disorder may have distorted thinking and behaviors. Changes in the brain's structure and function are what cause people to have intense cravings, changes in personality, abnormal movements, and other behaviors. Brain imaging studies show changes in the areas of a patient's brain that relate to judgment, decision making, learning, memory, and behavioral control. Repeated substance use can also cause changes in how the brain functions.

这些变化在物质的直接影响消失后，或者换句话说，在药物清除后，仍会持续很长时间。每种物质的中毒症状不同。当患上物质使用障碍时，患者通常会对物质产生耐受性，意味着他们需要更多的物质才能感受到效果。

These changes can last long after the immediate effects of the substance wears off, or in other words, after the period of intoxication. Intoxication symptoms are different for each substance. When someone has a substance use disorder, they usually build up a tolerance to the substance, meaning they need larger amounts to feel the effects.

美国药物滥用研究所指出，人们开始吸毒的原因有很多，包括为了获得快感——愉悦、"兴奋"或"陶醉"的感觉；为了获得安慰——缓解压力、

According to the National Institute on Drug Abuse, people begin taking drugs for a variety of reasons, including to feel good—feeling of pleasure,

忘记问题或感觉麻木；为了变得更强——提高表现或思维；或是因为好奇心、同伴压力或实验。除了物质，人还可能对赌博等行为上瘾。

有物质使用和行为成瘾的人可能会意识到他们的问题，但即使他们想要并尝试停止，也会无法停止。成瘾可能会导致身心问题，以及与家人、朋友和同事的人际关系问题。酒精和毒品使用已经是全美范围内导致可预防性疾病和早逝的主要原因之一。

（三）进食障碍 Eating Disorder[8]

进食障碍是严重的内科疾病，其特征是个体的饮食行为出现严重紊乱。对食物、体重和体型的痴迷可能是出现进食障碍的迹象。这会影响个体的身心健康。有时，还可能会危及生命。进食障碍会影响所有年龄、种族、民族、体重和性别的人。

"high" or "intoxication", to feel better—relieve stress, forget problems, or feel numb, to do better—improve performance or thinking, or curiosity, peer pressure or experimenting. In addition to substances, people can also develop addiction to behaviors, such as gambling.

People with substance use and behavioral addictions may be aware of their problem but not be able to stop even if they want and try to. The addiction may cause physical and psychological problems, as well as interpersonal problems such as with family members and friends or at work. Alcohol and drug use are one of the leading causes of preventable illnesses and premature deaths nationwide.

Eating disorders are serious medical illnesses marked by severe disturbances to a person's eating behaviors. Obsessions with food, body weight and shape may be signs of an eating disorder. These disorders can affect a person's physical and mental health. Sometimes they can be life-threatening. Eating disorders can affect people of all ages,

尽管进食障碍通常出现在青少年时期或成年早期，但也可能发生在童年时期或成年晚期（40岁及以上）。进食障碍患者可能看起来很健康，但实际上病得很重。进食障碍的确切原因尚不完全清楚，但研究表明，遗传、生物、行为、心理和社会综合因素会加大个体患上进食障碍的风险。

神经性厌食症是一种常见的进食障碍。患有神经性厌食症的人会避免进食，严格限制食物，或只吃很少量的某些食物。即使他们的体重严重不足，他们也可能认为自己超重。他们也可能反复称重。神经性厌食症有两种亚型：限制性亚型和暴食/催吐亚型。患有神经性厌食症限制性亚型的人对他们食用的食物数量和类型有严格的限制。患有神经性厌食症暴食/催吐亚型的人也严格限制他们食用的食物数量和类型。此外，他们可能有暴饮暴食和催吐行为（如呕吐、使用泻药和利尿剂等）。

racial/ethnic backgrounds, body weights, and genders.

Although eating disorders often appear during the teen years or young adulthood, they may also develop during childhood or later in life (40 years and older). People with eating disorders may appear healthy, yet be extremely ill. The exact cause of eating disorders is not fully understood, but research suggests a combination of genetic, biological, behavioral, psychological, and social factors can raise a person's risk.

Anorexia nervosa is one of the common eating disorders. People with anorexia nervosa avoid food, severely restrict food, or eat very small quantities of only certain foods. Even when they are dangerously underweight, they may see themselves as overweight. They may also weigh themselves repeatedly. There are two subtypes of anorexia nervosa: a restrictive subtype and a binge-purge subtype. People with the restrictive subtype of anorexia nervosa place severe restrictions on the amount and type of food they consume. People with the binge-purge subtype of anorexia nervosa also place severe restrictions on the amount and type of food they consume. In addition, they may have binge eating and purging behaviors (such as vomiting, use of laxatives and diuretics, etc.).

症状包括极度受限的饮食、剧烈和过度运动、极度瘦削（消瘦）、对瘦身的不懈追求和不愿意保持正常或健康的体重、对体重增加的强烈恐惧和对身体形象的扭曲态度、受体重和体型看法严重影响的自尊心、对低体重严重性的否认。

Symptoms include extremely restricted eating and/or intensive and excessive exercise, extreme thinness (emaciation), a relentless pursuit of thinness and unwillingness to maintain a normal or healthy weight, intense fear of gaining weight and distorted body image, a self-esteem that is heavily influenced by perceptions of body weight and shape, or a denial of the seriousness of low body weight.

随着时间的推移，患者还可能出现骨质减少或骨质疏松症，轻度贫血和肌肉萎缩无力，头发和指甲变脆，皮肤干燥发黄，全身细毛生长，严重便秘，低血压，呼吸和脉搏减慢，心脏结构和功能受损，体温下降因此时常感到寒冷、嗜睡、呆滞或时常感到疲倦，不孕症，脑损伤和多器官功能衰竭。

Over time, patients may also develop osteopenia or osteoporosis, mild anemia and muscle wasting and weakness, brittle hair and nails, dry and yellowish skin, growth of fine hair all over the body, severe constipation, low blood pressure, slowed breathing and pulse, damage to the structure and function of the heart, drop in internal body temperature, causing a person to feel cold all the time, lethargy, sluggishness, or feeling tired all the time, infertility, brain damage and multiorgan failure.

5 口译注释与学习资源

5.1 口译注释

Therapist vs. Psychologist vs. Psychiatrist

上面三个词的意思分别是治疗师、心理学家和精神科医生。请阅读下面关于三者区别的中英对照材料。

One of the most notable difference between a psychologist and a psychiatrist is that psychologists are not medical doctors. They do not have a medical degree and are not trained in general medicine or in prescribing medications. Practicing psychologists must earn an undergraduate major, a master's, and a doctorate in psychology. Additionally, most states require a two-year internship. Practicing psychologists may earn a PhD or PsyD.

心理学家和精神科医生之间最显著的区别之一就是心理学家不是医生。他们没有医学学位，也没有接受过一般医学或药物处方方面的培训。职业心理学家必须获得心理学专业的本科、硕士和博士学位。此外，大多数州还要求完成为期两年的实习。职业心理学家可以获得哲学博士学位或心理学博士学位。

Unlike psychologists, psychiatrists are medical doctors, or physicians, with a degree in medicine. Psychiatrists must complete an undergraduate and medical degree, plus a four-year residency in psychiatry. They may then choose to complete a fellowship in a sub-specialty. As medical doctors, psychiatrists can prescribe medication, and while they may provide some counseling, a psychiatrist might refer a patient to a

与心理学家不同，精神科医生是拥有医学学位的医生或医师。精神科医生必须获得本科学位和医学学位，以及完成四年的精神科住院医师培训。然后他们可以选择完成一项亚专科培训。作为医师，精神科医生可以开药，虽然他们可能会提供一些心理咨询，但更可能会将患者转介给心理学家或治疗师，以使患者可以进一步咨询或接受治疗。治疗师需要获取硕士学位并获得资格委员会的批准才能在心理

psychologist or therapist for additional counseling or therapy. Therapists require master degrees and approval of their licensing boards to practice in the mental health field.

健康领域执业。

5.2　学习资源

登录中国大学 MOOC（慕课），学习"医疗口译"课程中"精神科"的口译实战示范视频。补充主题包括：（1）Steps to Becoming a Psychiatrist 成为精神科医生的步骤；（2）Your First Appointment with a Psychiatrist 第一次看精神科医生；（3）What's the Difference Between a Psychologist and psychiatrist? 心理学家和精神科医生有什么区别？（4）Psychotherapist（Therapist）VS. Psychologist—What Is the Difference? 心理治疗师与心理学家的区别有哪些？（5）What Is Depression? 什么是抑郁症？（6）Generalized Anxiety Disorder（GAD）—Causes，Symptoms & Treatment 广泛性焦虑症——原因、症状和治疗；（7）Can Adults Have ADHD? A Psychiatrist Explains the Symptoms 成年人会患多动症吗？精神科医生来解释其症状。

参考文献

［1］American Psychiatric Association.（n. d.）. *What is psychiatry?*. Retrieved November 13，2021，from https：//www. psychiatry. org/patients-families/what-is-psychiatry-menu.

［2］U. S. Department of Health and Human Services. National Institute of Mental Health.（n. d.）. *Brain stimulation therapies*. Retrieved November 13，2021，from https：//www. nimh. nih. gov/health/topics/brain-stimulation-therapies/brain-stimulation-therapies.

［3］Mayo Foundation for Medical Education and Research.（2021，October 29）. *Mood disorders*. Retrieved November 13，2021，from https：//www. mayoclinic. org/diseases-conditions/mood-disorders/symptoms-causes/syc－20365057.

［4］Mayo Foundation for Medical Education and Research.（2018，May 4）. *Anxiety disorders*. Retrieved November 13，2021，from https：//www. mayoclinic. org/diseases-conditions/anxiety/symptoms-causes/syc－20350961.

［5］Sharma，A.，Madaan，V.，& Petty，F. D.（2006）. *Exercise for mental health.* Primary care companion to the Journal of clinical psychiatry. Retrieved November 13, 2021, from https://www.ncbi.nlm.nih.gov/pmc/articles/PMC1470658/.

［6］Cleveland Clinic. (n.d.). *Schizophrenia: Symptoms, causes, treatments.* Retrieved November 13, 2021, from https://my.clevelandclinic.org/health/diseases/4568－schizophrenia.

［7］American Psychiatric Association. (n.d.). *Addiction and Substance Use Disorders.* Retrieved November 13, 2021, from https://www.psychiatry.org/patients-families/addiction.

［8］U.S. Department of Health and Human Services. National Institute of Mental Health. (n.d.). *Eating disorders: About more than food.* Retrieved November 13, 2021, from https://www.nimh.nih.gov/health/publications/eating-disorders.

第十四章

眼　科

第十四章

序論

1　导读

　　本章的重点为口译技巧之双语转换（2）和眼科的 6 篇"口译实战"练习。口译实战练习中英译汉、汉译英各 3 篇，内容涵盖眼科、白内障、青光眼、年龄相关性黄斑变性、糖尿病视网膜病变和屈光不正。请结合本章口译技巧练习 6 篇口译实战文本。

2　口译技巧——双语转换（2）

　　双语转换的变换是指词性转换，例如将英语中的名词转换为汉语中的动词。

　　双语转换的调序主要是指将英语的后置定语或修辞成分变为汉语的前置定语或修辞成分。

　　在适当调整定语位置的同时兼顾顺句推动的原则，即尽量不对原语句序做大幅调整，以减轻短期记忆的压力，尤其是在认知资源比较紧张的同传中。

　　下面示例中，同样的英语原文，可以在交传和同传中出现不同句序（交传的策略是将英语的后置定语前置，中心词后置；同传是使用同位语进行顺句推动），但意思基本一致，因此，口译的最大优势就是灵活。

　　例 1：英汉交传

Psychiatry is the branch of medicine focused on the diagnosis, treatment and prevention of mental, emotional and behavioral disorders.	精神科是专注于诊断、治疗和预防精神、情绪和行为异常的医学分支。

　　例 2：英汉同传

Psychiatry is the branch of medicine focused on the diagnosis, treatment and prevention of mental, emotional and behavioral disorders.	精神科这个医学分支，主要是诊断、治疗和预防精神、情绪和行为异常。

3 口译词汇

3.1 英译汉

（一）Ophthalmology 眼科

ophthalmologist 眼科医生

optometrist 验光师

optician 配镜师

ophthalmic medical assistant 眼科医疗助理

strabismus/pediatric ophthalmology 斜视/小儿眼科

glaucoma 青光眼

neuro-ophthalmology 神经眼科

retina 视网膜

uveitis 葡萄膜炎

anterior segment 眼前节

cornea 角膜

oculoplastics 眼整形

orbit 眼眶

ocular oncology 眼肿瘤科

general ophthalmologist 普通眼科医生

residency in ophthalmology 眼科住院医师培训

microsurgery 显微外科

exquisite hand-eye coordination 精湛的手眼协调

suture 缝合线

unaided eye 肉眼

intraocular surgery 眼内手术

strabismus（crossed eyes）surgery 斜视（斗鸡眼）手术

optic nerve damage and visual field loss 视神经损伤和视野丧失

visual pathways 视觉通路

eye-movement patterns 眼球运动模式

optic nerve disease 视神经疾病

systemic neurological diseases with visual manifestations 具有视觉表现的系统性神经疾病

vitreous 玻璃体

surgical and laser treatment 手术和激光治疗

retinal detachment 视网膜脱落

diabetic retinopathy 糖尿病视网膜病变

corneal transplantation 角膜移植

refractive eye surgery（vision correction）屈光手术（视力矫正）

aesthetic，plastic and reconstructive surgery 美容、整形和重建手术

the face，orbit，eyelids，and lacrimal system 面部、眼眶、眼睑和泪道系统

conjunctival melanoma 结膜黑色素瘤

periorbital area 眶周区域

（二）Cataract 白内障

cloudy area 浑浊区域

blurry，hazy，or less colorful 模糊、朦胧或失去部分色彩

holo 光晕

double 重影

clouded lens 混浊晶（状）体

artificial lens 人工晶状体

intraocular lens 眼内透镜

contact lenses 隐形眼镜

local anesthetic 局部麻醉剂

（三）Glaucoma 青光眼

high intraocular pressure 高眼压

vision loss 视力下降，视力损伤

blindness 失明

aqueous humor 房水

iris 虹膜

open-angle glaucoma 开角型青光眼

angle-closure glaucoma 闭角型青光眼

congenital glaucoma 先天性青光眼

low- or normal-tension glaucoma 低眼压或正常眼压青光眼

severe eye pain and blurry vision 严重眼痛和视力模糊

blind spots 盲点

slow loss of peripheral（side）vision 周边（侧面）视力的缓慢丧失

reduced or cloudy vision 视力减退或视力模糊

3.2　汉译英

（一）年龄相关性黄斑变性 Age-related Macular Degeneration（AMD）

黄斑变性 macular degeneration

老化 aging

黄斑 macula

中心视力 central vision

湿性年龄相关性黄斑变性 wet AMD

干性年龄相关性黄斑变性 dry AMD

出血、渗出和瘢痕 bleeding, leaking, and scarring

玻璃膜疣 drusen

视网膜下微小的黄色或白色沉积物 tiny yellow or white deposits under the retina

永久性阅读障碍和精细或近距离视力受损 permanent impairment of reading and fine or close-up vision

（二）糖尿病视网膜病变 Diabetic Retinopathy

散瞳检查 dilated eye exam

玻璃体 vitreous

自行清除 clear up on their own

妊娠期糖尿病 gestational diabetes

蜘蛛网 cobweb

检测光线 detect light

（三）屈光不正 Refractive Error

近视 nearsightedness（myopia）

远视 farsightedness（hyperopia）

散光 astigmatism

老视 presbyopia

强光周围看见眩光或光晕 seeing a glare or halo around bright lights

眯眼 squinting

眼球长度 eyeball length

角膜形状问题 problems with the shape of the cornea

晶状体老化 aging of the lens

激光眼科手术 laser eye surgery

4　口译实战

4.1　英译汉

（一）Ophthalmology 眼科[1]

Ophthalmologists are physicians specializing in the comprehensive medical and surgical care of the eyes and vision. Optometrists provide vision tests, prescribe lenses and treat certain eye conditions. Opticians fit eyeglasses and contact lenses. Ophthalmic medical assistants help physicians examine and treat patients.

眼科医生是专门从事眼睛和视力相关疾病的内外科综合治疗的医生。验光师从事视力检查，开具配镜处方，进行某些眼部疾病的治疗。配镜师负责配制框架眼镜和隐形眼镜。眼科医疗助理帮助医生检查和治疗患者。

Ophthalmologists are the practitioners medically trained to diagnose and treat all eye and visual problems and provide treatment and prevention of medical disorders of the eye including surgery. Ophthalmology encompasses many different subspecialties, including strabismus/pediatric ophthalmology, glaucoma, neuro-ophthalmology, retina/uveitis, anterior segment/cornea, oculoplastics/orbit, and ocular oncology.

眼科医生受过专业医疗训练，可以诊断和治疗所有眼部疾病，解决视力问题，从事包括手术在内的眼部疾病治疗和预防的专业人员。眼科有许多不同的亚专科，包括斜视/小儿眼科、青光眼、神经眼科、视网膜/葡萄膜炎、眼前节/角膜、眼整形/眼眶和眼肿瘤科。

To become a general ophthalmologist, the specialty requires four years of postgraduate specialty training after the completion of a medical degree (MD). This requirement includes a three-year residency in ophthalmology in an approved surgical residency program, following at least a one-year internship. An ophthalmology residency involves training in the fundamentals of all the above subspecialty fields of ophthalmology.

This training period prepares you for a thriving practice (academic or private) with surgical cases that involve fascinating and challenging microsurgery. Ophthalmic surgery requires exquisite hand-eye coordination and surgical skill. As ophthalmologists, one routinely uses sutures that can't easily be visualized with the unaided eye. Cataract surgery and basic glaucoma surgery are two of the more common procedures an ophthalmologist routinely performs that requires such skill. One can further subspecialize after finishing an ophthalmology residency. This requires one to two years of additional training.

Strabismus/pediatric ophthalmology mainly deals with eye diseases in

要成为一名普通眼科医生，需要在完成医学学位（MD）后接受四年的毕业后专科培训。此要求包括在至少一年的实习期之后，按获得批准的外科住院医师计划完成三年眼科住院医师培训。眼科住院医师培训涉及上述所有眼科的亚专科基础知识的学习。

这一培训会为你在成熟机构（学术机构或私人机构）完成令人难忘且具有挑战性的显微外科手术案例做好准备。眼科手术需要精湛的手眼协调和手术技巧。眼科医生经常使用肉眼无法轻易看到的缝合线。两种常见的眼科手术——白内障手术和基本的青光眼手术，就需要此类技能。眼科医生在完成眼科住院医师培训后，还可以进一步细分专业。这需要一到两年的额外培训。

斜视/小儿眼科主要治疗儿童眼病，可以开展所有眼内手术以及斜视

children, involving all intraocular surgery as well as strabismus (crossed eyes) surgery, which incorporate detailed eye muscle surgery. Glaucoma is an area of ophthalmology that focuses on medical and surgical treatment of diseases that result in optic nerve damage and visual field loss.

Neuro-ophthalmology deals with the eye as it relates to neurological disease. It is a complex and intricate subspecialty that requires knowledge of the visual pathways, eye-movement patterns, optic nerve disease, and systemic neurological diseases with visual manifestations. Retina/uveitis concentrates on diseases, often systemic or inflammatory, involving the retina and vitreous (posterior aspect of the eye). This includes surgical and laser treatment of diseases such as retinal detachments, diabetic retinopathy, and others. It also requires proficiency of challenging microsurgical techniques.

In addition to routine cataract surgery, cornea/anterior segment specialists are skilled in corneal transplantation and one of the most exciting areas of medicine, refractive surgery (vision correction). Another

（斗鸡眼）手术，包括细致的眼肌手术。青光眼科是专注于导致视神经损伤和视野丧失的各类疾病的内外科治疗的眼科领域。

神经眼科专注于与神经系统疾病有关的眼病。这是一个错综复杂的亚专科，需要了解视觉通路、眼球运动模式、视神经疾病和具有视觉表现的系统性神经疾病。视网膜/葡萄膜炎通常涉及系统性或炎症性疾病，影响视网膜和玻璃体（眼睛后部）。医生要对视网膜脱落、糖尿病视网膜病变等疾病进行手术和激光治疗，还需要熟练掌握具有挑战性的显微外科技术。

除了常规的白内障手术，角膜/眼前节专家还擅长角膜移植和最令人兴奋的医学技术之一——屈光手术（视力矫正）。眼科的另一个亚专科是眼科整形和重建手术，该亚专科培训包括面部、眼眶、眼睑和泪道系统的美

subspecialty field of ophthalmology is ophthalmic plastic and reconstructive surgery. The fellowship of this ophthalmology encompasses aesthetic, plastic and reconstructive surgery of the face, orbit, eyelids, and lacrimal system. This includes learning techniques to remove tumors in the orbit, and on the surface of the eye, such as conjunctival melanoma, as well as repairing bony fractures of the periorbital area and face.

容、整形和重建手术，包括学习去除眼眶和眼睛表面肿瘤（如结膜黑色素瘤）的技术，以及修复眶周区域和面部的骨折。

（二）Cataract 白内障[2-3]

A cataract is a cloudy area in the lens of your eye. Cataracts are very common as you get older. In fact, more than half of all Americans aged 80 or older either have cataracts or have had surgery to get rid of cataracts. At first, you may not notice that you have a cataract. But over time, cataracts can make your vision blurry, hazy, or less colorful. You may have trouble reading or doing other everyday activities. The good news is that surgery can get rid of cataracts. Cataract surgery is safe and corrects vision problems caused by cataracts.

白内障是眼睛晶状体中出现的浑浊区域改变。随着年龄增大，白内障会十分常见。事实上，在所有80岁或更年长的美国人当中，有一半以上的人都患有白内障，或者已经做过手术来消除白内障。起初，你可能没有注意到你有白内障。但是随着时间推移，白内障会使你的视线变得模糊、朦胧，看东西时色彩变淡。你可能在阅读或做其他日常活动时遇到困难。好消息是手术可以消除白内障。白内障手术是安全的，并能解决白内障引起的视力问题。

Most cataracts are age-related—they happen because of normal changes in

大多数白内障都与年龄有关，是眼睛随着年龄的增长而出现的正常变

your eyes as you get older. But you can get cataracts for other reasons—for example, an eye injury or surgery for another eye problem (like glaucoma). No matter what type of cataract you have, the treatment is always surgery. You might not have any symptoms at first, when cataracts are mild. But as cataracts grow, they can cause changes in your vision. For example, your vision is cloudy or blurry. Colors look faded. You can't see well at night. Lamps, sunlight, or headlights seem too bright. You see a halo around lights. You see double (this sometimes goes away as the cataract gets bigger). And you have to change the prescription for your glasses often. These symptoms can be a sign of other eye problems, too. Be sure to talk to your eye doctor if you have any of these problems. Over time, cataracts can lead to vision loss.

Talk with your eye doctor about whether surgery is right for you. Most eye doctors suggest considering cataract surgery when your cataracts begin to affect your quality of life or interfere with your ability to perform normal daily activities, such as reading or driving at night. Cataract surgery involves removing the

化。但是你也可能会因为其他原因患上白内障，例如因为眼外伤或做了其他眼科手术（比如青光眼手术）。不管你患有什么类型的白内障，治疗方案都是手术。起初，当白内障较轻微时，你可能没有任何症状。但是随着白内障的发展，它会引起视力的变化。例如，视线朦胧或模糊，颜色看起来变淡，晚上会视力不好，灯、阳光或大灯看起来会很刺眼，在灯光周围会看到光晕，出现重影（这种情况有时会随着白内障的增大而消失），得经常换眼镜。这些症状也可能是其他眼部问题的征兆。如果有任何问题，一定要和眼科医生沟通。随着时间推移，白内障会导致视力下降。

与眼科医生讨论手术是否适合你。当白内障开始影响你的生活质量或干扰你正常的日常活动（例如夜间阅读或开车）时，大多数眼科医生会建议考虑进行白内障手术。白内障手术要摘除混浊晶体并用透明的人工晶状体替换。人工晶状体又称为眼内透镜，被置于与自然晶状体相同的位置。它

clouded lens and replacing it with a clear artificial lens. The artificial lens, called an intraocular lens, is positioned in the same place as your natural lens. It remains a permanent part of your eye. For some people, other eye problems prohibit the use of an artificial lens. In these situations, once the cataract is removed, vision may be corrected with eyeglasses or contact lenses.

Cataract surgery is generally done on an outpatient basis, which means you won't need to stay in a hospital after the surgery. During cataract surgery, your eye doctor uses local anesthetic to numb the area around your eye, but you usually stay awake during the procedure. Cataract surgery is generally safe, but it carries a risk of infection and bleeding. Cataract surgery also increases the risk of retinal detachment. After the procedure, you'll have some discomfort for a few days. Healing generally occurs within eight weeks. If you need cataract surgery in both eyes, your doctor will schedule surgery to remove the cataract in the second eye after you've healed from the first surgery.

将成为眼睛的永久部分。对于某些人来说，其他的眼睛问题会令其无法使用人工晶体。在这种情况下，摘除白内障后，可以佩戴框架眼镜或隐形眼镜来矫正视力。

白内障手术通常在门诊进行，这意味着手术后无须住院。在白内障手术期间，眼科医生会使用局部麻醉剂麻醉眼周区域，但你通常能在手术过程中保持清醒。白内障手术一般是安全的，但也有感染和出血的风险。白内障手术还会增加视网膜脱落的风险。你会在手术后的几天内感到不适。八周内一般能够痊愈。如果你的双眼都需要进行白内障手术，医生会在你第一次手术痊愈后再安排去除第二只眼睛白内障的手术。

（三）Glaucoma 青光眼[4-5]

Glaucoma is a group of diseases that affect the optic nerve, which transmits images from the eye to the brain. Glaucoma often results from high intraocular pressure. The condition causes vision loss and can lead to blindness. In a healthy eye, a clear fluid (aqueous humor) fills the front of the eye and normally flows in and out through channels where the iris and cornea meet.

Because glaucoma often results from high intraocular pressure, anything that blocks or slows the flow of this fluid increases pressure. Glaucoma has the following major types. Open-angle glaucoma: More than 90 percent of adults have glaucoma of this type. In open-angle glaucoma, fluid pressure inside the eye increases slowly over a long time, and patients often do not notice a change. As pressure on the optic nerve increases, it can damage the nerve and cause vision loss such as blind spots.

Angle-closure glaucoma: This type occurs when the fluid suddenly becomes blocked, leading to a quick, dramatic pressure increase inside the eye. Angle-closure glaucoma usually causes

青光眼是一组影响视神经的疾病，而视神经负责将图像从眼睛传输到大脑。青光眼常由高眼压引起，会导致视力下降，并可能导致失明。在健康的眼睛里，透明液体（房水）充满了眼睛的前部，通常通过虹膜和角膜交汇处的通道流入流出。

因为青光眼通常由高眼压引起，任何阻碍或减缓这种液体流动的东西都会导致眼压增加。青光眼有如下主要类型：开角型青光眼。超过90%的成人青光眼患者是这种类型。开角型青光眼患者眼内的液体压力在很长一段时间内缓慢增加，患者通常不会注意到任何变化。视神经压力的增加会损伤神经，造成盲点等视力损伤。

闭角型青光眼。当房水突然阻塞并导致眼内压力迅速急剧升高时，就会发生这种类型的青光眼。闭角型青光眼通常会引起立即的、明显的症状，如严重眼痛和视力模糊。这种类型的

immediate, noticeable symptoms such as severe eye pain and blurry vision. This type of glaucoma is a medical emergency and requires immediate treatment to prevent blindness.

青光眼情况紧急，需要立即治疗，以防止失明。

Low- or normal-tension glaucoma: Some people with normal eye pressure can develop this type of glaucoma, a form of open-angle glaucoma. Congenital glaucoma: Some babies are born with a defect in the eye that slows the normal fluid drainage. Congenital glaucoma usually causes noticeable symptoms and signs very early. Prompt surgery provides children with an excellent chance for good vision.

低眼压或正常眼压青光眼。一些眼压正常的人会形成这种类型的青光眼，它是一种开角型青光眼。先天性青光眼。有些婴儿出生时眼睛有缺陷，会减慢正常的液体排出。先天性青光眼通常很早就会引起明显的症状和体征，及时手术能为儿童提供拥有良好视力的良机。

Symptoms of glaucoma can include slow loss of peripheral (side) vision, sudden, severe pain in one eye, reduced or cloudy vision, nausea or vomiting, visions of halos around lights, redness or swelling of the eye, sensitivity to light and cloudy appearance in the front of the eye.

青光眼的症状包括周边（侧面）视力的缓慢丧失，单眼的突然剧烈疼痛，视力减退或视力模糊，恶心或呕吐，感觉灯光周围有光晕，眼睛红肿，对光线敏感，以及眼睛前部出现混浊。

4.2 汉译英

（一）年龄相关性黄斑变性 Age-related Macular Degeneration（AMD）[5-6]

黄斑变性，通常被称为年龄相关性黄斑变性，是一种与老化相关的眼

Macular degeneration, often called age-related macular degeneration（AMD），

部疾病，导致锐利和中心视力受损。中心视力对于清晰地看到物体以及进行阅读、驾驶等日常活动来说都是必需的。年龄相关性黄斑变性会影响黄斑，黄斑是视网膜的中心部分，可以让眼睛看到非常细微的细节。年龄相关性黄斑变性有干性和湿性两种类型。

湿性年龄相关性黄斑变性是指视网膜后面的异常血管开始在黄斑下生长，最终导致血液和液体渗出。这些血管的出血、渗出和瘢痕会造成损伤，并导致中心视力迅速降低。湿性年龄相关性黄斑变性的早期症状是直线看上去呈波浪状。

黄斑随着年龄的增长而逐渐变薄，会出现干性年龄相关性黄斑变性，使中心视力逐渐下降。干性年龄相关性黄斑变性更常见，占年龄相关性黄斑变性病例的70%～90%，其进展比湿性年龄相关性黄斑变性慢。随着时间推移以及黄斑功能的减弱，患眼的中心视力将逐渐丧失。

干性年龄相关性黄斑变性通常会影响双眼。干性年龄相关性黄斑变性

is an eye disorder associated with aging and results in damaging sharp and central vision. Central vision is needed for seeing objects clearly and for common daily tasks such as reading and driving. AMD affects the macula, the central part the retina that allows the eye to see fine details. There are two forms of AMD—wet and dry.

Wet AMD occurs when abnormal blood vessel behind the retina start to grow under the macula, ultimately leading to blood and fluid leakage. Bleeding, leaking, and scarring from these blood vessels cause damage and lead to rapid central vision loss. An early symptom of wet AMD is that straight lines appear wavy.

Dry AMD occurs when the macula thins overtime as part of aging process, gradually blurring central vision. The dry form is more common and accounts for 70% - 90% of cases of AMD and it progresses more slowly than the wet form. Over time, as less of the macula functions, central vision is gradually lost in the affected eye.

Dry AMD generally affects both eyes. One of the most common early

最常见的早期症状之一是玻璃膜疣。玻璃膜疣是视网膜下微小的黄色或白色沉积物。常见于 60 岁及以上的人群。小玻璃膜疣的存在是正常的，不会导致视力下降。然而，较大和较多的玻璃膜疣会增加患上严重干性年龄相关性黄斑变性或湿性年龄相关性黄斑变性的风险。

据估计，40 岁及以上的美国人中有 180 万人患有年龄相关性黄斑变性，另外 730 万有较大玻璃膜疣的人有患上年龄相关性黄斑变性的巨大风险。据估计，到 2020 年，年龄相关性黄斑变性患者人数将达到 295 万。年龄相关性黄斑变性是导致 65 岁及以上人群永久性阅读障碍和精细或近距离视力受损的主要原因。

（二）糖尿病视网膜病变 Diabetic Retinopathy [7]

糖尿病视网膜病变是一种可导致糖尿病患者视力损伤和失明的眼部疾病。它影响视网膜的血管。如果你有糖尿病，那要确保每年至少做一次全面的散瞳检查。糖尿病视网膜病变一开始可能没有任何症状，但及早发现可以帮助你采取措施保护视力。控制糖尿病——通过运动、健康饮食、吃

signs of dry AMD is drusen. Drusen are tiny yellow or white deposits under the retina. They are often found in people aged 60 and older. The presence of small drusen is normal and does not cause vision loss. However, the presence of large and more numerous drusen raises the risk of developing advanced dry AMD or wet AMD.

It is estimated that 1.8 million Americans aged 40 years and older are affected by AMD and an additional 7.3 million with large drusen are at substantial risk of developing AMD. The number of people with AMD is estimated to reach 2.95 million in 2020. AMD is the leading cause of permanent impairment of reading and fine or close-up vision among people aged 65 and older.

Diabetic retinopathy is an eye condition that can cause vision loss and blindness in people who have diabetes. It affects blood vessels in the retina. If you have diabetes, it's important for you to get a comprehensive dilated eye exam at least once a year. Diabetic retinopathy may not have any symptoms at first, but

药，也可以帮助预防或延缓视力下降。

糖尿病视网膜病变早期通常没有任何症状。有些人会注意到他们的视力发生变化，比如阅读困难或看不到远处的物体。这些变化可能时有时无。在疾病的后期，视网膜中的血管开始流血至玻璃体（眼睛中央的胶状液体）。如果发生这种情况，你可能会看到像蜘蛛网的黑色浮动斑点或条纹。有时，斑点会自行清除，但立即接受治疗很重要。如果不治疗，出血可能再次发生，情况会恶化或造成瘢痕。

任何类型的糖尿病患者都可能患上糖尿病视网膜病变，包括 1 型、2 型和妊娠期糖尿病患者。患糖尿病的时间越长，风险就越大。超过五分之二的美国糖尿病患者出现了某个阶段的糖尿病视网膜病变。好消息是你可以通过控制糖尿病来降低患糖尿病

finding it early can help you take steps to protect your vision. Managing your diabetes—by staying physically active, eating healthy, and taking your medicine—can also help you prevent or delay vision loss.

The early stages of diabetic retinopathy usually don't have any symptoms. Some people notice changes in their vision, like trouble reading or seeing faraway objects. These changes may come and go. In later stages of the disease, blood vessels in the retina start to bleed into the vitreous (gel-like fluid in the center of the eye). If this happens, you may see dark, floating spots or streaks that look like cobwebs. Sometimes, the spots clear up on their own—but it's important to get treatment right away. Without treatment, the bleeding can happen again, get worse, or cause scarring.

Anyone with any kind of diabetes can get diabetic retinopathy, including people with type 1, type 2, and gestational diabetes. The longer you have diabetes the higher your risk of getting diabetic retinopathy is. More than 2 in 5 Americans with diabetes have

视网膜病变的风险。

患妊娠期糖尿病的妇女患糖尿病视网膜病变的风险很高。糖尿病视网膜病变源于糖尿病引起的高血糖。随着时间的推移，血液中的糖分过多会损害视网膜。视网膜是眼睛中检测光线并通过视神经向大脑发送信号的组织。

（三）屈光不正 Refractive Error[8]

屈光不正是一种视力问题，使眼睛很难看清。当眼睛形状使光线无法正确聚焦在视网膜上时，就会发生屈光不正。屈光不正是最常见的视力问题。如果你有屈光不正，眼科医生可以帮你配框架眼镜或隐形眼镜来帮助你看清楚。

有4种常见的屈光不正：近视使远处的物体看起来模糊；远视使近处的物体看起来模糊；散光使远处和近处的物体都看起来模糊或扭曲；老视使中老年人很难近距离观察事物。最

some stage of diabetic retinopathy. The good news is that you can lower your risk of developing diabetic retinopathy by controlling your diabetes.

Women who develop gestational diabetes are at high risk for getting diabetic retinopathy. Diabetic retinopathy is caused by high blood sugar due to diabetes. Over time, having too much sugar in your blood can damage your retina—the part of your eye that detects light and sends signals to your brain through optic nerve.

Refractive errors are a type of vision problem that makes it hard to see clearly. They happen when the shape of your eye keeps light from focusing correctly on your retina. Refractive errors are the most common type of vision problem. If you have a refractive error, your eye doctor can prescribe eyeglasses or contact lenses to help you see clearly.

There are 4 common types of refractive errors: Nearsightedness (myopia) makes far-away objects look blurry. Farsightedness (hyperopia) makes nearby objects look blurry. Astigmatism can make far-away and

常见的症状是视力模糊。其他症状包括复视、视力模糊、强光周围看见眩光或光晕、眯眼、头痛、眼睛疲劳以及阅读或看电脑时无法集中注意力。

有些人可能不会注意到屈光不正的症状。定期进行眼科检查很重要，这样你的眼科医生就能确保你看得尽可能清楚。如果你已经戴了框架眼镜或隐形眼镜，但仍然有这些症状，那你可能需要换新的了。如果你的视力现在就有问题，那可以和眼科医生谈谈，做个眼科检查。

任何人都可能出现屈光不正，但如果你的家人戴框架眼镜或隐形眼镜，你的风险会更高。大多数类型的屈光不正，如近视，通常始于儿童时期。老视常见于 40 岁及以上的成年人。屈光不正可由眼球长度、角膜形状问题和晶状体老化引起。眼科医生可以用框架眼镜或隐形眼镜矫正屈光不正，或通过手术修复屈光不正。

nearby objects look blurry or distorted. Presbyopia makes it hard for middle-aged and older adults to see things up close. The most common symptom is blurry vision. Other symptoms include double vision, hazy vision, seeing a glare or halo around bright lights, squinting, headaches, eye strain, and trouble focusing when reading or looking at a computer.

Some people may not notice the symptoms of refractive errors. It's important to get eye exams regularly, so your eye doctor can make sure you're seeing as clearly as possible. If you wear glasses or contact lenses and still have these symptoms, you might need a new prescription. Talk to your eye doctor and get an eye exam if you are having trouble with your vision.

Anyone can have refractive errors, but you're at higher risk if you have family members who wear glasses or contact lenses. Most types of refractive errors, like nearsightedness, usually start in childhood. Presbyopia is common in adults aged 40 and older. Refractive errors can be caused by eyeball length, problems with the shape of the cornea and aging of the lens. Eye doctors can correct refractive errors with glasses or contact lenses, or fix the refractive error with surgery.

佩戴眼镜是矫正屈光不正的最简单、最安全的方法。眼科医生会挑选合适的镜片，让你获得尽可能清晰的视力。将隐形眼镜贴在眼球表面也能矫正屈光不正。眼科医生会为你配合适的隐形眼镜，并向你展示如何安全地清洗和佩戴隐形眼镜。某些类型的手术，如激光眼科手术，可以改变角膜的形状以修复屈光不正。您的眼科医生可以帮助您确定手术是否适合您。

Wearing eyeglasses is the simplest and safest way to correct refractive errors. Your eye doctor will prescribe the right eyeglass lenses to give you the clearest possible vision. Contact lenses sit on the surface of your eyes and correct refractive errors. Your eye doctor will fit you for the right lenses and show you how to clean and wear them safely. Some types of surgery, like laser eye surgery, can change the shape of your cornea to fix refractive errors. Your eye doctor can help you decide if surgery is right for you.

5 口译注释与学习资源

5.1 口译注释

镜片种类

矫正老视（老花眼，presbyopia），有三种镜片可选择：（1）单光镜（single vision lens），单光镜只能用于看近处或阅读，看远处时需要摘掉眼镜；（2）双光镜（bifocal lens），双光镜可以用同一副眼镜看远、看近，但是在配镜之后可能会出现中间视力模糊的情况；（3）渐进多焦镜（varifocal/multifocal lens），通过渐进多焦镜同一个镜片的不同区域可以看到近、中、远距离的物体，该镜片能解决双光镜中间视力模糊的问题，是目前为止比较理想的矫正老视的方法。

5.2 学习资源

登录中国大学 MOOC（慕课），学习"医疗口译"课程中"眼科"的口译实战示范视频。补充主题包括：（1）Dry Eye Disease：Overview 干眼症：概览；（2）Presbyopia 老视；（3）Keratitis 角膜炎；（4）Intraocular Lens（IOL）Implant 人工晶体植入；（5）Myopia 近视；（6）Diabetic Eye Disease 糖尿病眼病；（7）Amblyopia 弱视。另外可以关注美国卫生研究院、美国眼科学会（American Academy of Ophthalmology）、美国外科医师学会（American College of Surgeons）、妙佑医疗国际、得克萨斯大学西南医学中心（University of Texas Southwestern Medical Center）等机构官网关于眼科和相关疾病的介绍。

参考文献

［1］ American Academy of Ophthalmology. (2021，April 7). *What is an ophthalmologist?*. Retrieved November 13，2021，from https：//www. aao. org/eye-health/tips-prevention/what-is-ophthalmologist.

［2］ U. S. Department of Health and Human Services. (n. d.). *Cataracts*. National Eye Institute. Retrieved November 13，2021，from https：//www. nei. nih. gov/learn-about-eye-health/eye-conditions-and-diseases/cataracts.

［3］ Johns Hopkins Medicine. (n. d.). *Cataracts*. Retrieved November 13，2021，from https：//www. hopkinsmedicine. org/health/conditions-and-diseases/cataracts.

［4］ Cleveland Clinic. (n. d.). Glaucoma: *Causes，symptoms，types，treatment & prevention*. Retrieved November 13，2021，from https：//my. clevelandclinic. org/health/diseases/4212 − glaucoma.

［5］ Centers for Disease Control and Prevention. (2020，June 3). *Common eye disorders and diseases*. Retrieved November 13，2021，from https：//www. cdc. gov/visionhealth/basics/ced/index. html.

［6］ U. S. Department of Health and Human Services. National Eye Institute. (n. d.). *Macular edema*. Retrieved November 13，2021，from https：//www. nei. nih. gov/learn-about-eye-health/eye-conditions-and-diseases/macular-edema.

［7］ U. S. Department of Health and Human Services. National Eye Institute. (n. d.). *Diabetic retinopathy*. Retrieved November 13，2021，from https：//www. nei. nih. gov/learn-about-eye-health/eye-conditions-and-diseases/diabetic-retinopathy.

［8］ U. S. Department of Health and Human Services. National Eye Institute. (n. d.). *Refractive errors*. Retrieved November 13，2021，from https：//www. nei. nih. gov/learn-about-eye-health/eye-conditions-and-diseases/refractive-errors.

第十五章

耳鼻喉科

1　导读

本章的重点为口译技巧之文化调解和耳鼻喉科的 6 篇"口译实战"练习。口译实战练习中英译汉、汉译英各 3 篇，内容涵盖耳鼻喉科、慢性鼻窦炎、听力损失（耳聋）、睡眠呼吸暂停、鼻炎和声带病变。请结合本章口译技巧练习 6 篇口译实战文本。

2　口译技巧——文化调解

口译是面对面的跨文化交际活动，受到各种社会文化和非语言因素的影响和制约。因此，译员在交际中除了需要注意语言和文化差异，还要遵守非语言和职业行为准则，才能良好地辅助完成交际的任务。以下是口译员在文化调解过程中需要注意的一些方面：

（1）身体语言。非语言交际行为包括姿态动作、目光接触、面部表情、身体距离、衣着打扮等。在不同文化中，非语言交际方式具有很大差异。例如，在谈话时，西方人习惯注视着对方，这被认为是诚实和尊重的表现；而东方人则会避免目光直视，因为看着对方的眼睛可能会令对方感到尴尬。在中国，人们竖起拇指表示"好"；而在美国，将拇指朝上可能表示要求搭便车。东方人比较含蓄，感情不容易外露；而西方人往往有着更丰富的面部表情。多数西方人在交谈时不喜欢靠得太近；而中国人可能觉得身体偶尔接触一下才显得亲近。

（2）准时守约。译员参加会见、会谈或谈判翻译时，应该至少提前半个小时到达指定场地，不能以任何理由迟到或缺席，因为涉外活动没有译员就无法开展。译员如果担心迟到，就早出发。如果有万不得已的原因，必须通知雇主，以便寻找替补译员。

（3）不犯禁忌。译员应尊重不同国家和民族特有的风俗习惯。例如，穆斯林不吃猪肉，印度教徒不吃牛肉，印度和印度尼西亚人不用左手传递东西，西方人可能不喜欢吃内脏。宴请西方人时尽量避免他们忌讳的数字"13"，如 13 日、13 楼、13 号包厢等。

（4）举止得体。译员听话时要注意聆听，做好口译笔记，说话时态度要自然真诚，语气要亲切和蔼，举止要落落大方，肢体语言不可过于夸张，遇急事也尽量不要慌张，不要放声大笑或高声喊人。

（5）注重仪表。译员在工作之前，应刷牙、梳头、刮脸、修剪指甲，女译员可化点淡妆。着装要整洁大方，与双方嘉宾的着装尽量保持一致或更加保守。不可随手乱扔果皮纸屑、随地吐痰；打喷嚏时说"Excuse me"，别人打喷嚏时说"Bless you"；工作餐不要吃大蒜等气味浓烈的食品。

（6）细致入微。译员可以随身带些小瓶装水或小包装零食，旅途中可以询问客人是否需要。译员平时可准备一些社交话术，避免在晚宴、冷餐会等场合出现冷场。译员的工作被赞扬和肯定时，不必受之有愧，直接回应"Thank you"或者"I appreciate your kind words"。实在需要谦虚，可说"I'm just doing my job"。

总而言之，译员必须多实践，不断发现和总结技巧和方法，全面提高自身修养和综合素质，才能掌握并熟练运用跨文化交际技能。

3 口译词汇

3.1 英译汉

（一）Otolaryngology 耳鼻喉科

otolaryngology-head and neck surgery 耳鼻喉及头颈外科

otolaryngologist（ear, nose, and throat doctor, ENT）耳鼻喉科医生

American Academy of Otolaryngology 美国耳鼻喉科学会

hearing loss 听力损失、耳聋

ear infection 耳部感染

balance disorder 平衡障碍

ear noise（tinnitus）耳鸣

nerve pain, and facial and cranial nerve disorder 神经疼痛以及面部和颅神经疾病

congenital（birth）disorder of the outer and inner ear 外耳和内耳的先天性疾病

care of the nasal cavity and sinuss 鼻腔和鼻窦的护理

allergy, sinusitis, smell disorder 过敏、鼻窦炎、嗅觉障碍

polyp 息肉

nasal obstruction due to a deviated septum 鼻中隔偏曲引起的鼻塞

correct the appearance of the nose（rhinoplasty surgery）矫正鼻子的外观（鼻整形术）

larynx 喉部

upper aero-digestive tract or esophagus 上消化道或食道

voice and swallowing disorder 构音和吞咽障碍

benign and malignant（cancerous）tumor 良性和恶性（癌性）肿瘤

facial trauma 面部创伤

deformity of the face 面部畸形

cosmetic plastic and reconstructive surgery 美容整形和重建手术

American Board of Otolaryngology 美国耳鼻喉科委员会

specialty training 专科培训

fellowship（亚）专科培训

（二）Chronic Sinusitis 慢性鼻窦炎

long-term inflammation of the sinuses 鼻窦的长期炎症

drain/drainage 引流

mucus 黏液

pus 脓液

tissue swelling caused by allergy 过敏引起的组织肿胀

increased sinus pressure and facial pain 鼻窦压力增加和面部疼痛

nasal swelling 鼻肿胀

allergies to inhaled dust, mold, pollen, or the spores of fungi 对吸入的灰尘、霉菌、花粉或真菌孢子过敏

histamine 组胺

inner lining of the nose 鼻子内壁

sinus drainage 鼻窦引流

nasal tumor and nasal fracture 鼻肿瘤和鼻骨折

nasal passage 鼻腔

people with asthma, cystic fibrosis, or immune system problems 患有哮喘、囊性纤维化或免疫系统问题的人

nasal corticosteroids 鼻用皮质类固醇

nasal spray 鼻腔喷雾剂

rinse with a solution of saline mixed with drops of budesonide 使用混合了布地奈德滴剂的生理盐水溶液进行冲洗

use nasal mist of the solution 使用溶液性鼻雾

saline nasal irrigation 生理盐水鼻腔冲洗

irritant and allergen 刺激物和过敏原

oral or injected 口服或注射

aspirin desensitization treatment 阿司匹林脱敏治疗

antifungal treatment 抗真菌治疗

lessen congestion 减轻充血

（三）Hearing Loss 听力损失（耳聋）

confused，unresponsive，or uncooperative 犯糊涂、没反应或不合作

hearing aids 助听器

inner ear or auditory nerve 内耳或听神经

sensorineural hearing loss 感音神经性听力损失（聋）

conductive hearing loss 传导性听力损失（聋）

earwax buildup 耳垢堆积

fluid or a punctured eardrum 积液或鼓膜穿孔

3.2 汉译英

（一）睡眠呼吸暂停 Sleep Apnea

阻塞性睡眠呼吸暂停 obstructive sleep apnea

中枢性睡眠呼吸暂停 central sleep apnea

打鼾或气喘 snoring or gasping

呼吸减少或消失 reduced or absent breathing

呼吸暂停事件 apnoea events

心房颤动（房颤）atrial fibrillation

胰腺癌、肾癌和皮肤癌 pancreatic，renal，and skin cancers

语言和视觉空间记忆 verbal and visuospatial memory

痴呆 dementia

动脉粥样硬化 atherosclerosis

青光眼 glaucoma

圆锥角膜 keratoconus

葡萄糖不耐受 glucose intolerance

发作次数 number of episodes

持续正压通气机 continuous positive air pressure（CPAP）machines

（二）鼻炎 Rhinitis

鼻塞、流鼻涕、打喷嚏和瘙痒 nasal congestion, runny nose, sneezing, and itching

急性鼻炎 acute rhinitis

过敏性或季节性鼻炎 allergic or seasonal rhinitis

非过敏性或全年性鼻炎 nonallergic or year-round rhinitis

过敏原 allergen

花粉 pollen

尘螨 dust mite

蟑螂排泄物 cockroach waste

动物皮屑 animal dander

烟雾和气味 fume and odor

局部喷鼻剂 topical nose spray

嘴呼吸 breathing through the mouth

加热、过滤或加湿空气 warm, filter, or humidify the air

抗组胺药 antihistamine

减充血剂 decongestant

（三）声带病变 Vocal Cord Lesion

声腔病变 vocal fold lesion

良性（非癌性）增生 benign (noncancerous) growth

结节、息肉和囊肿 nodule, polyp and cyst

反复过度使用或误用 repetitive overuse or misuse

歌者结节或小结 singer's nodule or node

血管化、血供丰富 vascularized

水疱 blister

息肉样心膜炎 polypoid carditis

囊 sac

黏液潴留囊肿 mucus retention cyst

表皮样（或皮脂腺）囊肿 epidermoid (or sebaceous) cyst

上呼吸道感染或喉炎 upper respiratory infection or laryngitis

声音嘶哑、气息声 hoarseness, breathiness

多音、音域丧失 multiple tones, loss of vocal range

声带疲劳或失声 vocal fatigue or loss of voice

难治性病变 refractory lesion

戒烟 smoking cessation

嗓音疗法 voice therapy

4 口译实战

4.1 英译汉

（一）Otolaryngology 耳鼻喉科[1]

Otolaryngology is a medical specialty which is focused on the ears, nose, and throat. It is also called otolaryngology-head and neck surgery because the specialists are trained in both medicine and surgery. An otolaryngologist is often called an ear, nose, and throat doctor, or an ENT for short. This medical specialty dates back to the 19th century, when doctors recognized that the head and neck contained a series of interconnected systems.

耳鼻喉科是专注于耳朵、鼻子和喉咙的医学专科。它也被称为耳鼻喉及头颈外科，因为该专科医生需要接受内科和外科的培训。耳鼻喉科医生通常被称为耳鼻喉医生，或简称 ENT。这个医学专科可以追溯到 19 世纪，当时医生们就认识到头部和颈部包含了一系列相互关联的系统。

Doctors developed techniques and tools for examining and treating problems of the head and neck, eventually forming a medical specialty. According to the American Academy of Otolaryngology, it is the oldest medical specialty in the United States. Otolaryngologists differ from many physicians in that they are qualified to perform many types of surgery

医生们还开发了检查和治疗头颈部问题的技术和工具，最终形成了该医学专科。根据美国耳鼻喉科学会的说法，它是美国最古老的医学专科。耳鼻喉科医生与其他医生的不同之处在于他们可以对头颈部脆弱而复杂的组织进行多种类型的手术。

on the delicate and complex tissues of the head and neck.

What do otolaryngologists treat? Ear：Otolaryngologists are trained in the medical and surgical treatment of hearing loss, ear infections, balance disorders, ear noise (tinnitus), nerve pain, and facial and cranial nerve disorders. They also manage congenital (birth) disorders of the outer and inner ear.

Nose：Care of the nasal cavity and sinuses is one of the primary skills of otolaryngologists. Otolaryngologists diagnose, manage and treat allergies, sinusitis, smell disorders, polyps, and nasal obstruction due to a deviated septum. They can also correct the appearance of the nose (rhinoplasty surgery).

Throat：Otolaryngologists have expertise in managing diseases of the larynx and the upper aero-digestive tract or esophagus, including voice and swallowing disorders. Head and Neck：In the head and neck area, otolaryngologists are trained to treat infectious diseases, both benign and malignant (cancerous) tumors, facial

耳鼻喉科医生治疗什么？耳：耳鼻喉科医生接受过听力损失、耳部感染、平衡障碍、耳鸣、神经疼痛以及面部和颅神经疾病的内科和外科治疗培训。他们还能治疗外耳和内耳的先天性疾病。

鼻：鼻腔和鼻窦的护理是耳鼻喉科医生的主要技能之一。耳鼻喉科医生诊断、管理和治疗过敏、鼻窦炎、嗅觉障碍、息肉和鼻中隔偏曲引起的鼻塞。他们还可以矫正鼻子的外观（鼻整形术）。

喉：耳鼻喉科医生在管理喉部，上呼吸道、消化道，以及食道疾病，包括构音和吞咽障碍方面具有专业知识。头颈：在头部和颈部区域，耳鼻喉科医生接受过治疗感染性疾病、良性和恶性（癌性）肿瘤、面部创伤和面部畸形的培训。他们还能进行美容整形和重建手术。

trauma, and deformities of the face. They can also perform both cosmetic plastic and reconstructive surgery.

How are otolaryngologist-head and neck surgeons trained? An otolaryngologist is ready to start practicing after completing up to 15 years of college and post-graduate training. To receive certification from the American Board of Otolaryngology, individuals must first complete college, medical school, and at least five years of specialty training. Next, the physician must pass the American Board of Otolaryngology examination. Some then pursue a one- or two-year fellowship for more training in a subspecialty area.

如何培训耳鼻喉及头颈外科医生？耳鼻喉科医生要在完成长达15年的大学和毕业后培训之后才能开始执业。要获得美国耳鼻喉科委员会的认证，必须首先完成大学和医学院的学习，接受至少5年的专科培训。接下来，必须通过美国耳鼻喉科委员会的考试。然后，有些人会继续进行一年或两年的亚专科培训，以便在亚专业领域接受更多训练。

（二）Chronic Sinusitis 慢性鼻窦炎[2-3]

Chronic sinusitis is a long-term inflammation of the sinuses. The sinuses are moist air spaces behind the bones of the upper face—between the eyes and behind the forehead, nose and cheeks. Normally, the sinuses drain through small openings into the inside of the nose.

慢性鼻窦炎是鼻窦的长期炎症。鼻窦是上面部骨骼后面的潮湿的含气空腔——在两眼之间，前额、鼻子和脸颊的后面。通常，鼻窦通过鼻子内部的小开口进行引流。

Anything that obstructs that flow can cause a buildup of mucus, and sometimes pus, in the sinuses. Drainage

任何阻塞这种流动的东西都会导致鼻窦中积聚黏液，有时甚至是脓液。鼻子结构异常、感染或过敏引起的组

from the sinuses can be obstructed by structural abnormalities of the nose, infection, or tissue swelling caused by allergies. The buildup of mucus leads to increased sinus pressure and facial pain.

In adults, chronic sinusitis is most often linked to nasal swelling caused by allergies, especially allergies to inhaled dust, mold, pollen, or the spores of fungi. These allergies trigger the release of histamine and other chemicals that cause the inner lining of the nose to swell and block sinus drainage.

Polyps, nasal tumors and nasal fractures can obstruct the sinus drainage, leading to chronic sinusitis. Chronic sinusitis can also be seen in people whose sinuses and nasal passages are structurally abnormally narrow. People with asthma, cystic fibrosis, or immune system problems develop chronic sinusitis more often than others.

Treatments for chronic sinusitis include the following options. Nasal corticosteroids. These nasal sprays help prevent and treat inflammation. If the sprays aren't effective enough, your doctor might recommend rinsing with a

织肿胀都会阻碍鼻窦的引流。黏液的堆积会导致鼻窦压力增加和面部疼痛。

在成人中，慢性鼻窦炎最常与过敏引起的鼻肿胀有关，尤其是对吸入的灰尘、霉菌、花粉或真菌孢子过敏。这些过敏会触发组胺和其他化学物质的释放，导致鼻子内壁肿胀并阻塞鼻窦引流。

息肉、鼻肿瘤和鼻骨折也会阻塞鼻窦引流，导致慢性鼻窦炎。慢性鼻窦炎也见于鼻窦和鼻腔结构异常狭窄的人。患有哮喘、囊性纤维化或免疫系统问题的人比其他人更容易患上慢性鼻窦炎。

慢性鼻窦炎的治疗方式包括以下几种：使用鼻用皮质类固醇。这类鼻腔喷雾剂有助于预防和治疗炎症。如果喷雾剂不够有效，医生可能会建议你使用混合了布地奈德滴剂的生理盐水溶液进行冲洗或使用其溶液性鼻雾。

solution of saline mixed with drops of budesonide or using a nasal mist of the solution. Saline nasal irrigation, with nasal sprays or solutions, reduces drainage and rinses away irritants and allergens.

Oral or injected corticosteroids. These medications are used to relieve inflammation from severe sinusitis, especially if you also have nasal polyps. Oral corticosteroids can cause serious side effects when used long-term, so they're used only to treat severe symptoms.

Allergy medications. If allergies are causing sinusitis, your doctor may recommend allergy medications.

Aspirin desensitization treatment, if you have reactions to aspirin that cause sinusitis and nasal polyps. Under medical supervision, you're gradually given larger doses of aspirin to increase your tolerance.

Antifungal treatment. If your infection is due to fungi, you may have antifungal treatment.

用鼻腔喷雾剂或溶液进行生理盐水鼻腔冲洗，可减少引流，并冲洗掉刺激物和过敏原。

口服或注射皮质类固醇。这些药物用于缓解严重鼻窦炎引起的炎症，尤其是如果你还患有鼻息肉。长期使用口服皮质类固醇会引起严重的副作用，因此它们仅用于缓解严重的症状。

抗过敏药物。如果过敏导致了鼻窦炎，那你的医生可能会推荐使用抗过敏药物。

阿司匹林脱敏治疗。如果你对阿司匹林有反应，从而导致了鼻窦炎和鼻息肉，那么在医生的指导下，你可以逐渐服用更大剂量的阿司匹林以增加耐受性。

抗真菌治疗。如果感染是由真菌引起的，那你可能需要抗真菌治疗。

Last but not least, medication to treat nasal polyps and chronic sinusitis. If you have nasal polyps and chronic sinusitis, medications may reduce the size of the nasal polyps and lessen congestion.

最后是治疗鼻息肉和慢性鼻窦炎的药物。如果你患有鼻息肉和慢性鼻窦炎，药物可以缩小鼻息肉并减轻充血。

（三）Hearing Loss 听力损失（耳聋）[4]

Hearing loss is a common problem caused by noise, aging, disease, and heredity. People with hearing loss may find it hard to have conversations with friends and family. They may also have trouble understanding a doctor's advice, responding to warnings, and hearing doorbells and alarms. Approximately one in three people between the ages of 65 and 74 has hearing loss, and nearly half of those older than 75 has difficulty hearing. But some people may not want to admit they have trouble hearing.

听力损失是由噪声、衰老、疾病和遗传引起的常见问题。听力损失者可能很难与朋友和家人交谈。他们也可能无法理解医生的建议、无法对警告做出反应，并且听不到门铃和警报声。65 至 74 岁的人中，约三分之一有听力损失，75 岁以上的人中有近一半有听力困难。但是，有些人可能不想承认他们有听力问题。

Older people who can't hear well may become depressed, or they may withdraw from others because they feel frustrated or embarrassed about not understanding what is being said. Sometimes, older people are mistakenly thought to be confused, unresponsive, or uncooperative because they don't hear well. Hearing problems that are ignored

听力不好的老年人可能会变得抑郁，他们可能会因为不理解别人所说的内容而感到沮丧或尴尬，从而疏远他人。有时，老年人会因为听力不佳而被错误地认为是犯糊涂、没反应或不合作。忽视听力问题，不进行治疗，会使听力问题变得更严重。如果你有听力问题，请去看医生。助听器、特殊训练、药物和手术都是可以提供帮

or untreated can get worse. If you have a hearing problem, see your doctor. Hearing aids, special training, certain medicines, and surgery are some of the treatments that can help.

Some people have a hearing problem and don't realize it. You should see your doctor if you have trouble hearing over the telephone, find it hard to follow conversations when two or more people are talking, often ask people to repeat what they are saying, need to turn up the TV volume so loud that others complain, have a problem hearing because of background noise, think that others seem to mumble, or can't understand when women and children speak to you.

Hearing loss comes in many forms. It can range from a mild loss, in which a person misses certain high-pitched sounds, such as the voices of women and children, to a total loss of hearing. There are two general categories of hearing loss: Sensorineural hearing loss occurs when there is damage to the inner ear or the auditory nerve. This type of hearing loss is usually permanent. Conductive hearing loss occurs when sound waves cannot reach the inner ear. The cause

助的治疗方法。

有些人有听力问题，却没有意识到。如果你在打电话时听不清，两个或更多人谈话时难以跟上谈话内容，经常要求别人重复他们说过的话，需要将电视音量调得很大以至于他人都要抱怨，觉得背景噪声干扰了听力，认为他人似乎在喃喃自语，或听不懂妇女和儿童对你说的话，那么你就应该去看医生。

听力损失有多种形式。它的范围从轻微的听力损失，听不到某些高音，比如妇女和儿童的声音，到完全丧失听力。听力损失可分为两大类：当内耳或听神经受损时，会发生感音神经性听力损失。这种类型的听力损失通常是永久性的。当声波无法到达内耳时，就会出现传导性听力损失。原因可能是耳垢堆积、积液或鼓膜穿孔。药物或手术通常可以治疗传导性听力损失。

may be earwax buildup, fluid, or a punctured eardrum. Medical treatment or surgery can usually restore conductive hearing loss.

4.2　汉译英

（一）睡眠呼吸暂停 Sleep Apnea[5-6]

睡眠呼吸暂停是一种常见现象。当上呼吸道在睡眠期间反复阻塞，使通过的气流减少或完全阻止气流通过时，就会发生这种情况。这被称为阻塞性睡眠呼吸暂停。如果大脑不发送呼吸所需的信号，那这种病情则被称为中枢性睡眠呼吸暂停。

Sleep apnea is a common condition. It can occur when the upper airway becomes blocked repeatedly during sleep, reducing or completely stopping airflow. This is known as obstructive sleep apnea. If the brain does not send the signals needed to breathe, the condition may be called central sleep apnea.

睡眠呼吸暂停的常见症状和体征包括睡眠时打鼾或气喘，呼吸减少或消失，这又称为呼吸暂停，以及困倦。睡眠呼吸暂停不诊断、不治疗会妨碍睡眠和休息，还会导致影响身体许多部位的并发症。

Common sleep apnea signs and symptoms are snoring or gasping during sleep; reduced or absent breathing, called apnea events and sleepiness. Undiagnosed or untreated sleep apnea prevents restful sleep and can cause complications that may affect many parts of your body.

睡眠呼吸暂停会增加你患以下疾病的风险：哮喘，心房颤动，癌症（例如胰腺癌、肾癌和皮肤癌），慢性肾病，以及认知和行为障碍（例如注意力、警惕性、专注力、运动技能和

Sleep apnea may increase your risk of the following disorders: asthma, atrial fibrillation, cancers (such as pancreatic, renal, and skin cancers), chronic kidney disease, and cognitive

语言和视觉空间记忆的降低）。

其他风险还包括老年人的痴呆和儿童的学习障碍，心血管疾病（如动脉粥样硬化、心脏病发作、心力衰竭、难以控制的高血压以及中风），眼睛疾病（如青光眼、干眼症、圆锥角膜），代谢紊乱（包括葡萄糖不耐受和 2 型糖尿病），以及妊娠并发症（包括妊娠期糖尿病、妊娠高血压，以及婴儿出生体重低）。

医疗服务人员可以通过睡眠研究来诊断睡眠呼吸暂停。他们会记录呼吸缓慢或停止的发作次数以及一小时内检测到的中枢性睡眠呼吸暂停发生的次数。他们还要确定在这期间血液中的氧含量是否较低。

呼吸设备，如持续正压通气（CPAP）机，以及生活方式的改变，

and behavioral disorders (such as decreases in attention, vigilance, concentration, motor skills, and verbal and visuospatial memory).

Other risks include dementia in older adults and learning disabilities in children, diseases of the heart and blood vessels (such as atherosclerosis, heart attacks, heart failure, difficult-to-control high blood pressure, and stroke), eye disorders (such as glaucoma, dry eye, or keratoconus), metabolic disorders (including glucose intolerance and type 2 diabetes), and pregnancy complications (including gestational diabetes and gestational high blood pressure, as well as having a baby with low birth weight).

Healthcare providers use sleep studies to diagnose sleep apnea. They record the number of episodes of slow or stopped breathing and the number of central sleep apnea events detected in an hour. They also determine whether oxygen levels in the blood are lower during these events.

Breathing devices such as continuous positive air pressure (CPAP)

是常见的睡眠呼吸暂停治疗方法。睡眠呼吸暂停不做诊断，不进行治疗，会导致严重的并发症，例如心脏病发作、青光眼、糖尿病、癌症以及认知和行为障碍。

machines and lifestyle changes are common sleep apnea treatments. Undiagnosed or untreated sleep apnea can lead to serious complications such as heart attack, glaucoma, diabetes, cancer, and cognitive and behavioral disorders.

（二）鼻炎 Rhinitis[7]

大多数类型的鼻炎是由炎症引起的，并与眼睛、耳朵或喉咙的症状有关。鼻炎有几种类型。最常见的是通常由病毒性疾病引起的急性鼻炎、过敏性或季节性鼻炎，以及非过敏性或全年性鼻炎。当空气中的过敏原触发体内组胺的释放时，就会引起过敏性鼻炎。组胺会导致鼻腔、鼻窦和眼睑的脆弱内壁出现瘙痒、肿胀和积液。

Most types of rhinitis are caused by an inflammation and are associated with symptoms in the eyes, ears, or throat. There are several types of rhinitis. The most common are acute rhinitis, which is usually caused by a viral illness, allergic or seasonal rhinitis, and nonallergic or year-round rhinitis. Allergic rhinitis is caused when allergens in the air trigger the release of histamine in the body. Histamine causes itching, swelling, and fluid to build up in the fragile linings of the nasal passages, sinuses, and eyelids.

鼻炎最常见的原因是树木和草释放的花粉、尘螨、霉菌、蟑螂排泄物、动物皮屑、烟雾和气味、温度、荷尔蒙变化、某些药物和局部喷鼻剂的过度使用、环境变化、吸烟，以及某些食物和香料。过敏性鼻炎可能与哮喘有关。然而，其相关性还没有被完全

The most common causes of rhinitis are pollen given off by trees and grass, dust mites, mold, cockroach waste, animal dander, fumes and odors, temperature, hormonal changes, certain medicines and overuse of topical nose sprays, changes in the environment,

理解。专家认为，由于鼻炎使人难以通过鼻子呼吸，鼻子更加难以发挥正常功能。在空气进入肺部之前，通过嘴呼吸不会加热、过滤或加湿空气。这会使哮喘症状恶化。控制过敏性鼻炎可能有助于控制某些人的哮喘。

鼻炎的症状包括打喷嚏，鼻塞，流鼻涕，鼻子、喉咙、眼睛和耳朵发痒，流鼻血，复发性耳朵感染，打鼾，嘴呼吸和疲倦。避免接触引起问题的过敏原是过敏性鼻炎的最佳治疗方法。鼻炎的治疗手段有抗组胺药、喷鼻剂、减充血剂、治疗哮喘症状的药物、抗过敏针，以及针对某些健康问题的手术。过敏性鼻炎的预防措施包括避开有大量灰尘、螨虫或霉菌的区域，避免接触宠物，避开已知的会导致你过敏的东西，以及对环境采取控制措施。

smoke, and certain foods or spices. Allergic rhinitis may be linked to asthma. However, this link is not fully understood. Experts think that since rhinitis makes it hard to breathe through the nose, it is harder for the nose to work normally. Breathing through the mouth does not warm, filter, or humidify the air before it enters the lungs. This can make asthma symptoms worse. Controlling allergic rhinitis may help control asthma in some people.

Symptoms of rhinitis include sneezing, stuffy nose, runny nose, itchy nose, throat, eyes, and ears, nosebleeds, ear infections that keep coming back, snoring, breathing through the mouth, and tiredness. Avoidance of the allergens that cause the problem is the best treatment for allergic rhinitis. Treatments for rhinitis may include antihistamines, nose sprays, decongestants, medicines for asthma symptoms, allergy shots and surgery for some health problems. Preventive measures for avoiding allergic rhinitis include avoiding areas where there is heavy dust, mites, or molds, avoiding pets, avoiding what you know you are allergic to and controls in your environment.

（三）声带病变 Vocal Cord Lesion[8]

声带病变，也称为声腔病变，是包括结节、息肉和囊肿在内的良性（非癌性）增生。所有这些都能导致声音嘶哑，并可能与声带过度使用或声带创伤有关。

Vocal cord lesions, also known as vocal fold lesions, are benign (noncancerous) growths that include nodules, polyps, and cysts. All can cause hoarseness and may be associated with vocal overuse or vocal cord trauma.

声带小结，有时也称为歌者结节或小结，是由于反复过度用嗓或用嗓不当造成的。这些茧状增生发生在声带的正中央。声带小结在显微镜下看起来像老茧，偶尔伴有异常血管。20至50岁的女性更容易患声带小结，但男性和女性都可能受到影响。

Vocal cord nodules, sometimes called singer's nodules or nodes, result from repetitive overuse or misuse of the voice. These callous-like growths develop in the midpoint of the vocal folds. Vocal cord nodules look like calluses under the microscope and are occasionally associated with abnormal blood vessels. Women between the ages of 20 and 50 are more prone to vocal cord nodules, but both men and women can be affected.

声带息肉与结节不同，因为它们出现在一侧声带上，也可以出现在两侧声带上。它们相比结节血供更丰富，这意味着它们有更多的血管并且呈红色。这些增生的大小和形状各不相同，但通常比结节大，类似于水疱。与声带小结一样，息肉源于过度用嗓或用嗓不当，但也可源于单次嗓音滥用（例如在体育赛事中尖叫）。另一种声带息肉，或者说息肉样声带炎，则几

Vocal cord polyps are different from nodules because they can occur on either one or both vocal cords. They tend to be more vascularized than nodules, meaning they have more blood vessels and appear reddish in color. These growths can vary in size and shape, but are usually larger than nodules and resemble blisters. Like vocal cord nodules, polyps can be caused by overuse or misuse of the voice,

乎仅与吸烟有关。

声带囊肿是一种囊状增生，中间是液体或半固体。它们不如声带小结和息肉常见。声带囊肿有两种类型，黏液潴留囊肿和表皮样（或皮脂腺）囊肿。囊肿通常与过度用嗓或声带创伤无关。

当一个人患有上呼吸道感染或喉炎时，用嗓也可能导致声带损伤。声带损伤可导致声音嘶哑、气息声、多音、音域丧失、声带疲劳或失声。通常可在语言病理学家的指导下采用嗓音疗法和行为矫正保守治疗结节。手术仅用于难治性病变或仅靠嗓音疗法无法满足发声需求的情况。与结节相反，嗓音疗法通常对息肉和囊肿收效甚微，最好通过手术方法进行治疗。

but can also be caused by a single episode of vocal abuse (such as yelling at a sports event). Another type of vocal cord polyp, polypoid carditis, is associated almost exclusively with smoking.

Vocal cord cysts are growths that have a sac around a fluid-filled or semisolid center. They are less common than vocal cord nodules and polyps. There are two types of vocal cord cysts, mucus retention cysts and epidermoid (or sebaceous) cysts. Cysts are not typically associated with overuse of the voice or vocal fold trauma.

Vocal cord lesions can also be caused by using the voice while one is sick with an upper respiratory infection or laryngitis. Vocal cord lesions can result in hoarseness, breathiness, multiple tones, loss of vocal range, vocal fatigue or loss of voice. Nodules are typically treated conservatively with voice therapy and behavioral modification under the guidance of a speech language pathologist. Surgery is reserved for refractory lesions or in situations where vocal needs are not being met with voice therapy alone. In contrast to nodules,

治疗影响嗓音的潜在健康问题，例如反流、过敏和鼻窦炎，可能有助于减轻声带病变的严重程度或降低其发生率。行为干预如戒烟、减压和提高用嗓意识也可以缓解嗓音问题。嗓音疗法通常会强化这些行为，并提供技术和策略来最大限度地提高发声效率和功能。

polyps and cysts do not typically respond to voice therapy and are best managed with a surgical approach.

Treatment of underlying medical problems that affect the voice, such as reflux, allergies, and sinusitis, may help lessen the severity or occurrence of vocal lesions. Behavioral intervention for smoking cessation, stress reduction, and improved vocal awareness may also ease voice problems. Voice therapy typically reinforces these behaviors and provides techniques and strategies to maximize vocal efficiency and function.

5　口译注释与学习资源

5.1　口译注释

图式记忆

我们知道视觉记忆比单纯的语言记忆更有效。下面以口鼻腔和咽喉区为例，大家可以根据下图对照记忆相关结构的中英词汇。

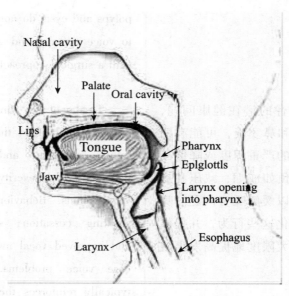

nasal cavity 鼻腔；palate 腭部；lips 嘴唇；jaw 下颌

nasal and oral pharynx ['færɪŋks] 鼻咽和口咽

isthmus ['ɪsməs] 峡部

epiglottis [ˌepɪ'glɒtɪs] 会厌

larynx ['lærɪŋks] 喉

esophagus [i'sɒfəgəs] 食道

5.2 学习资源

登录中国大学 MOOC（慕课），学习"医疗口译"课程中"耳鼻喉科"的口译实战示范视频。补充主题包括：（1）Sinus Pain 鼻窦痛；（2）Dizziness 头晕；（3）Ear Ache 耳痛；（4）Nose Bleed 流鼻血；（5）Difficulty in Swallowing 吞咽困难；（6）Mouth Breathing 口呼吸；（7）Sore Throat 喉咙痛。另外还可以关注美国卫生研究院、美国耳鼻喉及头颈外科学会（American Academy of Otolaryngology-Head and Neck Surgery，AAO-HNS）、妙佑医疗国际、克利夫兰诊所、哥伦比亚大学医学中心，约翰斯·霍普金斯大学医学院、哈佛医学院等机构官网的耳鼻喉科介绍。

参考文献

［1］Columbia University Department of Otolaryngology Head and Neck Surgery.（2015，December

4）. *What is otolaryngology?*. Retrieved November 13, 2021, from https://www. entcolumbia. org/about-us/what-otolaryngology.

[2] Harvard Health. (2019, March 19). *Chronic sinusitis*（*in adults*）. Retrieved November 13, 2021, from https://www. health. harvard. edu/a_ to_ z/chronic-sinusitis-in-adults-a－to-z.

[3] Mayo Foundation for Medical Education and Research. (2021, July 16). *Chronic sinusitis*. Retrieved November 13, 2021, from https://www. mayoclinic. org/diseases-conditions/chronic-sinusitis/diagnosis-treatment/drc－20351667.

[4] U. S. Department of Health and Human Services. National Institute on Aging. (n. d.). *Hearing loss: A common problem for older adults*. Retrieved November 13, 2021, from https://www. nia. nih. gov/health/hearing-loss-common-problem-older-adults.

[5] U. S. Department of Health and Human Services. National Heart, Lung and Blood Institute. *Sleep apnea*. Retrieved November 13, 2021, from https://www. nhlbi. nih. gov/health-topics/sleep-apnea.

[6] Cleveland Clinic. (n. d.). *Sleep apnea: Causes, symptoms, tests & treatments*. Retrieved November 13, 2021, from https://my. clevelandclinic. org/health/diseases/8718－sleep-apnea.

[7] Johns Hopkins Medicine. (n. d.). *Rhinitis*. Retrieved November 13, 2021, from https://www. hopkinsmedicine. org/health/conditions-and-diseases/rhinitis.

[8] Cleveland Clinic. (n. d.). *Vocal cord nodules, Polyps & Cysts: Treatment & Prevention*. Retrieved November 13, 2021, from https://my. clevelandclinic. org/health/diseases/15424－vocal-cord-lesions-nodules-polyps-and-cysts.

第十六章

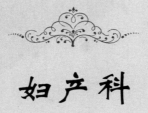

妇产科

1　导读

　　本章重点为口译技巧之应急技巧和妇产科的6篇"口译实战"练习。口译实战练习中英译汉、汉译英各3篇，内容涵盖妇产科介绍、子宫肌瘤、羊水栓塞、多囊卵巢综合征、宫颈癌筛查与预防、高龄孕妇孕前孕期健康保健。请结合本章口译技巧练习6篇口译实战文本。

2　口译技巧——应急技巧

　　口译员在接到口译任务时，应评估自己是否能够胜任后再选择是否接受。在接受口译任务后，口译员应做好充分的准备。前两个步骤可最大限度地减少口译活动中口译员能力不足可能造成的风险。但无论口译员一方准备得多充分，口译活动作为多方参与的交流活动，总会出现无法预知的情况，因此需要口译员随机应变、合理应对。口译应急技巧能在一定程度上帮助口译员应付现场的突发情况。突发情况大致可分为以下三类，每一类都有相应的应急技巧。

2.1　理解困难

　　口译员遇到没听懂的生词、术语，或者对讲话者的口音和讲话逻辑不熟悉，就会出现理解困难的情况。医疗口译中这类问题尤其突出，因为医疗场景中术语繁多，患者来自不同地方，有不同文化背景。除医学类国际会议外，医疗口译多为交替传译，因此，口译员可以：（1）询问讲话者，再次确认信息。如果医学术语难以理解，可以请医生用普通人能够理解的方式再次表达。（2）请教现场其他专家或者陪同人员。现场如有其他双语人士，可就个别专业词汇进行请教。如果患者由于病情讲话不清楚，可以询问其陪同家属。（3）查询词典或网络。如果实在有术语无法用简单语言表述，应及时在现场查询。除非是急救，否则医疗口译中还是有一定的时间可以就个别关键词进行查询。

2.2　表达困难

　　由于医学术语的词根词缀有规律可循，有可能出现译员能听懂但无法在译入语中找出对应术语的情况，或者是能找到对应术语但患者无法听懂医学术语的情况。此时，口译员可以参照上述应对理解困难的技巧予以处理。在得到帮助后需道谢，在查询术语耽搁医疗进程时需表达歉意。

2.3　决策困难

在医疗口译中译员有时会对如何应对一些意外的情况产生疑问，例如：该不该翻译患者家属的讨论或者医务人员的讨论？如何应付对口译员业务能力的质疑？口译员该不该帮忙做语言服务外的工作？患者询问口译员自身对医疗方案的意见或者对医生的评价时该如何回应？这些突发情况与口译员职业伦理、职业素养及跨文化交际技巧相关。口译员应本着促进医患双方友好交流的原则，将生命安全放在首要位置，做出相应的决策。

需要特别注意的是，医疗口译不同于其他内容的口译，其准确性与患者的生命安全和基本权利息息相关，口译员需谨慎使用其他口译场合下的应急技巧，如省略、解释、猜测等。本章口译实战部分的篇章中医学术语类生词较多，适合模拟练习应急技巧。

3　口译词汇

3.1　英译汉

（一）Obstetrics and Gynecology 妇产科

obstetrics 产科

gynecology 妇科

postpartum 产后的

physiology 生理学

fetal cardiac ultrasound 胎儿心脏超声

genetic screening and testing 基因筛查

percutaneous umbilical cord sampling 经皮脐带穿刺取样检测

ectopic pregnancy 异位妊娠

placenta 胎盘

preeclampsia 先兆子痫

delivery through cesarean section 剖宫产

gestational diabetes 妊娠期糖尿病

ailment 不适、小病

uterus 子宫

fallopian tubes 输卵管

cervix 子宫颈

ovary 卵巢

vagina 阴道

pelvic and uterine fibroid tumor 盆腔子宫纤维瘤

cervical dysplasia 宫颈非典型增生

cervical cancer 宫颈癌

endometriosis 子宫内膜异位症

fallopian tube cancer 输卵管癌

galactorrhea 乳溢

gestational trophoblastic diseases 妊娠性滋养细胞疾病

human papillomavirus（HPV）人乳头状瘤病毒

menstrual abnormalities 月经异常

menopause 更年期

incontinence 失禁

pelvic organ prolapse 盆腔器官脱垂

ovarian cancer 卵巢癌

polycystic ovarian syndrome 多囊卵巢综合征

primary and secondary amenorrhea 原发性和继发性闭经

sexually transmitted infections 性传染病

uterine cancer 子宫内膜癌

vaginal cancer 阴道癌

vulvar cancer 外阴癌

birth control pill 避孕药

intrauterine contraception device（IUD）宫内节育器

long-acting contraceptive injection 长效避孕针

tubal ligation 输卵管结扎

hysterectomy 子宫切除术

oophorectomy 卵巢切除术

salpingectomy 输卵管切除术

cone biopsy 锥形活检

pap test 宫颈涂片检查（Papanicolaou Test）

maternal-fetal medicine 母胎医学

reconstructive surgery 修复外科（手术）、重建手术

reproductive endocrinology 生殖内分泌学

（二）Hysteromyoma 子宫肌瘤

uterine fibroid 子宫纤维瘤

fibromyoma 纤维肌瘤

leiomyoma 平滑肌瘤

intramural fibroid 肌壁间肌瘤

subserosal fibroid 浆膜下肌瘤

submucosal fibroid 黏膜下肌瘤

pedunculated fibroid 带蒂子宫肌瘤

gonadotropin-releasing hormone（GnRH）agonists 促性腺激素释放激素激动剂（又称 GnRH 激动剂）

estrogen 雌激素

progesterone 黄体酮、孕激素

progestin-releasing 释放黄体酮的

tranexamic acid 氨甲环酸

Lysteda 利斯替达

Cyklokapron 赛克洛卡普朗

nonsteroidal anti-inflammatory drugs（NSAIDs）非甾体抗炎药

MRI-guided focused ultrasound surgery（FUS）磁共振引导超声聚焦手术

uterine artery embolization 子宫动脉栓塞手术

radio frequency ablation 射频消融术

laparoscopic myomectomy 腹腔镜肌瘤切除术

hysteroscopic myomectomy 宫腔镜肌瘤切除术

endometrial ablation 子宫内膜切除术

（三）Amniotic Fluid Embolism 羊水栓塞

cardiovascular collapse 心血管坍塌

disseminated intravascular coagulopathy 弥散性血管内凝血

amniotic cavity 羊膜腔

opening of sinusoid 血窦开放

rupture of fetal membrane 胎膜破裂

elderly primipara 高龄初产妇

multipara 经产妇，非初产妇

cervical laceration 宫颈撕裂

uterine rupture 子宫破裂

hydramnios 羊水过多

multiple gestation 多胎妊娠

premature ruptured membrane 胎膜早破

placenta previa 胎盘前置

curettage 清宫术

vital signs 生命体征

oxygen saturation 氧饱和度

oxygen inhalation through masks 面罩给氧

tracheal intubation 气管插管

artificial auxiliary ventilator 人工辅助呼吸机

cardiac arrest 心搏骤停

hemodynamics 血流动力学

cardiac output 心排血量

dobutamine 多巴酚丁胺

phosphodiesterase type 5 inhibitor 磷酸二酯酶-5 抑制剂

dilate 扩张

glucocorticoid 糖皮质激素

coagulation dysfunction 凝血功能障碍

postpartum hemorrhage 产后出血

coagulation factor 凝血因子

cryoprecipitate 冷沉淀

fibrinogen 纤维蛋白原

3.2　汉译英

（一）多囊卵巢综合征 Polycystic Ovary Syndrome（PCOS）

雄激素 androgen

月经紊乱 irregular periods

经量过少 light period

皮赘 skin tag

（二）宫颈癌筛查与预防 Cervical Cancer Screening and Prevention

宫颈癌 cervical cancer

宫颈病变 cervical lesion

宫颈脱落细胞 cervical exfoliated cell

宫颈细胞学检查 cervical cytology examination

二价疫苗 2-valent vaccine

外阴尖锐湿疣 vulvar condyloma acuminatum

肛门癌 anal cancer

外阴癌 vulva cancer

生殖器疣 genital wart

（三）高龄孕妇孕前孕期保健 Maternal Healthcare for Elderly Pregnancy

围产期的 perinatal

高龄孕妇 elderly pregnant women

既往生育史 past fertility history

辅助生殖治疗 assisted reproductive therapy/treatment

受孕 conception

胎儿染色体异常 fetal chromosomal abnormality

胎儿畸形 fetal malformation

妊娠期糖尿病 gestational diabetes mellitus（GDM）

胎儿生长受限 limited fetal growth（FGR）

早产 premature birth

死胎 stillbirth

叶酸 folic acid

复合维生素 multivitamins

产前筛查 prenatal screening

胎儿颈项皮肤褶皱厚度 fetal nuchal translucency（NT）

鼻骨 nasal bone

胎儿神经管缺陷 fetal neural tube defect（NTD）

无创产前基因检测 non-invasive prenatal testing（NIPT）

胎儿染色体非整倍体异常 fetal chromosome aneuploidy abnormality

绒毛穿刺取样术 chorionic villus sampling（CVS）

羊膜腔穿刺术 amniocentesis

胎儿染色体核型分析 karyotype analysis of fetal chromosomes

染色体微阵列分析 chromosomal microarray analysis（CMA）

4 口译实战

4.1 英译汉

（一）Obstetrics and Gynecology 妇产科[1-3]

Obstetrics and gynecology are medical specialties that focus on two different aspects of the female reproductive system. Obstetrics（OB）includes complete care for pregnant women from early symptoms through postpartum. Gynecology is the branch of physiology and medicine which deals with the functions and diseases specific to women and girls, especially those affecting the reproductive system.

产科和妇科是专注于女性生殖系统的两个不同方面的医学专科（专业）。产科（OB）包括从孕早期到产后对孕妇的全面护理。妇科是生理学和医学的交叉学科，主要关注与妇女生殖系统有关的生理功能和疾病。

Obstetricians provide medical services including pregnancy routine checks, diagnostic ultrasound evaluations, chorionic villus sampling, fetal cardiac ultrasound, fetal heart rate monitoring, genetic screening and testing, labor and delivery, and percutaneous umbilical cord sampling, etc. Obstetricians are also trained to handle pregnancy complications, such as ectopic pregnancy, in which the fetus grows outside of the uterus, placenta issues,

产科医生提供的医疗服务包括孕常规检查、诊断性超声评估、绒毛取样、胎儿心脏超声、胎儿心率监测、基因筛查、分娩生产、经皮脐带穿刺取样检测等。产科医生的职责还包括处理妊娠并发症，如异位妊娠（胎儿生长在子宫外部）、胎盘问题、先兆子痫、剖宫产、孕吐、妊娠期糖尿病等。

preeclampsia, delivery through cesarean section, morning sickness, gestational diabetes, etc.

A gynecologist (GYN) provides the diagnosis and management of the reproductive system and disorders that may affect the reproductive health. Gynecology deals with any ailment concerning the female reproductive organs: uterus, fallopian tubes, ovaries and vagina.

Gynecologists treat conditions including benign pelvic and uterine fibroid tumors, cervical dysplasia, cervical cancer, endometriosis, fallopian tube cancer, galactorrhea, gestational trophoblastic diseases, human papillomavirus (HPV)-related disorders, menstrual abnormalities, menopause, incontinence and pelvic organ prolapse, ovarian cancer, polycystic ovarian syndrome, primary and secondary amenorrhea, sexually transmitted infections, uterine cancer, vaginal cancer, vulvar cancer and so on.

Gynecologists may provide medical services such as modern contraceptive care including birth control pills, intrauterine contraception devices (IUDs), long-acting contraceptive injections and implants, HPV

妇科医生（GYN）诊断并管理生殖系统和可能影响生殖健康的疾病。妇科治疗包括子宫、输卵管、卵巢和阴道在内的女性生殖器官疾病。

妇科医生治疗的病症包括良性盆腔子宫肌瘤、宫颈非典型增生、宫颈癌、子宫内膜异位症、输卵管癌、乳溢、妊娠性滋养细胞疾病、人乳头状瘤病毒（HPV）相关疾病、月经异常、更年期、失禁和盆腔器官脱垂、卵巢癌、多囊卵巢综合征、原发性和继发性闭经、性传染病、子宫内膜癌、阴道癌、外阴癌等。

妇科医生可以提供现代避孕措施等医疗服务，如提供避孕药、宫内节育器、长效避孕针和植入体，还可以提供 HPV 疫苗接种等。

vaccination, etc.

Gynecology encompasses specific surgical procedures related to female reproductive organs. The most common procedures are: tubal ligation—a permanent form of birth control, hysterectomy—the removal of the uterus, oophorectomy—the removal of the ovaries, salpingectomy—the removal of the fallopian tubes, cone biopsy—the removal of precancerous cells in the cervix identified during a pap test, and surgical termination of pregnancies.

There are four subspecialties for an OB/GYN: The first is gynecologic oncology. This OB/GYN subspecialty involves treating tumors located in a female's reproductive organs. Gynecologic oncologists are specially trained in techniques used to provide the best possible treatment for patients with gynecologic tumors.

The second is maternal-fetal medicine. OB/GYNs who practice maternal-fetal medicine are experts in high-risk pregnancies. They can address health concerns for both the mother and baby, and also help manage complications that arise during pregnancy.

妇科医生可以做与女性生殖器官相关的外科手术。最常见的有：输卵管结扎术，这是一种永久性的节育；子宫切除术，也就是去掉整个子宫；卵巢切除术，也就是去掉卵巢；输卵管切除术，也就是切除输卵管；锥形活检，也就是切除在宫颈涂片检查中查出的宫颈癌前细胞；以及终止妊娠手术。

妇产科下有四个方向。第一个方向是妇科肿瘤学。这个亚专科涉及治疗位于女性生殖器官的肿瘤。妇科肿瘤医生接受技术培训，为妇科肿瘤患者提供最佳治疗。

第二个方向是母胎医学。此方向的妇产科医生是高危妊娠方面的专家。他们主攻母婴健康问题和孕期并发症。

The third is female pelvic medicine and reconstructive surgery. Physicians who specialize in this subspecialty provide medical and surgical treatment to women with pelvic floor disorders. These specialists treat conditions like urinary incontinence, pelvic organ prolapse, and an overactive bladder.

第三个方向是女性盆腔医学和修复外科。专门从事这一亚专科的医生为患有盆腔疾病的妇女提供药物和手术治疗。这些医生治疗尿失禁、盆腔器官脱垂、膀胱过度活动症等疾病。

The last is reproductive endocrinology and infertility. Reproductive endocrinologists are OB/GYNs who evaluate and treat fertility issues for both men and women. Their expertise is valuable for those facing reproductive health issues, such as endometriosis.

最后是生殖内分泌学和不孕症方向。生殖内分泌学家主攻评估和治疗两性生育方面的问题。他们的专业知识对于面临生殖健康问题（如子宫内膜异位症）的人来说是有价值的。

（二）Hysteromyoma 子宫肌瘤 [4-5]

The hysteromyoma (a disease also called a uterine fibroid, a fibromyoma, a leiomyoma) is a tumor of high-quality character which is shown in the muscular layer of a uterus called a myometrium. Myoma is a peculiar ball in which smooth muscle fibers chaotically intertwine among themselves, and the roundish node as a result is formed.

子宫肌瘤（一种疾病，也称为子宫纤维瘤、纤维肌瘤、平滑肌瘤）是一种具有高质量特征的肿瘤，因为它通常生长在子宫的肌肉层（又称子宫肌层）中。肌瘤是一种特殊的球形瘤，光滑的肌肉纤维无序交织在一起，最终形成球形瘤体。

Such nodes sometimes reach especially big sizes and can even weigh several kilograms. Diameter of such

这种肌瘤有时可以达到相当大的尺寸，重达几公斤。肌瘤的直径从几毫米到几厘米大小不等。子宫肌瘤是

nodes makes from several millimeters to the size in several centimeters. The tumor is hormone-dependent and arises in women at the reproductive age. Most often women from 30 to 45 have higher chances to develop this tumor. Today hysteromyoma makes about thirty percent of all diseases of gynecologic character.

Classification according to growth of nodes and their localization is as follows: intramural fibroids which grow within the muscular walls of your uterus, subserosal fibroids which grow on the outside of your uterus, submucosal fibroids which grow into your uterine cavity, and pedunculated fibroids which, unlike the previous three types growing within tissues, develop on stalk-like structures that come out from tissue, almost like mushrooms.

There's no single best approach to uterine fibroid treatment. Many treatment options exist. (1) Watchful waiting. Many women with uterine fibroids experience no signs or symptoms, or have only mildly annoying signs and symptoms that they can live with. In that case, watchful waiting could be the best option, because fibroids aren't

一种激素依赖性疾病，在育龄妇女中较为常见。30 到 45 岁的女性有更高的患病风险。目前，妇科疾病中约有 30% 与子宫肌瘤相关。

根据其生长和定位，子宫肌瘤可分为下述类型：生长在子宫肌壁内的肌壁间肌瘤、生长在子宫外壁的浆膜下肌瘤、向子宫腔内生长的黏膜下肌瘤，以及带蒂肌瘤。带蒂肌瘤与前三种生长在组织内的肌瘤不同，它外形像蘑菇，常发于从组织生长出来的茎状结构上。

子宫肌瘤的治疗没有哪种单一疗法是最佳方案，有许多治疗方案可供选择：（1）不做处理，注意观察。许多患子宫肌瘤的妇女没有症状，或只有轻微的、可以忍受的不适。在这种情况下，不做治疗，注意观察可能是最好的选择，因为肌瘤不是癌变，很少影响怀孕。子宫肌瘤常常生长缓慢，或是长期不长大，在进入更年期后，

cancerous. They rarely interfere with pregnancy. They usually grow slowly—or not at all—and tend to shrink after menopause, when levels of reproductive hormones drop.

（2）Medications for uterine fibroids target hormones that regulate the menstrual cycle, treating symptoms such as heavy menstrual bleeding and pelvic pressure. They don't eliminate fibroids, but may shrink them. For example, gonadotropin-releasing hormone（GnRH）agonists treat fibroids by blocking the production of estrogen and progesterone, putting the patient into a temporary menopause-like state. As a result, menstruation stops, fibroids shrink and anemia often improves. Many women have significant hot flashes while using GnRH agonists, so they are typically used for no more than three to six months. Symptoms may return when the medication is stopped, but long-term use of GnRH agonists can cause loss of bone.

Another option is progestin-releasing intrauterine device（IUD）which can relieve heavy bleeding caused by fibroids, but it provides symptom relief only and doesn't shrink fibroids or make

当生殖激素水平下降时，它们往往会变小。

（2）针对调节月经周期激素的治疗子宫肌瘤的药物可以治疗经期严重出血和盆腔压力过大。这类药物不能消除肌瘤，但可以使之缩小。例如，促性腺激素释放激素激动剂（又称GnRH激动剂）可通过阻止雌激素和黄体酮的产生，使患者临时进入类似更年期的状态，以此来治疗子宫肌瘤。在此方案下，患者出现停经，子宫肌瘤得以缩小，并且贫血的状况往往得到改善。许多妇女在使用GnRH激动剂时出现明显的潮热，因此用药通常不超过三到六个月。停药后，可能复发，但长期用药可能导致骨量流失。

另一种选择是释放黄体酮的宫内避孕器（IUD），它可以缓解由肌瘤引起的大量出血，但它只能缓解症状，不能缩小肌瘤或让肌瘤消失。氨甲环酸（比如利斯替达和赛克洛卡普朗）

them disappear. Tranexamic acid (Lysteda, Cyklokapron), which is nonhormonal medication, is taken to ease heavy menstrual periods. Nonsteroidal anti-inflammatory drugs (NSAIDs) may also be effective in relieving pain related to fibroids, but they don't reduce bleeding caused by fibroids.

属于非激素类药物，服用这类药物可以减少经期出血量。非甾体抗炎药（NSAIDs）也可以有效地缓解与肌瘤相关的疼痛，但它不能减少肌瘤引起的出血。

Besides medication, there are other options, such as MRI-guided focused ultrasound surgery (FUS), uterine artery embolization, radio frequency ablation, laparoscopic myomectomy, hysteroscopic myomectomy, and endometrial ablation.

除了药物治疗，还有其他选择，如磁共振引导超声聚焦手术（FUS）、子宫动脉栓塞术、射频消融术、腹腔镜肌瘤切除术、宫腔镜肌瘤切除术和子宫内膜切除术。

（三）Amniotic Fluid Embolism 羊水栓塞[6-7]

Amniotic fluid embolism is a rare but serious condition that occurs when amniotic fluid—the fluid that surrounds a baby in the uterus during pregnancy—or fetal material, such as fetal cells, enters the mother's bloodstream. Amniotic fluid embolism is most likely to occur during delivery or in the immediate postpartum period.

羊水栓塞比较罕见，但当羊水（怀孕期间子宫内包裹胎儿的液体）或者胎儿组织（比如胎儿细胞）进入母体血液中时，情况就会非常危急。羊水栓塞最有可能发生在分娩期间或产后很短的时间内。

Amniotic fluid embolism might develop suddenly and rapidly. Signs and symptoms might include sudden shortness

羊水栓塞发病突然，病情进展迅速。其症状包括突然呼吸困难、肺部积液（肺水肿）、血压骤低、急性心

of breath, excess fluid in the lungs (pulmonary edema), sudden low blood pressure, sudden failure of the heart (cardiovascular collapse), life-threatening blood clotting (disseminated intravascular coagulopathy), bleeding from the uterus, rapid heart rate or disturbances in the rhythm of the heart rate, seizures, loss of consciousness, and fetal distress, such as a slow heart rate, or other fetal heart rate abnormalities.

The specific cause of amniotic fluid embolism is not clear, which may be related to the following factors: (1) Excessive high pressure of amniotic cavity; (2) Opening of sinusoid; (3) Rupture of fetal membrane. The common inducing factors are elderly primipara, multipara, cervical laceration, uterine rupture, hydramnios, multiple gestation, uterine contraction, emergency delivery, premature ruptured membranes, placenta previa, cesarean section, and curettage. Most of these factors can directly or indirectly induce amniotic fluid embolism.

Once amniotic fluid embolism occurs, the consequences are severe.

力衰竭（心血管坍塌）、危及生命的血栓（弥散性血管内凝血）、子宫出血、心率过快或不齐、癫痫发作、意识丧失，以及胎儿不适，如心率缓慢，或其他胎儿心率异常。

羊水栓塞的具体病因目前尚未明确，可能与下列因素有关：一是羊膜腔压力过高；二是血窦开放；三是胎膜破裂。其常见诱发因素有高龄初产妇、经产妇、宫颈裂伤、子宫破裂、羊水过多、多胎妊娠、子宫收缩过强、急产、胎膜早破、胎盘前置、剖宫产术和清宫术。这些诱因可以直接或间接诱发羊水栓塞。

羊水栓塞一旦发生，后果严重。因此，一旦怀疑羊水栓塞，应立即按

Therefore, once amniotic fluid embolism is suspected, it is necessary to carry out rescue immediately according to the first aid process of amniotic fluid embolism. The treatment principle of amniotic fluid embolism is to maintain vital signs and protect organ function. Specific treatment includes the following aspects:

First, increase oxygen saturation and keep the respiratory tract unobstructed with oxygen inhalation through masks, tracheal intubation or artificial auxiliary ventilator to avoid respiratory and cardiac arrest. Second, provide hemodynamic support to stabilize cardiac output and blood pressure. Dobutamine and phosphodiesterase type 5 inhibitor can strengthen the heart and dilate the pulmonary artery simultaneously, which is the first choice of treatment, because it can maintain stable hemodynamics.

Third, provide antiallergic treatment. At present, the early use of high-dose glucocorticoid treatment is still worthy of reference. Fourth, correct coagulation dysfunction, such as active treatment of postpartum hemorrhage, a timely supplement of coagulation factors,

照羊水栓塞急救流程实施抢救，分秒必争。羊水栓塞的处理原则是维持生命体征和保护器官功能。具体处理包括以下几方面：

一是增加氧饱和度，保持呼吸道通畅，使用面罩给氧、气管插管或人工辅助呼吸机维持氧供，以避免呼吸和心搏骤停。二是提供血流动力支持，保证心排血量和血压稳定。多巴酚丁胺、磷酸二酯酶-5抑制剂可在强心的同时扩张肺动脉，是治疗的首选，可维持血流动力稳定。

三是抗过敏治疗。目前认为，早期使用大剂量糖皮质激素的治疗还是值得参考的。四是纠正凝血功能障碍，比如积极处理产后出血，及时补充凝血因子，包括输注新鲜血浆、冷沉淀、纤维蛋白原等，以及静脉滴注氨甲环酸。五是全面监测生命体征变化，关

including infusion of fresh plasma, cryoprecipitate, fibrinogen, etc., and intravenous drip of tranexamic acid. Fifth, monitor vital signs comprehensively and pay attention to coagulation function.

注凝血功能。

4.2　汉译英

（一）多囊卵巢综合征 Polycystic Ovary Syndrome [8-9]

多囊卵巢综合征（PCOS）是一种卵巢产生了过多的雄激素的情况，而正常情况下，女性仅分泌少量的雄激素。排卵是卵子成熟并从卵巢中释放出来的过程。排出的卵子遇到男性精子就完成了受精。如果卵子没有受精，它会在经期排出身体。有些女性不能产生足够的排卵所需的激素。

Polycystic ovary syndrome （PCOS） is a condition in which the ovaries produce an abnormal amount of androgens. Male sex hormones are usually present in women in small amounts. Ovulation occurs when a mature egg is released from an ovary. This happens so it can be fertilized by a male sperm. If the egg is not fertilized, it is sent out of the body during the period. In some cases, a woman doesn't make enough of the hormones needed to ovulate.

患有多囊卵巢综合征的妇女通常具有高水平雄激素。这可能导致女性月经周期出现更多问题。患有多囊卵巢综合征的妇女更有可能出现某些严重的健康问题，包括 2 型糖尿病、高血压、心脏和血管问题以及子宫内膜癌。患有多囊卵巢综合征的妇女往往怀孕困难。

Women with PCOS often have high levels of androgens. This can cause more problems with a woman's menstrual cycle. Women with PCOS are more likely to develop certain serious health problems, including type 2 diabetes, high blood pressure, problems with the heart and blood vessels, and uterine cancer. Women with PCOS often have problems with their ability to get pregnant.

多囊卵巢综合征的症状可能包括：（1）停经、月经紊乱，或经量过少；（2）卵巢较大或有多个囊肿；（3）体毛浓密，胸部、腹部和背部的毛发过多；（4）体重增加，腹部脂肪堆积；（5）痤疮或油性皮肤；（6）男性型脱发或头发稀疏；（7）颈部或腋下出现多余的小块皮肤（皮赘）；（8）颈后部、腋窝和乳房下部出现深色斑片或皮肤变厚。

The symptoms of PCOS may include： （1）Missed periods，irregular periods，or very light periods；（2）Ovaries that are large or have many cysts；（3）Excess body hair on the chest，stomach，and back；（4）Weight gain，especially around the belly（abdomen）；（5）Acne or oily skin；（6）Male-pattern baldness or thinning hair；（7）Small pieces of excess skin on the neck or armpits（skin tags）；（8）Dark or thick skin patches on the back of the neck，in the armpits，and under the breasts.

导致多囊卵巢综合征的确切原因尚不清楚。早诊断、早治疗以及减肥可以降低不孕、流产或早产、子宫异常出血、2 型糖尿病、心脏病等长期并发症的风险。多囊卵巢综合征的治疗取决于多种因素，包括年龄、症状严重程度、患者整体健康状况。治疗方案也取决于患者短期是否有怀孕计划。

The exact cause of PCOS is unknown. Early diagnosis and treatment along with weight loss may reduce the risk of long-term complications such as infertility， miscarriage or premature， abnormal uterine bleeding， type 2 diabetes， and heart disease. Treatment for PCOS depends on a number of factors. These may include age， severity of the symptoms， and the patients' overall health. The type of treatment may also depend on whether the patient wants to become pregnant in the near future.

如果患者计划怀孕，建议的治疗方案为改变饮食和活动习惯，这样可以帮助身体更有效地使用胰岛素，降低血糖水平，且有助于排卵。促排卵药物可以帮助卵巢正常释放卵子。这些药物也有一定的风险。它们可能增大怀上多胞胎（双胞胎或更多）的概率，并对卵巢产生过度刺激。如果你不打算怀孕，避孕药有助于控制月经周期，降低雄激素水平和减少痤疮。

If the patient is planning a pregnancy, the treatment is suggested as a change in diet and activities that can help the body use insulin more efficiently, lower blood glucose levels, and may help ovulation. Medications to cause ovulation can help the ovaries to release eggs normally. These medications also have certain risks. They can increase the chance for a multiple birth (twins or more). And they can cause ovarian hyperstimulation. If you don't plan to become pregnant, birth control pills help to control menstrual cycles, lower androgen levels and reduce acne.

（二）宫颈癌筛查与预防 Cervical Cancer Screening and Prevention[10]

宫颈癌是一种发生在宫颈细胞中的癌症。大多数宫颈癌是由 HPV 的多种亚型造成的，该病毒可通过性传播感染。宫颈癌的早期发现主要靠筛查。早检查相当于给宫颈安上了一个监视器。一旦有癌症发生，就能够及时地发现，把宫颈癌控制在萌芽阶段。

Cervical cancer is a type of cancer that occurs in the cells of the cervix. Various strains of the human papillomavirus (HPV), a sexually transmitted infection, play a role in causing most cervical cancer. Early detection of cervical cancer depends mainly on screening. Early detection is just like installing a monitor on the cervix. Once there is cancer, it can be found in time, and cervical cancer can be controlled in the budding stage.

宫颈病变早期筛查一般是检查宫

Early detection of cervical lesions is

颈的脱落细胞。宫颈细胞学检查是宫颈癌筛查的核心。我们建议所有的女性从 21 岁开始，只要是已婚或者是有了性生活，都应该进行宫颈癌筛查。21 岁以下的女性一般是不需要进行筛查的，除非有一些特殊的情况，因为这个年龄段的年轻女性一般来说免疫力都比较强，即使发生了 HPV 感染，她们也可以靠自己的免疫力自行清除掉。

对于 21～29 岁的女性，我们推荐每三年进行一次细胞学检查。30～65 岁的女性推荐每三年进行一次宫颈细胞学检查，每五年进行一次联合筛查。对于 65 岁以上的女性，如果说过去多次检查都是正常的，那么就不需要再进行常规的筛查了。曾经患过宫颈癌的女性，即使治疗成功之后，也仍然要继续进行为期 20 年的筛查。

目前已经成功推广上市的 HPV 疫苗主要有三种：二价、四价和九价。宫颈癌疫苗的价是指能够覆盖的病毒

often done by examining cervical exfoliated cells. Cervical cytology examination is the core of cervical cancer screening. We recommend cervical cancer screening for all women from the age of 21, as long as they are married or have had sex. Women under the age of 21 do not need to be screened unless there are some particular circumstances, because young women of this age group generally have strong immune resistance. Even if an HPV infection occurs, they can clear it by their own immunity.

For women aged 21 – 29, we recommend a cytological examination every three years. For those aged 30 – 65, cervical cytology examination is recommended every three years, and package screening is recommended every five years. For women over 65 years old, if multiple tests in the past are normal, there is no need for routine screening. If a woman suffered from cervical cancer, even after successful treatment, she still needs to continue the routine screening for 20 years.

At present, there are three kinds of preventive HPV vaccines: 2-valent, 4-valent, and 9-valent. The valent of

种类。二价宫颈癌疫苗主要适用于 9 ~ 25 岁的女性。这种疫苗可以预防接近 70% 的宫颈癌。四价宫颈癌疫苗适用于 20 ~ 45 岁的女性，可以预防接近 70% 的宫颈癌和 90% 左右的外阴尖锐湿疣。九价疫苗适用于 9 ~ 45 岁的人群。我国大陆目前获批的九价疫苗适用于 16 ~ 25 岁的年轻女性，可以预防 90% 的宫颈癌、85% 的阴道癌、80% 的宫颈病变、90% 的尖锐湿疣以及 95% 的肛门癌、外阴癌、生殖器疣，以及由 HPV 引起的持续性感染、癌前病变等。

cervical cancer vaccine refers to the type of virus that can be covered. 2-valent HPV vaccines are mainly suitable for women aged 9 - 25. The vaccine can prevent nearly 70% of cervical cancer. 4-valent HPV vaccine, ideal for women aged 20 - 45, can prevent almost 70% of cervical cancer and 90% of vulvar condyloma acuminatum. 9-valent vaccine is suitable for people from 9 to 45 years old. The currently approved 9-valent vaccine in China mainland is ideal for young women aged 16 - 25. It can prevent 90% of cervical cancer, 85% of vaginal cancer, 80% of cervical lesions, 90% of condyloma acuminatum, and about 95% of anal cancer, vulva cancer, genital warts as well as persistent infection and precancerous lesions caused by HPV.

（三）高龄孕妇孕前孕期保健 Maternal Healthcare for Elderly Pregnancy[11]

孕前保健和孕期保健是降低孕产妇和围产儿并发症发生率及死亡率、减少出生缺陷的重要措施，能够及早防治妊娠期并发症，及时发现胎儿异常，评估孕妇及胎儿的安危，确定分娩时机和分娩方式，保障母婴安全。

Pre-pregnancy and pregnancy health care is an important measure to reduce the incidence and mortality of maternal and perinatal complications, reduce birth defects, prevent and treat pregnancy complications early, detect fetal abnormalities in a timely manner, assess the safety of pregnant women and fetuses, determine the timing and mode of

对高龄孕妇，需仔细询问孕前病史，重点询问是否患有糖尿病、慢性高血压、肥胖、肾脏及心脏疾病等，还应询问既往生育史，本次妊娠是否为辅助生殖治疗受孕，两次妊娠的间隔时间。医生需明确并记录高危因素。

同时，还需评估并告知高龄孕妇的妊娠风险，包括流产、胎儿染色体异常、胎儿畸形、妊娠期高血压、妊娠期糖尿病（GDM）、胎儿生长受限（FGR）、早产和死胎等。产妇应规范补充叶酸或含叶酸的复合维生素，并及时规范补充钙剂和铁剂，根据情况可考虑适当增加剂量。

delivery, and ensure the safety of mothers and babies.

As for elderly pregnant women, it is necessary for the doctor to carefully inquire about the history of pre-pregnancy, focusing on whether they have diabetes, chronic hypertension, obesity, kidney and heart disease, etc. It is necessary to ask about past fertility history, whether this pregnancy is assisted reproductive conception, the interval between two pregnancies. The doctor should identify and record high-risk factors.

At the same time, assessment and communication need to be done on pregnancy risks for elderly pregnant women, including miscarriage, fetal chromosomal abnormalities, fetal malformations, hypertension during pregnancy, gestational diabetes mellitus (GDM), limited fetal growth (FGR), premature birth and stillbirth. Supplementation of folic acid or folic acid-containing multivitamins, calcium and iron need to be standardized and regulated in a timely manner. An appropriate increase in dose is necessary in consideration of the specific conditions.

高龄孕妇是产前筛查和产前诊断的重点人群。重点检查项目如下：（1）妊娠 11～13 周$^{+6}$应进行孕早期超声筛查，筛查胎儿颈项皮肤褶皱厚度（NT）、有无鼻骨缺如、胎儿神经管缺陷（NTD）等。

Elderly pregnant women are the target group for prenatal screening and diagnosis. Key examinations and tests are as follows：（1）Ultrasound screening in early pregnancy should be done between week 11 and week 13 plus 6 for fetal nuchal translucency（NT），nasal bones，fetal neural tube defect（NTD），etc.

（2）预产期年龄在 35～39 岁而且仅年龄为高危因素，签署知情同意书可先行无创产前基因检测（NIPT）进行胎儿染色体非整倍体异常的筛查；预产期年龄在 40 岁以上的孕妇，建议行绒毛穿刺取样术或羊膜腔穿刺术，进行胎儿染色体核型分析和（或）染色体微阵列分析（CMA）。

（2）If the mother's age is between 35 and 39 years old on the date of delivery，and age is the single risk factor during pregnancy，upon the signing of the informed consent non-invasive prenatal testing（NIPT）can be done for the purpose of fetal chromosome aneuploidy abnormalities. If the mother's age is above 40 on the date of delivery，chorionic villus sampling（CVS）and amniocentesis are suggested for karyotype analysis of fetal chromosomes and/or chromosomal microarray analysis（CMA）.

（3）妊娠 20～24 周，进行胎儿系统超声筛查和宫颈长度测量。（4）重视妊娠期糖尿病筛查、妊娠期高血

（3）Systematic fetal ultrasound screening and cervical length measurement are performed at 20－24 weeks of pregnancy. （4）Attention

压和胎儿生长受限的诊断。（5）40 岁以上的孕妇，应加强胎儿监护，妊娠 40 周前适时终止妊娠。

needs to be paid to screening GDM, hypertension during pregnancy, and the diagnosis of FGR. （5）For pregnant women above 40, fetal monitoring needs to be strengthened and the pregnancy should be terminated at the appropriate time before the 40th week.

5　口译注释与学习资源

5.1　口译注释

（一）Lysteda

该词是药物商品名称，其主要成分为氨甲环酸，又名传明酸。主要成分是氨甲环酸的药物有很多，文中的 Cyklokapron 也是主要成分为氨甲环酸的药物商品名称。

（二）elderly

该词原义为"上了年纪的""过了中年的""老龄的、高龄的"。在日常英语中，通常使用"the elderly"指称"老年人"。在日常生活语境下，这一词语多用于指称 60 岁及以上的人群。但在妇产科医学中，一般认为妇女的最佳生育年龄是 25 岁到 30 岁，30 岁以后妇女的生育能力开始衰退，35 岁以上的产妇被认为有高危孕产风险，因此是高龄产妇，使用"elderly pregnancy"（高龄怀孕）一词。此外还有"elderly primigravida"（高龄初产妇）等。

5.2　学习资源

登录中国大学 MOOC（慕课），学习"医疗口译"课程中"妇产科"的口译实战示范视频和补充材料：（1）大英百科全书"妇产科"词条；（2）全国妇联"两癌"（乳腺癌、宫颈癌）防治科普宣教系列视频；（3）医疗科普网站"中国医疗"科普文章《孕产妇致命点——羊水栓塞》。

参考文献

[1] Encyclopædia Britannica, inc. (n. d.). *Obstetrics and gynecology*. Retrieved November 14,

2021, from https://www.britannica.com/science/obstetrics.

[2] St. George's University. (2021, October 21). *What is an OB/GYN?. A look at the doctors specializing in women's health.* Retrieved November 14, 2021, from https://www.sgu.edu/blog/medical/what-is-an-ob-gyn/.

[3] Healthcare Business Today. (2020, June 8). *What is the difference between Obstetrics & Gynecology?.* Retrieved November 14, 2021, from https://www.healthcarebusinesstoday.com/what-is-the-difference-between-obstetrics-gynecology/.

[4] Mayo Foundation for Medical Education and Research. (2021, September 16). *Uterine fibroids.* Retrieved November 14, 2021, from https://www.mayoclinic.org/diseases-conditions/uterine-fibroids/diagnosis-treatment/drc－20354294.

[5] Medicalmed. us. (n. d.). *Hysteromyoma.* Retrieved November 14, 2021, from https://medicalmed.us/mioma-matki.htm.

[6] Mayo Foundation for Medical Education and Research. (2020, August 18). *Amniotic fluid embolism.* Retrieved November 14, 2021, from https://www.mayoclinic.org/diseases-conditions/amniotic-fluid-embolism/symptoms-causes/syc－20369324.

[7] 中国医疗. 孕产妇致命点——羊水栓塞 [EB/OL]. [2021－07－18]. http://med.china.com.cn/content/pid/283106/tid/1026.

[8] Johns Hopkins Medicine. (n. d.). *Polycystic ovary syndrome (PCOS).* Retrieved November 14, 2021, from https://www.hopkinsmedicine.org/health/conditions-and-diseases/polycystic-ovary-syndrome-pcos.

[9] Mayo Foundation for Medical Education and Research. (2020, October 3). *Polycystic ovary syndrome (PCOS).* Retrieved November 14, 2021, from https://www.mayoclinic.org/diseases-conditions/pcos/symptoms-causes/syc－20353439.

[10] 全国妇联. "两癌"（乳腺癌，宫颈癌）防治科普宣教系列视频（十二集）[EB/OL]. [2020－12－19]. https://www.bilibili.com/video/BV1L54y1t74Z? p=11&spm_id_from=pageDriver.

[11] 中华医学会. 孕前和孕期保健指南（2018）[EB/OL]. [2021－09－19]. https://max.book118.com/html/2018/0827/8124117114001121.shtm.

第十七章

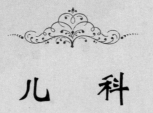

儿　科

1 导读

本章重点为口译技巧之译前准备和儿科的 6 篇"口译实战"练习。口译实战练习中英译汉、汉译英各 3 篇，内容涵盖儿科介绍、佝偻病、小儿脑炎、脊髓灰质炎、注意力缺陷多动障碍和先天性心脏病。请结合本章口译技巧练习 6 篇口译实战文本。

2 口译技巧——译前准备

为了提供高质量的口译服务，口译员除了需要长期进行知识储备和技巧训练以外，在承担具体某次口译任务之前，还需要因地制宜地做好译前准备。这既是出色完成口译任务的必要前提条件，也是口译员职业道德规范的要求。口译的译前准备主要分为语言主题准备、服务协调准备和心理素质准备三个方面。

第一，语言主题准备。在医疗会议口译开始前，首先，口译员应主动询问主办方或者发言人有无讲稿及其他与讲话有直接关联的资料，如 PPT、印刷品等其他视觉辅助材料。如果有，最好能做一到两遍视译，醒目标注难点和重点，并对难句进行笔译。其次，在准备专业术语和生词时，应制作词汇表。词汇表可按照一定的顺序进行排列（可按首字母或拼音、出现先后等顺序）以方便查找。在此基础上，做好口译主题背景及关联主题的准备。在医疗场合开展口译活动时，应提前了解患者背景、具体疾病、医疗方案、设备等背景知识，熟记相关术语。如生词术语较多，则应制作易拿取的精简术语表。除此之外，口译员需要对讲话者的口音特征提前做准备，以避免在口译活动中由于不熟悉口音引起听解困难。

第二，服务协调准备。在翻译医学国际会议时，首先需了解服务对象的姓名、职务，最好制作发言人及出席嘉宾名单及职务中英对照表。如有可能，对其供职的机构也做相应的背景了解。其次，熟悉口译服务的日程和场地，并及时做调整，如增加桌面立式话筒架、协调口译员座位等。另外，注意口译服务规范，准备好备用纸笔，着装需大方得体。在进行医疗场景口译语言服务时，应提前与患者沟通，了解其诉求，熟悉医疗场景及设备，注意遵守医疗口译职业伦理规范，比如对患者病情保密、不向患者提供医疗相关的专业建议等。

第三，心理素质准备。医学口译实践术语多、专业知识难度大、涉及生命健康安全，因此对口译员的心理素质要求较高。口译员要有过硬的心理素质，给自己积极的心理暗示，克服怯场，并做到即使出错也能迅速调整心态完成好剩余的工作。

对口译员来说，长期坚持进行知识储备和译前准备是保障口译任务顺利完成的前提条件。在日常训练中可以从语言主题、服务协调和心理素质三个方面进行相应的准备，尤其需要注意语言主题方面的准备，因为语言能力的增长是一个日积月累的过程。在日常练习中有以下两点需要特别注意。

第一，积累医学专业术语需要建立在理解的基础上，也就是说医学基础知识的补充是术语准备的重要一环。比如在记忆有关病变的中英文名称时，可以补充相关的病理知识，扩大阅读量。同时，对于医学词根词缀，可分门别类地做规律性的总结记忆。

第二，在语音准备方面，译员不仅需要适应不同国家和地区的英语口音，还需要适应中国的地方口音。适应不同的语音要求口译学习者"耳听八方"，即保证听足够时长的非标准英语国家和地区的语料，可在每次或者每隔一次的练习中涉及一两篇非标准英语材料，包括非英语国家和地区讲话者语料和英语国家的非标准英语讲话者语料。以"听、复述、总结发音规律"的步骤，逐步提高听解不同语音讲话者的能力。中国地域辽阔，有丰富的方言种类，口译学习者也需要下意识地安排相应的时间适应。

3 口译词汇

3.1 英译汉

（一）Pediatrics 儿科

preventive health care 预防保健

congenital conditions 先天性疾病

developmental delays 发育迟缓

neonate 新生儿

（二）Rickets 佝偻病

phosphorus 磷

celiac disease 脂肪泻

inflammatory bowel disease 炎症性肠道疾病

cystic fibrosis 囊性纤维化

growth plate 生长板

skeletal deformity 骨骼畸形

breastbone projection 胸骨外翻

melanin 黑色素

antiretroviral medication 抗逆转录病毒药物

premature birth 早产

exclusive breast-feeding 纯母乳喂养

（三）Pediatric Encephalitis 小儿脑炎

encephalitis 脑炎

spinal cord 脊髓

measles 麻疹

mumps 腮腺炎

rubella 风疹

herpes simplex virus 单纯疱疹病毒

West Nile virus 西尼罗河病毒

Lyme disease 莱姆病

syphilis 梅毒

toxoplasmosis 弓形虫病

hallucination 幻觉

glycine 甘氨酸

amino acid 氨基酸

meningitis 脑膜炎

Epstein-Barr virus 爱泼斯坦 - 巴尔病毒（又称巴尔病毒或者 EB 病毒）

prion disease 朊蛋白病

stool test 粪便检测

sputum culture 痰培养

electroencephalogram （EEG）脑电图

lumbar puncture 腰椎穿刺

3.2 汉译英

（一）脊髓灰质炎 Poliomyelitis

麻痹 paralysis

粪－口途径 fecal-oral route

僵化 immobilize

腹膜炎 paresthesia

灭活脊髓灰质炎疫苗 inactivated poliovirus vaccine（IPV）

口服脊髓灰质炎疫苗 oral poliovirus vaccine（OPV）

（二）注意力缺陷多动障碍 Attention Deficit Hyperactivity Disorder（ADHD）

神经发育障碍 neurodevelopmental disorder

烦躁 fidget

注意力缺陷障碍表现型 predominantly inattentive presentation

活跃过度的 hyperactive

易冲动的 impulsive

（三）先天性心脏病 Congenital Heart Disease（CHD）

损伤 lesion

胎儿 fetus

先天性心血管畸形 congenital cardiovascular malformation

发病率 incidence

心脏杂音 heart murmur

超声心动图 ultrasound cardiogram

嗜睡 sleepiness

自愈 clear without treatment

心力衰竭 heart failure

心内膜炎 endocarditis

血栓 thrombosis

拔牙 tooth extraction

扁桃体切除术 tonsillectomy

心律不齐 arrhythmia

心肌病 cardiomyopathy

4 口译实战

4.1 英译汉

(一) Pediatrics 儿科[1]

Pediatrics is the specialty of medical science concerned with the physical and mental health of children from birth to young adulthood. Pediatric care encompasses a broad spectrum of health services ranging from preventive health care to the diagnosis and treatment of acute and chronic diseases. The word "pediatrics" means "healer of children". Pediatrics is a relatively new medical specialty, developing only in the mid-19th century. Abraham Jacobi (1830–1919) is known as the father of pediatrics.

The aim of the study of pediatrics is to reduce infant and child rate of deaths, control the spread of infectious disease, promote healthy lifestyles for a long disease-free life and help ease the problems of children and adolescents with chronic conditions. Pediatricians diagnose and treat several conditions among children, including injuries, infections, genetic and congenital conditions, cancers, organ diseases and

儿科是一个医学分支学科，涉及儿童从出生到成年早期的成长过程中的身体与精神健康。儿科包含从预防保健到急性病和慢性病的诊断和治疗的一系列健康服务。"pediactrics"（儿科）一词的字面意思是"儿童治愈者"。儿科是一个相对较新的医学专业，直到19世纪中叶才发展起来。亚伯拉罕·雅各比（1830—1919）被称为儿科之父。

儿科的目标是降低婴儿和儿童的死亡率，控制传染病的传播，宣传健康的生活方式以远离病痛，延长寿命，并帮助缓解儿童和青少年慢性病的问题。儿科医生主要诊断和治疗的儿童疾病包括创伤、感染、遗传和先天性疾病、癌症、器官疾病和功能障碍。

dysfunctions.

Pediatrics is concerned not only about immediate management of the ill children but also the long-term influence on children's quality of life, disability and survival. Pediatricians are involved with the prevention, early detection, and management of problems including developmental delays and disorders, behavioral problems, functional disabilities, mental disorders including depression and anxiety disorders, etc.

儿科不仅帮助患儿快速得到治疗，还关注儿童长期的生活质量、残疾和生存状况。儿科医生参与预防、早期发现和管理以下问题：发育迟缓和紊乱、行为问题、功能障碍、精神障碍（包括抑郁症和焦虑症）等。

Pediatrics is a collaborative specialty. Pediatricians need to work closely with other medical specialists and healthcare professionals and subspecialists of pediatrics to help children with problems. The pediatricians include primary care pediatricians, pediatric medical subspecialists, and pediatric surgical specialists

儿科是一个需要协作的医学专科。儿科医生需要与其他医学专家、医疗保健专业人员和儿科下辖细分方向的医生密切合作，帮助有问题的儿童。儿科医生包括初级保健儿科医生、儿内科医生和儿外科医生。

Pediatrics is different from adult medicine in more ways than one, because children differ from adults anatomically, physiologically, immunologically, psychologically, developmentally, and metabolically. We can get the difference

儿科在很多方面与成人医学不同，因为儿童在解剖、生理、免疫、心理、发育和代谢上与成人有所差异。我们可以一目了然地发现，婴儿、新生儿或儿童在生理上与成人有很大不同，因此医治儿童不能看作医治缩小版的成人。

at a glance that the smaller body of an infant, a neonate or a child is substantially different physiologically from that of an adult, so treating children is not like treating a miniature adult.

Congenital defects, genetic variance, and developmental issues are of greater concern to pediatricians than physicians treating adults. In addition, there are several legal issues in pediatrics. Children are minors and, in most jurisdictions, cannot make decisions for themselves. The issues of guardianship, privacy, legal responsibility and informed consent should be considered in every pediatric procedure.

与治疗成人不同，先天缺陷、遗传差异和发育问题更受儿科医生的关注。此外，儿科中还存在一些法律问题。儿童是未成年人，在大多数司法管辖领域没有自我决定权。监护、隐私、法律责任和知情同意等问题应在每个儿科医治程序中加以考虑。

（二）Rickets 佝偻病[2]

Rickets is the softening and weakening of bones in children, usually because of an extreme and prolonged vitamin D deficiency. Not enough vitamin D makes it difficult to maintain proper calcium and phosphorus levels in bones, which can cause rickets. Vitamin D deficiency may due to lack of sunlight exposure or food sources such as fish oil, egg yolks, salmon etc. It can also be problems with absorption.

佝偻病是儿童骨骼的软化和弱化，通常是由于长期极度缺乏维生素 D 造成的。维生素 D 不足，难以维持骨骼中适当的钙和磷水平，也就导致了佝偻病。维生素 D 的缺乏可能是由缺乏阳光照射，或缺乏鱼油、蛋黄、鲑鱼等食物来源造成的。它也可能与吸收问题相关。

Some children are born with or develop medical conditions that affect the way their bodies absorb vitamin D, such as celiac disease, inflammatory bowel disease, cystic fibrosis, and kidney problems. Signs and symptoms of rickets may include delayed growth, delayed motor skills, pain in the spine, pelvis and legs, and muscle weakness. Because rickets softens the areas of growing tissue at the ends of a child's bones (growth plates), it can cause skeletal deformities such as bowed legs or knock knees, thickened wrists and ankles, and breastbone projection.

Risk factors that can increase a child's risk of rickets are as follows: (1) Dark skin. Dark skin has more of the pigment melanin, which lowers the skin's ability to produce vitamin D from sunlight. (2) Northern latitudes. Children who live in geographical locations where there is less sunshine are at higher risk of rickets. (3) Medications. Certain types of anti-seizure medications and antiretroviral medications which are used to treat HIV infections, appear to interfere with the body's ability to use vitamin D.

有些儿童自出生起或者在成长发育中出现健康状况而影响其身体吸收维生素 D，比如患有脂肪泻、炎症性肠道疾病、囊性纤维化、肾脏疾病。佝偻病的症状包括生长迟缓，运动技能延迟，脊椎、骨盆和腿部疼痛，肌肉无力。佝偻病使儿童骨骼末端的生长组织区域（生长板）软化，从而可能导致骨骼畸形，如弓形腿或膝盖内扣，手腕和脚踝出现骨突，胸骨外翻。

可能增加儿童患佝偻病的风险因素如下：（1）深肤色。深色皮肤含有更多的黑色素，从而降低了皮肤在阳光下产生维生素 D 的能力。（2）靠北高纬度。生活在阳光较少的地理位置的儿童患佝偻病的风险较高。（3）药物。某些类型的抗癫痫药物和过去用于治疗艾滋病病毒感染的抗逆转录病毒药物，会干扰身体使用维生素 D 的能力。

（4）Premature birth. Babies born before their due dates tend to have lower levels of vitamin D because they had less time to receive the vitamin from their mothers in the wombs. （5）Mother's vitamin D deficiency during pregnancy. （6）Exclusive breast-feeding. Breast milk doesn't contain enough vitamin D to prevent rickets.

Most cases of rickets can be treated with vitamin D and calcium supplements. Adding vitamin D or calcium to the diet generally corrects the bone problems associated with rickets. But too much vitamin D can be harmful. When rickets is due to another underlying medical problem, additional medications or other treatment are needed. Some skeletal deformities caused by rickets may require corrective surgery.

Exposure to sunlight provides the best source of vitamin D. During most seasons, 10 to 15 minutes of exposure to the sun near midday is enough. Make sure your child eats foods that contain vitamin D naturally—fatty fish such as salmon and tuna, fish oil and egg yolks—or that have been fortified with vitamin D, such as infant formula, cereal bread, milk etc.

（4）早产。早产儿的维生素 D 水平往往较低，因为他们在子宫里从母体获得维生素的时间更短。（5）怀孕期间母亲缺乏维生素 D。（6）纯母乳喂养。母乳中没有足够的维生素 D 来预防佝偻病。

佝偻病在大多数情况下可以通过补充维生素 D 和钙来加以治疗。在饮食中加入维生素 D 或钙通常可以纠正佝偻病相关的骨骼问题。但是，维生素 D 过量对人体也是有害的。当佝偻病是由其他潜在的健康问题引起时，需要使用额外的药物或其他治疗手段。一些由佝偻病引起的骨骼畸形需要进行矫正手术。

晒太阳是补充维生素 D 的最佳方式。在大多数季节，中午晒 10 到 15 分钟的太阳便可以获得足够的维生素 D。让孩子吃天然富含维生素 D 的食物，比如鲑鱼和金枪鱼这类富含天然脂肪的鱼，以及鱼油和蛋黄，或让孩子吃添加维生素 D 的食物，如婴儿配方奶粉、添加维生素 D 的谷物面包和牛奶等。

It is recommended that all infants receive 400 IU of vitamin D a day. Because human milk contains only a small amount of vitamin D, infants who are exclusively breast-fed should receive supplemental vitamin D daily. Some bottle-fed infants may also need vitamin D supplements if they aren't receiving enough from their formula.

建议所有婴儿每天摄入 400IU 的维生素 D。由于母乳中只含有少量维生素 D，纯母乳喂养的婴儿应每天补充维生素 D。对于一些非母乳喂养的婴儿来说，如果配方奶粉没有足够的维生素 D，也需要通过补充剂补充。

（三）Pediatric Encephalitis 小儿脑炎[3]

Pediatric encephalitis (encephalopathy) is a term used to describe inflammation of the membranes that surround the brain and spinal cord. This condition causes problems with the brain and spinal cord function. The inflammation causes the brain to swell, which leads to changes in the child's neurological condition, including mental confusion and seizures. The cause of encephalitis varies with the season, the area of the country, and the exposure of the child.

小儿脑炎（脑病）是用来描述覆盖小儿大脑和脊髓的膜出现炎症的专有词汇。这种疾病会导致大脑和脊髓功能性问题。炎症导致大脑肿胀，引起儿童神经方面的变化，如精神错乱和癫痫发作。脑炎的病因有多种，与季节、地区和患儿暴露情况相关。

Viruses are the leading cause of encephalitis. Although vaccines for many viruses, including measles, mumps, rubella, and chickenpox have greatly lowered the rate of encephalitis from these diseases, other viruses can cause

病毒感染是导致脑炎的主要原因。虽然许多病毒的疫苗，比如麻疹、腮腺炎、风疹和水痘的疫苗，大大降低了这些疾病导致脑炎的发病率，但其他病毒也有可能导致脑炎，如单纯疱疹病毒、西尼罗河病毒（由蚊子携

encephalitis. These include herpes simplex virus, West Nile virus (carried by mosquitoes) and rabies (carried by a number of different animals).

In most cases, babies and children with encephalitis experience mild flu-like symptoms, including fever, headache, fatigue, loss of appetite, nausea and vomiting, increased irritability, body stiffness. In more severe cases, babies and children with encephalitis experience confusion, hallucinations, loss of consciousness, loss of sensation or paralysis in certain regions of the face or body, problems with speech or hearing, and seizures.

Pediatric encephalopathy may be caused by several factors. In infants, it is usually a genetic condition involving high levels of glycine (amino acid) in the brain. Other causes of encephalopathy include bacterial meningitis, Epstein-Barr virus (the virus that causes mononucleosis, chicken pox and shingles), enteroviruses, Hashimoto's disease, herpes simplex virus 1 and 2, Lyme disease, measles, mosquito-borne viruses, mumps, West Nile virus, tick-borne viruses, rabies,

带）和狂犬病病毒（由许多不同的动物携带）。

在大多数情况下，患有脑炎的婴幼儿会出现轻微的流感样症状，包括发烧、头痛、疲劳、食欲不振、恶心、呕吐、烦躁不安、身体僵硬。在更严重的情况下，患有脑炎的婴幼儿会出现意识混乱、幻觉、意识丧失、脸部或身体的某些部位知觉丧失或瘫痪、语言或听觉障碍以及癫痫发作。

小儿脑病可能由多个因素引起。婴儿患小儿脑炎往往由一种遗传性疾病造成，涉及大脑中甘氨酸（氨基酸）浓度过高。脑炎的其他发病原因包括细菌性脑膜炎、爱泼斯坦－巴尔病毒（这种病毒往往造成单核细胞增多症状、水痘和皮肤疱疹）、肠道病毒、桥本病、1 型或 2 型单纯疱疹病毒、莱姆病、麻疹、蚊虫传播型病毒、腮腺炎、西尼罗河病毒、虱子传播型病毒、狂犬病、朊蛋白病（蛋白质紊乱）、产前用药不慎、维生素 B_1 缺乏、高血压、感染和肾衰竭。

prion diseases (protein disorders), prenatal drug exposure, vitamin B1 deficiency, high blood pressure, infection, and kidney failure.

Diagnostic tests that may be performed to confirm the diagnosis of encephalitis may include X-ray, magnetic resonance imaging (MRI), computed tomography scan (CT or CAT scan), blood tests, urine and stool tests, sputum culture, electroencephalogram (EEG), lumbar puncture (spinal tap) and in rare cases brain biopsy.

The key to treating encephalitis is early detection and treatment. A child with encephalitis requires immediate hospitalization and close monitoring. The goal of treatment is to reduce the swelling in the head and to prevent other related complications. Medications to control the infection, seizures, fever, or other conditions may be used.

脑炎确诊检测手段有 X 光检测、核磁共振成像（MRI）、计算机断层扫描（CT 或 CAT 扫描）、血液检测、尿液和粪便检测、痰培养、脑电图（EEG）、腰椎穿刺（脊柱穿刺）。在极少数情况下使用脑活检。

治疗脑炎的关键是早发现、早治疗。患有脑炎的儿童需要立即住院接受密切监测。治疗的目标是减少脑部肿胀，并防止相关并发症。可使用控制感染、癫痫发作、发烧或其他情况的药物。

4.2 汉译英

（一）脊髓灰质炎 Poliomyelitis[4]

小儿麻痹症或者说脊髓灰质炎，是一种由脊髓灰质炎病毒引起的致残和危及生命的疾病。该病毒入侵神经系统，可在数小时内导致患者完全麻

Polio, or poliomyelitis, is a disabling and life-threatening disease caused by the poliovirus. It invades the nervous system, and can cause total

痹。该病毒主要通过粪－口途径传播，实现人传人，偶尔也可通过其他媒介（例如受污染的水或食物）传播，并在肠道中繁殖。

最初的症状有发烧、乏力、头痛、呕吐、颈部僵硬和四肢疼痛。每200例感染中约有1例导致不可逆的麻痹（通常是腿部麻痹）。在该病致瘫痪的患者中，有5%至10%的人由于呼吸肌麻痹而死亡。脊髓灰质炎的患者主要是5岁以下的儿童。

约有72%感染脊髓灰质炎病毒的人不会有任何明显的症状。大约四分之一的感染者会有类似流感的症状，比如喉咙痛、发烧、疲倦、恶心、头痛、胃痛。这些症状通常持续2至5天，然后自行消失。脊髓灰质炎病毒感染者中，有一小部分会出现其他影响大脑和脊髓的更严重症状，如感觉异常。

paralysis in a matter of hours. The virus is transmitted from person to person through the fecal-oral route or, less frequently, by other vehicles (for example, contaminated water or food) and multiplies in the intestine.

Initial symptoms are fever, fatigue, headache, vomiting, stiffness of the neck and pain in the limbs. About 1 in 200 infections leads to irreversible paralysis (usually in the legs). Among those paralyzed, 5% to 10% die when their breathing muscles become immobilized. Polio mainly affects children under 5 years of age.

About 72% of people who get infected with poliovirus will not have any visible symptoms. About 1 out of 4 people with poliovirus infection will have flu-like symptoms that may include sore throat, fever, tiredness, nausea, headache, stomach pain. These symptoms usually last 2 to 5 days, and then go away on their own. A smaller proportion of people with poliovirus infection will develop other more serious symptoms that affect the brain and spinal cord such as paresthesia.

脑膜炎是覆盖脊髓或大脑的膜的感染，每 25 名脊髓灰质炎病毒感染者中约有 1 人会出现脑膜炎。每 200 名脊髓灰质炎病毒感染者中，约有 1 人会出现手臂和腿部麻痹或肌力降低的症状，或两种症状兼有。麻痹是脊髓灰质炎最严重的症状，因为它可能导致永久性残疾和死亡。每 100 名因脊髓灰质炎病毒感染而瘫痪的人中，有 2 至 10 人会死亡，因为病毒会影响帮助他们呼吸的肌肉。

脊髓灰质炎病毒具有很强的传染性，接触感染者的粪便、喷嚏或咳嗽中的飞沫均可造成感染。感染者可在症状出现前或者症状出现后的两周内，将病毒传播给他人。病毒可以在感染者的粪便中存活数周。在不卫生的环境中，它会污染食物和水。没有症状的人也可以将病毒传染给他人，造成他人患病。

有两种疫苗可以预防脊髓灰质炎：一种是灭活脊髓灰质炎疫苗（IPV），通常根据患者年龄，在腿部或手臂部

Meningitis is infection of the covering of the spinal cord or brain, and it occurs in about 1 out of 25 people with poliovirus infection. Paralysis or weakness in the arms, legs, or both, occurs in about 1 out of 200 people with poliovirus infection. Paralysis is the most severe symptom associated with polio, because it can lead to permanent disability and death. Between 2 and 10 out of 100 people who have paralysis from poliovirus infection die, because the virus affects the muscles that help them breathe.

Poliovirus is very contagious and the transmission can be through contact with the feces of an infected person or droplets from a sneeze or cough. An infected person may spread the virus to others immediately before and up to 2 weeks after symptoms appear. The virus can live in an infected person's feces for many weeks. It can contaminate food and water in unsanitary conditions. People who don't have symptoms can still pass the virus to others and make them sick.

There are two types of vaccine that can prevent polio. One is inactivated poliovirus vaccine (IPV), which is

位注射。另一种是口服脊髓灰质炎疫苗（OPV），它在世界各地被广泛使用。99%的接种了推荐剂量的灭活脊髓灰质炎疫苗的儿童，都将得到保护，免受脊髓灰质炎的感染。

given as an injection in the leg or arm, depending on the patient's age. The other is oral poliovirus vaccine (OPV) which is used throughout the world. 99 percent of children who get the recommended doses of the inactivated polio vaccine will be protected from this disease.

（二）注意力缺陷多动障碍 Attention Deficit Hyperactivity Disorder (ADHD)[5]

注意力缺陷多动障碍（多动症）是儿童时期最常见的神经发育障碍之一。多动症首次确诊通常是在儿童时期，病程可持续到成年。患多动症的儿童通常过于活跃，注意力难以集中，也很难控制冲动行为，也就是说他们的行动往往不考虑后果。

Attention deficit hyperactivity disorder (ADHD) is one of the most common neurodevelopmental disorders of childhood. It is usually first diagnosed in childhood and often lasts into adulthood. Children with ADHD may be overly active, have trouble paying attention, and feel difficult to control impulsive behaviors, namely they may act without thinking about what the result will be.

患有多动症的孩子常常异想天开，经常忘事或者丢东西，乱动或烦躁不安，多话，常因粗心而犯错误或冒不必要的风险，难以抵抗诱惑，也很难和他人相处。

A child with ADHD may daydream a lot, forget or lose things a lot, squirm or fidget, talk too much, make careless mistakes or take unnecessary risks, have a hard time resisting temptation, and have difficulty getting along with others.

根据患儿最突出的症状来划分，多动症有三种不同类型：第一种类型的多动症主要表现为注意力缺陷障碍。

There are three different types of ADHD, depending on which types of symptoms are strongest in the individual.

患儿很难组织或完成一项任务，难以注意事物的细节或遵循指示。这类孩子很容易分心或忘记日常生活的细节。

第二种类型的多动症主要表现为活跃过度及易冲动。患儿通常烦躁不安，爱不停说话。低龄幼儿常爱跑、跳、攀爬。他们很难有秩序意识，也不太听管教。第三种类型的多动症是混合型多动症，也就是上述两种类型的症状在患儿身上都有出现。

儿童多动症有别于儿童好动、调皮。好动、调皮是孩子的天性，但是，如果孩子的肢体活动明显比同龄儿童多，且自控力差，不能安静下来，就要警惕孩子是否患有多动症。研究发现，多动症患儿与淘气好动的儿童有着四点本质区别：

第一，注意力方面，调皮孩子对

The first type of ADHD is predominantly inattentive presentation. It is hard for the child to organize or finish a task, to pay attention to details, or to follow instructions. The child is easily distracted or forgets details of daily routines.

The second type is predominantly hyperactive-impulsive presentation: The child fidgets and talks a lot. Smaller children may run, jump or climb constantly. It is hard for them to wait their turn or listen to directions. The third type is combined presentation: Symptoms of the above two types are equally present in the person.

Children with ADHD are different from active and naughty children. Being active and naughty is in the nature of children, but if the child's physical activity is significantly more than that of his peers, and he has difficulty in self-control and quieting down, we should be alerted to consider whether the child has ADHD. Research has found that children with ADHD and naughty children have four essential differences.

Firstly, for attention, naughty

感兴趣的事物能聚精会神，还讨厌别人干扰，而患多动症的孩子玩什么都心不在焉，做事也无法有始有终；第二，自控力方面，调皮孩子在陌生的环境里、在要求下能约束自己，而多动症患儿根本坐不住，静不下来；

children can concentrate on things of their interests and hate other people's interference when they concentrate, but children with ADHD are always absent-minded in everything and cannot conclude things orderly. Secondly, for self-control, naughty children can discipline themselves in an unfamiliar environment or upon request, but children with ADHD are always restless and cannot quiet themselves down.

第三，行为活动方面，调皮孩子的好动行为一般有原因、有目的，而多动症患儿的行为多具有冲动性，缺乏目的性；第四，生理方面，调皮孩子思路敏捷、动作协调，没有记忆辨认方面的缺陷，而多动症患儿则有明显生理上的不足。

Thirdly, for behaviors in activities, naughty children's active behaviors generally have a reason or a purpose, but children with ADHD conduct behaviors impulsively and aimlessly. Fourthly, for the physiological aspect, naughty children are quick in mind, can coordinate their movements, and don't have defects in memory and recognition, but children with ADHD have obvious deficiencies physiologically.

（三）先天性心脏病 Congenital Heart Disease[6]

先天性心脏病指的是母亲在怀孕期间，由各种原因导致胎儿的心脏或血管发育异常所造成的心脏血管的功能障碍。因为出生时就存在，所以称为先天性心血管畸形，也叫先天性心脏病，简称先心病。先心病是新生儿

Congenital heart disease refers to the lesions of the heart vessels in the fetus caused by the fetus' abnormal development of the heart or heart vessels due to various reasons during the mother's pregnancy. Because it exists since birth,

和婴儿死亡最主要的原因之一。

据统计，先天性心脏病是中国发病率最高的出生缺陷疾病。约有千分之六到千分之八的新生儿患有先天性心脏病。一般有先天性心血管疾病的患儿，常有喂奶困难、营养不良的表现，易发生反复肺部感染。大多数先天性心脏血管病具有特殊的心脏杂音，参考胸部 X 光片或超声心动图，一般不难诊断。

先心病的体征和症状取决于特定缺陷的类型和严重程度。有些缺陷可能很少或不会导致出现体征或症状。其他缺陷可能导致婴儿指甲或嘴唇呈蓝色，呼吸急促或困难，进食时困乏以及嗜睡。先心病中有少数轻症病例可以自愈，但纠正心脏血管畸形一般需做手术。

it is called congenital cardiovascular malformation or congenital heart disease, for short CHD. CHD is one of the leading causes of the newborn and infant deaths.

According to statistics, CHD is the birth defect with the highest disease incidence in China. About 6 to 8 out of one thousand newborns suffer from the disease. Children with congenital cardiovascular disease often have difficulties in feeding, and they are often malnourished and prone to repeated lung infections. Most congenital cardiovascular diseases have special presentation such as heart murmurs, which makes the diagnosis not that difficult with reference to chest X-rays or ultrasound cardiograms.

Signs and symptoms for CHD depend on the type and severity of the particular defects. Some defects might have few or no signs or symptoms. Others might cause a baby to have blue-tinted nails or lips, fast or troubled breathing, tiredness when feeding, and sleepiness. A few mild cases of CHD can clear without treatment, but surgery is generally required to correct cardiac vascular malformation.

学龄前儿童期是施行手术的合适时期，但如若病情严重，即使是婴儿也应立即施行手术。未施行手术、暂不宜手术或病情好转而不考虑施行手术的病人，宜根据病情避免过度劳累、预防感染，以免引起心力衰竭、感染性心内膜炎或血栓。凡先心病患者，在施行任何其他手术前后，包括拔牙、切除扁桃体等，都要预防性使用抗生素以预防感染性心内膜炎。

即使患者病情通过治疗得到改善，心脏缺陷也已经修复，许多先心病患者也不能够说完全治愈了。先心病患者可能会随着时间的推移而出现其他健康问题，这取决于其心脏缺陷的类型、数量以及严重程度。

可能出现的一些其他健康问题包括心律失常，也就是心跳不规则；由心肌感染而导致的感染性心内膜炎；

Preschool childhood is the appropriate age for surgery, but surgeries need to be performed immediately even in infancy when the conditions are severe. Patients who have not undergone surgeries, are not suitable for surgeries or do not need surgeries because of the improvement of their conditions, should avoid overwork and prevent infection according to their condition, so as not to cause heart failure, infectious endocarditis or thrombosis. All patients with this disease should preventively apply antibiotics to prevent infectious endocarditis before and after any other surgeries, including tooth extraction, tonsillectomy, etc.

Even when the conditions have improved and the patients' heart defects have been repaired with treatments, many people with CHD are not cured entirely. People with CHD can develop other health problems over time, depending on the type, number and severity of their heart defects.

Some other health problems that might develop include arrhythmia which means irregular heartbeats, infective

心肌病，可使心脏虚弱。先心病患者需按时去看心内科医生，进行规范检查，以尽可能保持健康。儿童做完第一次手术后，可能需要进一步手术。对先心病患者来说，定期去看医生很重要，他们需要和医生沟通其健康状况，包括他们的心脏状况。

endocarditis which is due to the infection in the heart muscles, or cardiomyopathy indicating weakness in the heart. People with CHD need routine checkups with a cardiologist to stay as healthy as possible. They also might need further operations after initial childhood surgeries. It is important for people with CHD to visit their doctors on a regular basis and discuss their health, including their specific heart condition, with their doctors.

5 口译注释与学习资源

5.1 口译注释

国际单位 IU

IU 是医学效价单位。一些药物如维生素、激素、抗生素、抗毒素类生物制品等的化学成分不稳定，或者目前还不能用理化方法检定其质量规格，因此往往采用生物实验方法并与标准品加以比较来检定其效价。通过这种生物检定，具有一定生物效能的最小效价单元就叫"单位"（U）；经由国际协商规定的标准单位，称为"国际单位"（IU）。

5.2 学习资源

登录中国大学 MOOC（慕课），学习"医疗口译"课程中"儿科"的口译实战示范视频。

参考文献

[1] American Academy of Pediatrics Committee on Pediatric Workforce, C. O. P., Rimsza, M. E., Hotaling, A. J., Keown, M. E., Marcin, J. P., Moskowitz, W. B., Sigrest, T. D., & Simon, H. K. (2015, April 1). *Definition of a pediatrician*. Retrieved November 13, 2021, from https://

publications. aap. org/pediatrics/article/135/4/780/33636/Definition-of-a－Pediatrician.

［2］ Mayo Foundation for Medical Education and Research. (2021, February 25). *Rickets*. Retrieved November 13, 2021, from https://www. mayoclinic. org/diseases-conditions/rickets/diagnosis-treatment/drc－20351949.

［3］ The Children's Hospital of Philadelphia. (2014, August 24). *Encephalitis in children*. Retrieved November 13, 2021, from https://www. chop. edu/conditions-diseases/encephalitis-children.

［4］ World Health Organization. (n. d.). *Poliomyelitis*. Retrieved November 13, 2021, from https://www. who. int/news-room/fact-sheets/detail/poliomyelitis.

［5］ Centers for Disease Control and Prevention. (2021, September 23). *What is ADHD?*. Centers for Disease Control and Prevention. Retrieved November 13, 2021, from https://www. cdc. gov/ncbddd/adhd/facts. html.

［6］ 人民网. 健康卫生频道. 先天性心脏病［EB/OL］.［2021－09－12］. http://health. people. com. cn/GB/119042/120259/index. html

第十八章

重症科

1　导读

本章重点为口译技巧之职业伦理（1）和重症科的 6 篇"口译实战"练习。口译实战练习中英译汉、汉译英各 3 篇，内容涵盖重症医学简介、重症监护中的药代动力学变化、重症监护中的麻醉镇静、热射病、败血症以及重症监护中的营养评估。请结合本章口译技巧思考医学口译中的规范性操作，并练习 6 篇口译实战文本。

2　口译技巧——职业伦理（1）

任何行业都有成文的职业伦理规范，或者不成文的、约定俗成的规矩，这些规范和规矩是行业内认可的指导从业者决策和行为的依据。口译行业也不例外。口译是语言服务行业的重要组成部分。作为新兴的服务行业，口译服务流通及市场化运作日趋成熟，许多多语言、多文化的国家和地区在近 50 年间相继出台了语言服务职业伦理规范以及细分领域（法律、医疗等）的口笔译职业伦理规范。医疗口译从业人员需要熟悉医疗口译职业伦理规范和标准化操作流程，以提供优质的口译服务，维护医患双方权利。医疗口译从业人员熟知相关的职业伦理规范也能够最大限度地保护自身的权利。

在不同国家和地区，医疗口译职业伦理规范细则略有不同，但总体来说都覆盖以下基本纲领要义。

2.1　准确

口译员应准确、完整地传达信息。由于医学场景中术语较多，当口译员不确定时，不应随意揣测信息，而应尽量求证。

2.2　中立

口译员保持立场中立，对医患双方一视同仁，不偏向病人或者医疗机构而向另一方施加压力，同时在职责和能力范围内尽最大努力帮助双方沟通。

2.3　正直

诚实、公正地对待口译活动各参与方，尊重他人，具有同理心，不收受礼物，回避利益相关的口译任务或人员。

2.4　保密

对口译工作保密，除司法介入或有其他紧急情况，如基本人权、国家安全受威胁等，不得透露口译内容，尤其是与病人病情相关的个人隐私信息。

2.5　专业

包括但不限于：及时更新知识储备；具有合作意识和良好的沟通能力；具有奉献精神及同理心；不承担超出自身能力范围的口译任务；不恶意低价竞争或在服务过程中无理由加价；不随意解释医嘱或向病人提供个人看法和医疗建议；不嘲笑、歧视或评判医务人员或病人；如利益相关，应回避口译任务。

口译员职业伦理规范是规范口译员行为、保护口译员利益、维护口译活动各方利益、促进口译市场健康发展的指导性纲领。在不同的国家地区、不同的口译领域，口译职业伦理规范也有差别。但在某些极端情况下，医学口译员有可能陷入伦理决策困难，如病人出现轻生倾向等有可能产生负面结果的情况和口译员职业伦理中的"保密"原则冲突。这时，口译员需本着"生命至上"的原则和向善的价值观做出相应决策和行动，不能一味照搬规范条款。

3　口译词汇

3.1　英译汉

（一）Critical Care Medicine 重症医学

hemodynamic 血流动力学的

intubation 插管

mechanical ventilation 机械通气

hemodialysis 血液透析

resuscitation 复苏术

defibrillation 除颤

pacemaker 起搏器

anesthesiologist 麻醉医师

anesthesia 麻醉

anesthesiology 麻醉学

catheterization 导管插入；插管

intensive care unit（ICU）重症监护病房

secondary injury 继发性损伤

electrocardiomonitor 心电监护仪

defibrillator 除颤仪

ventilator 呼吸机

bronchoscope 支气管镜

extracorporeal membrane oxygenation（ECMO）体外膜肺

intra-aortic balloon pump（IABP）主动脉内球囊反搏泵

（二）Pharmacokinetic Changes in ICU 重症监护中的药代动力学变化

pharmacokinetics 药物代谢动力学

vasoactive 血管活性的

gastrointestinal 胃肠道的

levothyroxine 左旋甲状腺素

subcutaneous injection 皮下注射

vasopressor 升压药

skin perfusion 皮肤灌注

hypoalbuminemia 低蛋白血症

capillary leak syndrome 毛细血管渗漏综合征

hydrophilic 亲水的

serum concentration 血清浓度

aminoglycosides 氨基甙类抗生素

gentamicin 庆大霉素

glycopeptides 糖肽类抗生素

vancomycin 万古霉素

beta-lactam antibiotics 内酰胺类抗生素

loading dose 负荷剂量

hepatic clearance 肝脏清除

renal clearance 肾脏清除

serum creatinine level 血清肌酐水平

maintenance dose 维持剂量

intravenous（IV）静脉内的

（三）Sedation in ICU 重症监护中的麻醉镇静

sedation 镇静

analgesia 镇痛

benzodiazepines 苯二氮䓬类药（镇静剂）

propofol 异丙酚

dexmedetomidine 右旋美托咪啶

intracranial 颅内的

status epilepticus 癫痫

tetanus 破伤风

hepatic microsomal oxidation 肝脏微粒体氧化

glucuronidation 葡萄糖醛酸化

bolus dose 单次剂量

bradycardia 心跳过缓

metabolic acidosis 代谢性酸中毒

rhabdomyolysis 横纹肌溶解

hyperkalemia 高钾血症

ketamine 氯胺酮

fospropofol 磷丙泊酚

3.2 汉译英

（一）热射病 Thermoplegia

热调节 thermoregulation

汗腺 sweat gland

电解质 electrolyte

发病机制 pathogenesis

痉挛 cramp

虚脱 exhaustion

体温过高 hyperthermia

后遗症 sequelae

蛋白质变性 protein denaturation

脂膜流动性变化 fluidity changes in lipid

线粒体 mitochondrion（pl. mitochodria）

多器官功能障碍综合征 multiple organ dysfunction syndrome（MODS）

乌司他丁 ulinastatin

预后效果 prognosis

血管内的 endovascular

血液净化 blood purification

多靶点治疗效果 multi-target therapeutic effect

肌红蛋白 myoglobin

胆红素 bilirubin

炎症介质 inflammatory mediator

体内平衡 homeostasis

细胞因子 cytokine

分泌 secretion

地塞米松 dexamethasone

甘露醇 mannitol

高压氧 hyperbaric oxygen

（二）败血症 Septicemia

败血症 septicemia/sepsis

金黄色葡萄球菌 Staphylococcus aureus

肺炎链球菌 Streptococcus pheumoniae

大肠埃希菌 Escherichia coli or E. coli

针刺 pinprick

变色 discoloration

（三）重症监护中的营养评估 Nutritional Assessment in ICU

营养评分 nutrition score

烧伤 empyrosis

高分解代谢的 hypercatabolic

营养风险筛查 nutrition risk screening

营养风险筛查评分简表 2002 Nutrition Risk Screening 2002 （NRS2002）

重症患者营养风险筛查评估等级表 Nutrition Risk in the Critically Ill Score （NUTRIC Score）

血清白蛋白替代水平 serum albumin replacement level

4 口译实战

4.1 英译汉

（一）Critical Care Medicine 重症医学[1]

The term "Critical Care Medicine" was created from the concept that life-endangered patients may have substantially better chances of survival if provided with professionally advanced minute-to-minute objective measurements. Such measurements were largely based on "real time" electronic monitoring of vital signs, hemodynamic and respiratory parameters, and complementary measurements on blood and body fluids. Intubation, mechanical ventilation, hemodialysis, resuscitation, defibrillation and pacemaker insertion are in general use.

重症医学创建依据的理念是对危重病人进行专业、先进的实时客观数据监测，以显著提高病人生存的概率。这些数据主要基于电子设备对生命体征、血流动力学和呼吸参数进行的"实时"监测，以及对血液和体液的补充检测。插管、机械通气、血液透析、复苏、除颤、起搏器植入是较常见的手段。

These individual techniques had progressively evolved over the preceding decades by anesthesiologists in the operating room and post anesthesia recovery units and by cardiologists in the catheterization laboratory. Conventional methods of observation based on physical examination and largely manual measurement of vital signs at the bedside were therefore increasingly superseded by electronic techniques of quantitative monitoring and measurements. These

在过去几十年中，这些技术手段在手术室及麻醉恢复室的麻醉医师和导管实验室的心脏病专家的推进下，有了很大的进步。因此，医护人员到病床边进行健康检查以及手动测量生命体征的传统观察方法正逐步被定量监测的电子技术取代。这些监测方法不仅成为可接受的做法，而且在名为重症监护室（ICU），或在某些欧洲国家被称为重症治疗室（ITU）的院内单位迅速推广实施。

methods of monitoring and measurements not only became acceptable practices but were also remarkably rapidly implemented by in-hospital sites which were designated intensive care units (ICUs) or in some European countries, intensive therapy units (ITUs).

The main purposes of ICU are to treat patients with serious or life-threatening illnesses, to support failure organ systems and prevent secondary injury, and to provide a highly specialized environment with a higher level of care than the normal ward. In major centers, specialized units were established in part contingent on the volume of patients eligible for specialized cardiac, respiratory, surgical, neurological, and later pediatric and neonatal care.

Nowadays the discipline became a recognized subspecialty in which continuing on-site medical diagnosis and management of immediately life-threatening diseases and/or injuries was provided with high priority by advanced specialists recruited from internal medicine, general surgery, anesthesiology, and pediatrics.

Contemporary ICUs vary not only

重症监护室的主要任务是治疗危重病人，为衰竭的器官系统提供支持，防止继发性损伤，并提供一个比正常病房护理水平更高的高度专业化护理环境。大型医疗机构先是根据需要心脏、呼吸、术后以及神经类特殊护理的患者数量设立了相应的院内单位，而后又应需设立了儿童及新生儿特殊护理相关单位。

如今，重症医学科已成为公认的医学分支专业，从内科、普通外科、麻醉科和儿科聘请高级专家，优先对即刻可危及生命的疾病和伤害进行现场医疗诊断和管理。

当代重症监护室不仅在设施外观

from hospital to hospital with respect to physical structure and locale, but also with respect to the services that are provided, the staffing and the level of expertise of the health care providers, and the table of organization. Some commonly seen ICU equipment includes electrocardiomonitor, defibrillator, ventilator, bronchoscope, extracorporeal membrane oxygenation (ECMO), intra-aortic balloon pump (IABP), etc.

和地理位置上因医院而异，而且在所提供的服务、人员配备和医护人员专门知识水平以及组织架构方面也各不相同。常见的重症监护室设备包括心电监护仪、除颤仪、呼吸机、支气管镜、体外膜肺、主动脉内球囊反搏泵等。

（二）Pharmacokinetic Changes in ICU 重症监护中的药代动力学变化[2]

The recommended dose for a drug is based on the average adult, and a few adjustments are made based on the patient's body weight or renal function. However, in the ICU, the patient isn't the average adult anymore. ICU patients are frequently hemodynamically unstable, so they require vasoactive support; and they have all sorts of tubes connected to them, like a mechanical ventilator. These can all influence pharmacokinetics.

一种药物的推荐剂量一般是根据普通成人情况而定，并根据患者的体重或肾脏功能适当调整。然而，在ICU，病人不再是普通成年患者。ICU中的病人通常因血流动力方面不稳定而需要血管活性支持，而且病人身体连接着各种管子，如机械通气装置。这些都可能影响药物代谢。

Gastrointestinal absorption is decreased in most ICU patients. The absorption of certain drugs, like levothyroxine, is also compromised. Absorption through subcutaneous injection is compromised by shock or the use of vasopressors, since they

大多数ICU的病人胃肠道吸收能力下降，因此某些药物，如左旋甲状腺素的吸收，也会相应减少。皮下注射药物的吸收也会因休克或使用升压药而受到影响，因为这两种情况会降低皮肤灌注能力。这意味着最好一开

reduce skin perfusion. This means the patients will be better off with IV from the beginning.

In a lot of ICU patients, total body water is increased through several intertwined processes. Excessive fluid administration, which is used for the initial treatment of shock, increases total body water by filling up not only the intravascular compartment, but also the interstitial space. This is especially so if the patient can't pee it all out (in severe renal failure), or can't keep the fluids in the intravascular compartment, which is the case in hypoalbuminemia and capillary leak syndrome.

An increase in total body water means that for hydrophilic drugs, the volume of distribution is increased, so it will take a lot longer for drugs to reach the optimal serum concentration. A lot of antibiotics, especially aminoglycosides like gentamicin, glycopeptides like vancomycin, and several beta-lactam antibiotics, are hydrophilic drugs. Therefore, in these patients, doctors need to administer a loading dose for these drugs.

For hydrophilic drugs, renal

始就对病人采取静脉注射的方式。

由于一些复杂的医疗程序，很多 ICU 患者身体里的总液体量增加。最初治疗休克时过量补液，导致血管和间质被过量液体充盈，从而使身体总液体量增加。这种情况在一些患者中尤甚，如严重肾衰竭患者不能通过排尿的方式排出体液，而低蛋白血症和毛细血管渗漏综合征患者不能将液体保留在血管内部。

身体总水量的增加意味着亲水类药物分布体积增加，也就是说，药物要达到最佳血清浓度需要更长的时间。许多抗生素，特别是氨基甙类抗生素，如庆大霉素，糖肽类抗生素，如万古霉素，以及一些内酰胺类抗生素都是亲水类药物。因此，在治疗这些患者时，医生需要使用这类药物的负荷剂量。

相较肝脏代谢排出，亲水类药物

clearance is the most relevant versus hepatic clearance. Renal failure is common in the ICU. But some ICU patients develop an increase in renal function and thus clearance. The patients with augmented renal clearance are the younger, fairly healthy ICU patients, with normal to high cardiac outputs, singular organ failure but not renal failure, and they arrive at the ICU with normal serum creatinine levels. As increased clearance leads to lower serum levels, this would imply that it is necessary to increase maintenance dose in these patients.

更依赖于肾脏代谢排出。肾衰竭在 ICU 病人中很常见。但有一些 ICU 病人肾功能亢进，从而肾脏代谢排出能力增强。这类肾脏代谢排出能力增强的患者是较为年轻、健康情况也相对较好的 ICU 病人。他们一般有正常或者较高的心排血量，或者有非肾衰竭的单器官衰竭，在送入 ICU 时维持了正常的血清肌酐水平。由于代谢能力增强通常导致血清水平降低，这可能就意味着有必要增加这些患者的药物维持剂量。

（三）Sedation in ICU 重症监护中的麻醉镇静[3]

Pain, agitation and delirium are termed the "ICU triad" and appropriate sedation-analgesic techniques must be adopted to mitigate the ill-effects of this triad. Recent ICU guidelines prefer the use of nonbenzodiazepine sedatives (either propofol or dexmedetomidine) over benzodiazepines for improving clinical outcomes in mechanically ventilated adult ICU patients.

疼痛、焦躁和精神错乱被称为"ICU 三联征"，必须采用适当的镇静镇痛方法来减轻其不良影响。最新的 ICU 指南更倾向于使用非苯二氮䓬类镇静剂（异丙酚或右旋美托咪啶）以改善 ICU 中采用机械通气的成年患者的临床效果。

Sedation has different levels. Minimal sedation is defined as a minimally depressed level of consciousness, which

镇静有不同的分级。轻度镇静的定义是最低程度的意识抑制，患者保留有独立持续保持气道通畅的能力，

retains the patient's ability to independently and continuously maintain an airway and to respond normally to tactile stimulation and verbal command. Moderate sedation (conscious sedation) is a drug induced depression of consciousness during which patients respond purposefully to verbal commands or light tactile stimulation, with patent airway and spontaneous ventilation.

Deep sedation is a drug induced depression of consciousness during which patients cannot be easily aroused, but can respond purposefully following repeated or painful stimuli. Patients may require assistance in maintaining a patent airway and the cardiovascular function is usually maintained. Deep sedation is required only in patients having severe respiratory failure, intracranial hypertension, status epilepticus, tetanus and concurrent use of muscle relaxants.

There is a wide choice of sedative medications which can be used to achieve the desired level of sedation. Benzodiazepines are metabolized in the liver by hepatic microsomal oxidation or glucuronidation. Their metabolism may be impaired in elderly and in patients with liver disease. Propofol is one of the most

并能正常地对触觉刺激和言语命令做出反应。中度镇静（也称"清醒镇静"）使用药物抑制知觉。在此期间，患者能有意识地回应言语命令或轻微的触觉刺激，患者的气道通畅，能自主呼吸。

深度镇静使用药物抑制知觉。在此期间，患者不容易被唤醒，但对反复的、有痛觉的刺激有反应。患者需要外界辅助以维持气道通畅和心血管功能。深度镇静只在有严重呼吸衰竭、高颅压、癫痫、破伤风并同时使用肌肉松弛剂的患者身上使用。

镇静药物的选择广泛，均可达到理想的镇静水平。苯二氮草类镇静剂通过肝脏微粒体氧化或葡萄糖醛酸化在肝脏中代谢。老年人和肝病患者对这类药物的代谢可能会减弱。异丙酚是 ICU 中最常用的静脉镇静剂之一。它的单次剂量为每千克体重 2 毫克，维持剂量为每分钟每千克体重 5～50

commonly used intravenous sedative in all ICUs. It can be given in a bolus dose of 2mg/kg followed by a maintenance infusion of 5-50 microgram/kg/min. Hypotension is a common side effect. Prolonged infusions can lead to propofol infusion syndrome, characterized by bradycardia, cardiac failure, metabolic acidosis, rhabdomyolysis and hyperkalemia.

Ketamine is a unique agent as it provides both sedation and analgesia. It has a quick onset of action (usually 30 seconds) and is suitable for procedural sedation in the ICU, especially in patients with reactive airway disease and those with depressed cardiac function. Its side effects include increase in intra-cranial pressures, oral/airway secretions and hallucinations. There are some newer agents like fospropofol, which is water soluble; dexmedetomidine, which is a specific alpha-2 agonist that acts centrally to inhibit nor-epinephrine release; and AnaConDa system, which is an inhalational anesthesia system and attached to the mechanical ventilators to recycle the anesthetic agents.

Sedation is important in the ICU to facilitate amnesia during critical illness,

微克。异丙酚常见的副作用为低血压。长时间输液可引发异丙酚输液综合征,其特征是心跳过缓、心脏衰竭、代谢性酸中毒、横纹肌溶解和高钾血症。

氯胺酮是一种独特的药剂,它既有镇静作用又可镇痛。它见效快(通常30秒),适用于ICU中的程序性镇静,特别适用于反应性气道疾病和心脏功能抑制的患者。氯胺酮的副作用包括颅压增高、口腔或气道产生分泌物,以及出现幻觉。还有一些较新的药物,如水溶性的磷丙泊酚,抑制降肾上腺素释放的α-2激动剂右旋美托咪啶。另外还有AnaConDa系统,这是一种吸入式麻醉系统,可连接到呼吸机上循环麻醉剂。

ICU中的镇静在以下几方面有着重要的作用:诱导病人遗忘危重疾病

to prevent delirious patients from causing harm to self and others, to facilitate invasive management, to promote ventilator-patient synchrony, to circumvent post-traumatic stress disorder and to relieve dyspnea. Sedation and analgesia go hand in hand in achieving success in management of critically ill patients.

期间的记忆，防止神志不清的患者伤害自己和他人，帮助侵入式健康管理手段的实施，促进呼吸机与患者同步，规避创伤后应激障碍，缓解呼吸困难。镇静和镇痛在危重病人的有效管理中相辅相成。

4.2　汉译英

（一）热射病 Thermoplegia[4]

中暑表现为在炎热、潮湿且无风的环境中，人体出现热调节功能障碍、汗腺衰竭、水和电解质的过度流失。根据发病机制和临床表现，重症中暑可分为热痉挛、热衰竭和热射病三种。这三种类型的中暑可能会依次发生，其中热射病最为严重。

Heat stroke is characterized by the dysfunction of thermoregulation, sweat gland failure, excessive loss of water and electrolytes, as a result of exposure to heat, humidity, and wind-free environments. Depending on the pathogenesis and clinical manifestations, severe forms of heat stroke could be divided into heat cramps, heat exhaustion, and thermoplegia. These conditions might develop sequentially amongst which thermoplegia is the most severe form.

热射病的特点是神经系统功能障碍、恶性体温过高（体温升高超过40℃）、全身炎症反应、凝血、肝功能障碍及其他多器官功能障碍。中暑死亡率高达40%~50%，约30%的幸存

Thermoplegia is characterized by the dysfunction of the nervous system and malignant hyperthermia (acute elevation of body temperature of more than 40℃), systemic inflammatory reactions,

患者康复后有神经系统或其他系统的后遗症。

热射病是最严重的中暑，发病原因是内外热负荷超过了身体散热能力，身体储存过多的热量，引发身体过热。身体中积累过多的热量会损害人体组织的细胞膜和细胞内结构，并伴有蛋白质变性、脂膜流动性变化，从而导致线粒体损伤及组织和细胞的大面积损伤，进而引发多器官功能障碍综合征。

降低体温和治疗并发症是成功治疗中暑的关键。在徐州中心医院的临床观察中，使用连续血液净化与乌司他丁相结合的方法治疗中暑取得了良好的结果。对于热射病的治疗，早期快速降温是最重要的干预疗法，其目

coagulation, liver dysfunction and other multi-organ dysfunction. The mortality rate of heat stroke is as high as 40% - 50%, with approximately 30% of the surviving patients recovering with sequelae to the nervous system or other systems.

Known as the most severe heat stroke, thermoplegia is considered to be induced by internal or external thermal load exceeding the corresponding heat dissipation capacity, in which excessive body heat storage leads to overheating. Excessive heat accumulation might damage the cell membrane and intracellular structures of human tissues. Excessive heat accumulation is also associated with protein denaturation and fluidity changes in lipid membrane. This can result in mitochondria injury and extensive damages of tissues and cells, and eventually leading to multiple organ dysfunction syndrome (MODS).

Lowering body temperature and a regimen against complications are the key to a successful treatment of heat stroke. Favorable outcomes were observed at Xuzhou Central Hospital in the clinical treatment of heat stroke by continuous

标是在两小时内将直肠温度降至38.5℃，并在 4 小时内保持在 34.5 ~ 35.5℃范围内，以达到理想的预后效果。

血管内降温是最新的降温方法。病床边持续的血液过滤可以显著降低患者的体温。连续血液净化是一种基于间歇性血液透析的血液净化新技术，具有多重治疗效果：能有效降温；有效去除肌红蛋白、胆红素和其他有毒物质；全面去除血液中的炎症介质，减少全身炎症反应，从而有助于重建体内平衡。

由于热射病和败血症的发病机制有诸多相似之处，有许多研究评估抗败血症药剂在热射病治疗中的价值，

blood purification (CBP) in combination with ulinastatin. For the treatment of thermoplegia, early rapid cooling strategy is the most important therapeutic intervention, with the goal of rectal temperature reduced to 38.5℃ within two hours and maintained in the range of 34.5 – 35.5℃ within four hours, so as to achieve favorable prognosis.

The endovascular cooling strategy is the latest cooling concept. Continuous bedside blood filtering method could reduce a patient's temperature with a remarkable efficacy. Continuous blood purification is a newly developed BP technology based on intermittent hemodialysis and has multi-target therapeutic effects as follows: effective temperature-lowering performance; effective removal of myoglobin, bilirubin, and other toxic substances; non-selective removal of inflammatory mediators in the blood, reduction of systemic inflammatory response, contributing to the reconstruction of homeostasis.

Since thermoplegia bears similar pathogenesis in many aspects with sepsis, there are many studies available to

比如减少炎症细胞因子和提高抗炎细胞因子分泌。对于中暑引起的神经系统损伤，结合使用地塞米松和甘露醇，并辅以结合高压氧与活性蛋白 C，可显著提高存活率。

investigate the value of anti-sepsis agents in the treatment of thermoplegia such as reduction of inflammatory cytokines and elevation of anti-inflammatory cytokines secretion. For nervous system injury induced by heat stroke, the administration of dexamethasone and mannitol in combination, and supplementation of hyperbaric oxygen in combination with activated protein C can significantly increase survival rate.

（二）败血症 Septicemia[5-6]

败血症，又称脓毒症，是临床上对血液中毒的指称。败血症是病菌进入血液中弥散开后造成的感染。造成感染的通常是细菌，比如金黄色葡萄球菌、肺炎链球菌和大肠埃希菌，但也可以是病毒或真菌。败血症是人体对感染最极端的反应。当败血症发展导致败血性休克时，死亡率可以高达 50%，具体取决于涉及的身体器官类型。

Septicemia, or sepsis, is the clinical name for blood poisoning. It is an infection that occurs when germs get into the bloodstream and spread. What causes sepsis is usually bacteria, such as Staphylococcus aureus, Streptococcus pheumoniae, and E. coli, but it can also be viruses or fungi. Sepsis is the body's most extreme response to an infection. When it progresses to septic shock, the mortality rate can be as high as 50%, depending on the type of organism involved.

败血症发展非常迅速。患者病情快速恶化，并可能出现发烧、恶心、食欲不振、心率加快、极度疼痛或不适，甚至出现昏迷。败血症患者通常

Sepsis develops very quickly. The person rapidly becomes very ill, and may become feverish and nauseated, lose appetite, have a high heart rate,

会出现出血性皮疹，也就是皮肤上聚集出现看起来像针刺后的出血点。如果不治疗，出血点范围会逐渐扩大，看起来像新的瘀斑。这些瘀斑相互连接形成更大的紫色皮肤损伤和变色区域。

任何人都有可能出现感染症状，但有些危险因素使人们患败血症的风险更高。这些危险因素包括患有慢性病（如糖尿病、癌症、肺病、免疫系统疾病和肾脏疾病），以及免疫系统薄弱。因感染而住院的人也属于高危人群。

败血症的治疗手段包括使用抗生素、控制流向器官的血液以及治疗感染源。许多人需要静脉注射和吸氧，以帮助血液流动和让氧气进入器官。根据患者具体情况，可能需要使用呼吸机帮助患者呼吸或肾脏透析。有时要实施手术去除感染损坏的组织。

complain of extreme pain or discomfort, or even experience a coma. People with sepsis often develop a hemorrhagic rash— a cluster of tiny blood spots that look like pinpricks in the skin. If untreated, these gradually get bigger and begin to look like fresh bruises. These bruises then join together to form larger areas of purple skin damage and discoloration.

An infection can happen to anyone, but there are certain risk factors that put people at higher risk for developing sepsis. These include chronic medical conditions such as diabetes, cancer, lung disease, immune system disorders, and kidney disease, and weak immune systems. It may also happen to people who have been hospitalized for an infection.

Treatment of sepsis includes using antibiotics, managing blood flow to organs, and treating the source of the infection. Many people need oxygen and IV fluids to help get blood flow and oxygen to the organs. Depending on the person, breathing with a ventilator or kidney dialysis may be needed. Surgery is sometimes used to remove tissue damaged by the infection.

败血症属于紧急医疗情况。患者需要注意体征，如有以下症状需尽快就医：高烧、发冷、虚弱、出汗或血压骤降。可以通过接种疫苗、保持伤口清洁且包扎良好、谨遵医嘱应对健康状况、定期洗手来减少患败血症的概率。

Septicemia is a medical emergency. Be aware of the signs, and go to the hospital if you have signs like high fever, chills, weakness, sweating or sudden drop in blood pressure. You can lessen the chances of developing septicemia by getting vaccines, keeping any wounds clean and covered, taking good care of any medical conditions by following medical instructions, and washing your hands regularly.

（三）重症监护中的营养评估 Nutritional Assessment in ICU[7]

营养评分在重症患者营养评估与监测中的应用并不是新生事物，但也不是陈旧的话题。不管是因烧伤、感染还是创伤，患者病情危急，他们都处于高分解代谢状态，代谢率增加将近150%。而且热量不足，蛋白质分解，因此体内蛋白质含量下降，影响了组织的修复、伤口的愈合和患者的免疫力。病人免疫功能失常以后，就难以控制感染。营养不良最后会发展成慢重症甚至会导致死亡。

The application of nutrition score in nutritional assessment and monitoring of critically ill patients is not newly emerged, but it is not outdated either. Patients in critical conditions with empyrosis, infection and trauma are all in the hypercatabolic state, and their metabolic rate increases by nearly 150%. Moreover, due to the lack of calories, protein decomposes, in which the abasement of protein affects the repair of tissues, wound healing and immunity. If the patient's immune system cannot function well, it will be difficult to control infection. Malnutrition will gradually lead to the chronic critical illness (CCI) or even death.

营养风险筛查是 ICU 病人特别需要的一种检查手段。目前广受认可的评估方式是营养风险筛查评分简表2002 （NRS2002）。此外，还有专门为ICU 病人设计的重症患者营养风险筛查评估等级表。NRS2002 总分大于 3分，病人就有营养不良的危险，大于5 分则为高危人群。

营养风险筛查首先需要考虑病人的 BMI 值是否小于 20.5，近三个月是否体重下降，过去一周是否摄食减少，以及是否有严重疾病，对于 ICU 病人来说，通常这几个问题的答案都是"是"。ICU 病人插着管，测体重不容易，因此 BMI 值的测量也是一个难题。但如果血清白蛋白替代水平小于30g/L，则直接评为 3 分。

Nutrition risk screening is a much-needed examination for ICU patients. Currently the well-recognized assessment is Nutrition Risk Screening 2002, NRS 2002 in short. Apart from this, Nutrition Risk in the Critically Ill Score (NUTRIC Score) is designed especially for ICU patients. If the patient is assessed at a total score higher than 3 points by the metrics of NRS2002, we believe the patient is at risk of malnutrition. If the result comes back with a score above 5 points, the patient is considered to be in the high-risk group.

In nutritional risk screening, the first thing is to measure whether the patient's BMI is less than 20.5; whether the patient has lost weight in the last three months; whether there has been a decrease in food intake in the past week; and whether there are any serious illnesses. For ICU patients, the answer to these questions is usually "yes". Because of intubation, it is usually not easy to weigh ICU patients, which makes measuring BMI a challenge. However, if the serum albumin replacement level is less than 30g/L, the patient should be rated directly as 3 points.

NRS2002 的其他评分项有病情严重程度、营养状态受损情况和年龄。研究证明，NRS2002 评分大于或等于 3 分的患者，临床给予营养支持治疗后，获得较好临床效果的比例增高。

According to NRS2002, other scoring items include severity of the disease, nutritional impairment, and age. Studies have shown that for patients with NRS2002 scores greater than or equal to 3 points, with clinical nutritional support, the proportion of good clinical outcomes has increased.

5 口译注释与学习资源

5.1 口译注释

症状描述

医学英语中症状的描述通常使用一般现在时。在英译汉时，一般现在时对应到汉语中，可以加上"通常""一般"等汉语中的频度副词，以使译文更加流畅。有时医学英语中在描述症状时会出现情态动词"may"，汉译时可以翻译成"可能出现"，也可以使用汉语中上述频度副词替代，有时也可以直接省略。如"the symptoms may include"，汉译为"症状为……"或者"可能出现以下症状"或者"通常出现以下症状"。

5.2 学习资源

登录中国大学 MOOC（慕课），学习"医疗口译"课程中"重症医学科"的口译实战示范视频。登录四川大学华西医院重症医学科网站（http://www.wchscu.cn/department_ zzyxk.html）了解更多重症医学相关信息。

参考文献

［1］ Besso Joseé, Lumb, P. D. ,& Williams, G. (2009). *Intensive and critical care medicine Wfsiccm world federation of societies of intensive and Critical Care Medicine.* Springer Milan.

［2］ Varghese, J. M. , Roberts, J. A. , & Lipman, J. （2010）. Pharmacokinetics and pharmacodynamics in critically ill patients. *Current Opinion in Anaesthesiology*,23（4）, 472 -

478. https://doi. org/10. 1097/aco. 0b013e328339ef0a

[3] Hariharan，U. & Rakesh, G. Sedation and analgesia in critical care. (2017). *Journal of Anesthesia & Critical Care: Open Access*，7（3），1 - 5. https://doi. org/10. 15406/jaccoa. 2017. 07. 00262

[4] Lu，B. , Li，M. Q. , & Cheng，S. L.（2014）. Clinical effectiveness of continuous blood purification in combination with ulinastatin in treating thermoplegia. *European review for medical and pharmacological sciences*, 18（22），3464 - 3467.

[5] Johns Hopkins Medicine.（n. d. ）. *Septicemia*. Retrieved November 13，2021，from https://www. hopkinsmedicine. org/health/conditions-and-diseases/septicemia.

[6] Cleveland Clinic.（n. d. ）. Septicemia(blood poisoning): *Causes*，*management*. Retrieved November 13，2021，from https://my. clevelandclinic. org/health/diseases/21539 - septicemia.

[7] 宋青. 首届东方重症医学学术会议暨首届中国重症消化学术论坛. ［EB/OL］. ［2017 - 08 - 15］. https://v. youku. com/v_ show/id_ XMjk3MTIwMDkyNA ══ . html?spm = a2hzp. 8253869. 0. 0.

第十九章

中国传统医学

1 导读

本章重点为口译技巧之职业伦理（2）和中国传统医学的 6 篇"口译实战"练习。口译实战练习中英译汉、汉译英各 3 篇，内容涵盖中国传统医学介绍、十种有"奇效"的中草药、针灸与艾灸、四季养生、中医预防暴雨洪灾后疾病和中医治疗跌打损伤。请结合本章口译技巧思考医学口译中的职业伦理道德意识塑造，并练习 6 篇口译实战文本。

2 口译技巧——职业伦理（2）

上一章中我们谈到了口译职业伦理规范中的五个常见原则，但口译活动是一项动态的、涉及多方参与且偶有干扰因素及突发状况的语言服务活动。成文的口译职业伦理规范无法完全预测口译员在口译任务中的所有场景；口译类型、场景、参与方、文化等因素都会使现有的口译职业伦理规范具有一定的局限性和滞后性。此外，口译员本身是其决策和行为后果的责任承担者，因此完全刻板地执行某个口译职业伦理规范，也具有一定的风险性。尤其是当遵守职业伦理规则会带来更严重的危害时，口译员将陷入紧急决策的伦理困境。而伦理困境在通常情况下都没有唯一的、标准的解决方式，译员的决策和行动与译员的哲学伦理观、个人道德责任感、临场应变能力以及利弊权重审视能力直接相关。

因此，医学口译员在上岗开展口译工作时，不但需要熟知口译职业伦理规范，还应该了解医学伦理规范及行业常规操作，积极配合医患双方，树立良好的职业操守，促进医学场景下的交流向医患双方都满意的、正义向善的结果发展。

3 口译词汇

3.1 英译汉

（一）Traditional Chinese Medicine（TCM）中国传统医学（中医）

inspection 望

auscultation/olfaction 闻

inquiry 问

palpation 切

herbal medicine 中草药

dietary therapy 饮食疗法

acupuncture 针灸

moxibustion 艾灸

cupping 拔罐

Tui Na 推拿

medicinal properties 药效

light dieting 轻食

stagnation 淤积；停滞

suction 吸力

nanotechnology 纳米技术

particle size 颗粒大小

alternative 替代的

complementary 补充的

（二）Ten Chinese Herbs That Work Wonders 十种有"奇效"的中草药

antioxidant 抗氧化物

zinc 锌

amino acid 氨基酸

ginsenoside 人参皂苷

phytoestrogen 植物雌激素

coumarin 香豆素

spasm 痉挛

Chinese wild yam 野生山药

moisturize 滋润

free radical 自由基

detoxify 排毒

（三）Acupuncture and Moxibustion 针灸与艾灸

acupuncture 针灸

moxibustion 艾灸

meridian 经络

spinal cord 脊髓

menstrual cramps 痛经

mugwort 艾蒿

stagnant 停滞的；不流动的

direct moxibustion 明灸

indirect moxibustion 隔物灸

moxa stick 艾条

3.2 汉译英

（一）四季养生 Seasonal Health Preservation

《黄帝内经》*Yellow Emperor's Canon of Medicine*

寒性病变 cold lesion

疟疾 malaria

痿厥 weakness in limbs

（二）中医预防暴雨洪灾后疾病 TCM Preventing Diseases after Rainstorm and Flooding

暴雨 torrential rain or rainstorm

自来水系统 water supply system

污水 sewerage

垃圾填埋 landfill

堆肥 compost

介水传染病 water-borne infectious disease

血吸虫病 schistosomiasis

霍乱 cholera

痢疾 dysentery

病原体 pathogen

黄连素 berberine

（三）中医治疗跌打损伤 TCM Treating External Injuries

肌肉拉伤 muscle strain/muscle pull

脱臼 dislocate

跌打损伤 external injury/injury from falls, fractures, contusions and strains

内服药 drugs for oral administration

外用药 drugs for external use

4　口译实战

4.1　英译汉

（一）Traditional Chinese Medicine 中国传统医学[1]

Traditional Chinese Medicine (TCM) is one of the oldest medical systems in existence. The philosophy of TCM is based on the Taoist view that human beings as part of the nature should live in harmony with the nature. Therefore the 5 basic elements in the nature, namely metal, wood, water, fire and earth, should coexist in a balanced manner. Illness develops when the balance is broken, such as one element being in deficiency while others are excessive.

中国传统医学（简称"中医"）是现存最古老的医学体系之一。中医的哲学基础源于道家思想，即人类作为自然的一部分，应该与自然和谐相处。因此，自然界中的金、木、水、火、土五大基本要素应该平衡共存。疾病的发生是由于这种平衡被打破，比如某个元素出现短缺而其他元素处于过剩的状态。

The concept of Yin and Yang, whose literal meanings are negativity and positivity, is adopted in description of major body organs. Liver, heart, spleen, pancreas, lungs and kidneys have the nature of Yin; while gallbladder, small and large intestines, stomach and bladder share the nature of Yang.

阴和阳的概念其字面意思是负和正。这一概念被用来描述主要身体器官。肝、心、脾、胰、肺、肾属阴，而胆囊、小肠、大肠、胃、膀胱属阳。

TCM practitioners have four traditional diagnostic methods: inspection, auscultation/olfaction, inquiry, and

中医有四种传统的诊断方法，即望、闻、问、切，以此来收集有关患者健康状况的信息。中医在治疗疾病、

palpation. These methods gather information about the health conditions of the patients. Traditional Chinese Medicine is distinctive in treating diseases and relieving symptoms. Herbal medicine, dietary therapy, acupuncture, moxibustion, cupping, Tui Na, and energy work such as Tai Chi and Qi Gong are commonly used.

Herbal medicine is the use of traditional herbs that have medicinal properties. Dietary therapy in TCM emphasizes light dieting, balance of the "hot" and "cold" nature of food, harmony of the five flavors of food, and consistency between dietary intake and different health conditions. Acupuncture entails stimulating various pressure points throughout the body with needles. Moxibustion is the burning of herbs above the skin. Cupping is used to freeing stagnation by imposing suction on the skin. Tui Na is a type of massage that applies pressure to acupoints, meridians and groups of muscles or nerves to remove blockages that prevent the free flow of Qi. Tai Chi and Qi Gong use exercise and breathing to help circulation in the body. The treatment in TCM is centered around balance within the body and balance between the body and the

缓解症状方面独具一格，常采用中草药疗法，饮食疗法，针灸，艾灸，拔罐，推拿及运功如太极拳、气功等。

中草药疗法使用具有药用特性的传统草药。中医饮食疗法强调轻食，追求食物的热性和凉性的平衡，五味和谐，根据不同健康状况调节饮食摄入。针灸需要用针刺激全身各处的穴位。艾灸则是在皮肤上方燃烧草药。拔罐通过对皮肤表面产生吸力疏通经络。推拿是一种对穴位、经络、肌肉群或神经施加压力的按摩，目的是消除阻碍，让体内的气能自由流动。太极和气功利用运动和呼吸技巧帮助体循环。中医的治疗围绕身体内部的平衡和身体与环境的平衡展开。

environment.

Nowadays, TCM incorporates a modern approach into the diagnosis and treatment of illnesses. Researchers in TCM in recent studies probe into the application of nanotechnology into TCM, because the pharmacodynamics of medical herbs depends not only on the constituents but also on their physical state such as particle size. The application of modern technology shows that TCM is inclusive and improves with the times.

In fact, TCM has gained more and more popularity worldwide in the past couple of years, as evidenced by Olympic athletes utilizing the technique of cupping at 2016 Rio Olympic Games and licensed acupuncture becoming legalized in 43 out of 50 states in U. S. since 2008. Traditional Chinese Medicine is an alternative and complementary treatment process for certain chronic illnesses, because it provides more individualized treatment, and emphasizes balance in the body more heavily compared to Western medicine.

如今，中医在疾病的诊断和治疗中采用了现代方法。中医研究人员在最近的研究中探讨了纳米技术在中药中的应用，因为中医草药的药理动力不仅取决于成分，还与它们的物理形态有关，比如药物颗粒的大小。现代科技的应用表明中医具有包容性，并且与时俱进。

事实上，近年来，中医在全球越来越受欢迎。2016 年里约奥运会运动员使用拔罐疗法以及自 2008 年以来美国 50 个州中有 43 个州持牌针灸合法化就是很好的说明。中医是某些慢性病的替代和补充治疗方式，因为中医的治疗更个性化，相较西医更强调身体的平衡。

（二）Ten Chinese Herbs That Work Wonders 十种有"奇效"的中草药[2]

Herbal medicine is an integral part of Chinese culture and the practice of traditional Chinese Medicine. The emperor Shen Nong is said to have tasted 100 herbs, which allowed him to teach the Chinese people how to use herbs in their diet and treatment for illness. Today we are going to look at ten useful Chinese herbs that many Chinese use or incorporate into their daily diets in order to stay health.

草药是中国文化和中医实践的重要组成部分。据说炎帝神农尝过100种药草，而后向华夏子民传授草药在饮食和治病中的作用。今天，我们来看看十种有用的中草药。许多中国人使用这些中草药或者将它们纳入日常饮食以保持健康。

（1）Goji Berries. Goji berries have high levels of antioxidants, which can protect our eyes and skin. Goji berries contain many nutrients, including Vitamin C, fiber, iron, vitamin A, and zinc. They also contain all the amino acids our bodies need. （2）Ginseng. Ginseng can help balance hormones and recharge our bodies. The ginsenoside in it controls inflammation. Besides, ginseng can enhance the cognitive function and the immune system, so drinking ginseng tea is popular in China.

（1）枸杞。枸杞含有较高浓度的抗氧化物，可以保护我们的眼睛和皮肤。枸杞含有多种营养物质，包括维生素C、纤维、铁、维生素A和锌。它还含有我们的身体需要的所有氨基酸。（2）人参。人参可以帮助平衡激素，补充精力。人参皂苷有消炎作用。此外，人参还可以增强认知功能、强化免疫系统，因此饮用人参茶在中国很流行。

（3）Dang Gui. Dang Gui helps with the balance of female hormones because phytoestrogens in it add to the

（3）当归。当归可以平衡女性激素，因为当归含有植物雌激素，可以补充人体雌激素不足。香豆素是当归

estrogen in the body. Coumarins, compounds found in Dang Gui, dilate blood vessels and prevent muscle spasms. They help women regulate their menstrual cycles.

（4）Chinese Wild Yam. Chinese wild yam can help to put an end to diarrhea and other common digestive ailments. Furthermore, Chinese wild yam relieves a chronic cough, and people with asthma will find it a relief because it moisturizes the lungs.

（5）Lotus Seed. Lotus seeds contain proteins, phosphorus, magnesium, and potassium. Lotus seeds treat other illnesses such as insomnia and restlessness. They dilate blood vessels, which in turn reduces blood pressure.
（6）White Peony Root. Peony root cures gastrointestinal infections. It also relieves common skin problems and gets rid of wrinkles. The ethanol and gallic extract in peony root prevent free radicals from forming. Therefore, it might aid in cancer prevention.

（7）Longan. Longan is not only a delicious fruit but also has healing properties. Longan fruit will help you

含有的一种化合物，有扩张血管、防止肌肉痉挛的作用，还可以治疗月经不调。

（4）野生山药。野生山药有止泻、治疗消化系统疾病的作用。此外，野生山药可镇咳平喘。哮喘患者服用，会感到症状缓解，因为野生山药有润肺的作用。

（5）莲子。莲子含有蛋白质、磷、镁和钾。莲子可治疗失眠、烦躁等症状。莲子可扩张血管，降低血压。
（6）白牡丹根。白牡丹根可治疗胃肠道感染。它还可缓解常见的皮肤问题，消除皱纹。牡丹根中的乙醇和大蒜提取物可抑制自由基的形成，因此可能有预防癌症的作用。

（7）桂圆。桂圆不仅是一种美味的水果，也具有疗效。桂圆可以安神，缓解疲劳，治疗割伤和擦伤。这种水

calm your nerves. It also reduces exhaustion. It's a cure for cuts and abrasions. This fruit arrests free radicals and prevents cancer. (8) Red Dates. Red dates increase the body's serum protein which helps the liver detoxify. Besides, it can add the element of fire to your body so as to assist the circulation of blood. Therefore, women with menstrual problems often take red dates to ease the pain and stay warm.

(9) Black Sesame. This herb has phytosterols that lower cholesterol and help to protect heart health. Black sesame is high in calcium, so eating some can improve health conditions of deficiency in calcium. (10) Wheatgrass. Wheatgrass is an antioxidant that purges free radicals. If you struggle with digestive issues, this is a Chinese herb you must try. Wheatgrass also speeds up weight loss by stimulating the thyroid gland.

（三）Acupuncture and Moxibustion 针灸与艾灸[3-5]

Acupuncture and moxibustion are forms of Traditional Chinese Medicine widely practiced in China and also found in regions of south-east Asia, Europe and the Americas. The theories of acupuncture and moxibustion hold that

果可抑制自由基并预防癌症。（8）红枣。红枣可以增加身体的血清蛋白，后者可帮助肝脏排毒。此外，红枣可以向身体补充中医所说的火元素，以帮助血液的循环。因此，月经不调的女性常服用红枣缓解痛经和保暖。

（9）黑芝麻。这种草本中的植物甾醇可以降低胆固醇，保护心脏健康。黑芝麻含钙量高，因此服用黑芝麻可以改善缺钙的状况。（10）小麦草。小麦草是一种能清除自由基的抗氧化物。如果你有消化问题，你可以尝试一下小麦草。小麦草还可以通过刺激甲状腺来加速瘦身。

针灸和艾灸是在中国随处可见的中医疗法，在东南亚、欧洲和美洲地区也能见到。根据针灸和艾灸的理论，人体是一个以各种通道连接起来的小宇宙，对这些通道加以物理刺激可以提升人体的自我调节功能，给患者带

the human body acts as a small universe connected by channels, and that by physically stimulating these channels the practitioner can promote the human body's self-regulating functions and bring health to the patient.

Traditional Chinese Medicine practitioners believe the human body has more than 2,000 acupuncture points connected by pathways or meridians. These pathways create an energy flow (Qi) through the body that is responsible for overall health. Disruption of the energy flow can cause disease. Applying acupuncture to certain points improves the flow of Qi, thereby improving health. Acupuncture is done using hair-thin needles. Most people report feeling minimal pain as the needle is inserted. The needle is inserted to a point that produces a sensation of pressure or ache. Needles may be heated during the treatment or mild electric current may be applied to them.

Acupuncture points are believed to stimulate the central nervous system. This, in turn, releases chemicals into the muscles, spinal cord, and brain. These biochemical changes may stimulate

来健康。

中医师认为人体有2 000多个以通道和经络相连的穴位。这些通道创造能量流（也称"气"），气流向全身以保证人体健康。能量流动的中断可导致疾病。针灸某些穴位可改善气的流通，从而改善健康状况。针灸所用的针仅有发丝粗细。当针插入人体时，大多数人会有轻微痛感。针插入穴位，产生压迫感或者痛感。治疗中，针灸用针可能会加热或者接通微量电流。

针灸穴位可以刺激中枢神经系统。中枢神经接受刺激后，将化学物质释放到肌肉、脊髓和大脑中。这些生物化学变化可以刺激身体的自愈能力，促进身心健康。研究表明，针灸是一

the body's natural healing abilities and promote physical and emotional well-being. Studies have shown that acupuncture is an effective treatment alone or in combination with conventional therapies to treat nausea caused by surgical anesthesia and cancer chemotherapy, headaches, menstrual cramps, tennis elbow, back pain and other types of chronic pain.

Moxibustion is a Traditional Chinese Medicine technique that involves the burning of mugwort to promote healing with acupuncture. The purpose of moxibustion is to strengthen the blood circulation, stimulate the flow of Qi, and maintain general health. Moxibustion is used on people who have a cold or stagnant condition. The practice expels cold and warms the meridians, which leads to smoother flow of blood and Qi.

Moxibustion is usually divided into direct and indirect moxibustion, in which either moxa cones are placed directly on points or moxa sticks are held and kept at some distance from the body surface to warm the chosen area. The more popular form of moxibustion is the

种有效的独立治疗手段，也可以结合传统疗法来治疗由手术麻醉和癌症化疗引起的恶心，以及头痛、痛经、网球肘、背痛和其他类型的慢性疼痛。

艾灸是一种传统的中医技术，通过燃烧艾蒿和针灸促进康复。艾灸的目的是增强血液循环，促进气的流通，保持人体健康。艾灸常用于感冒或经脉不通的患者。它可以驱寒气、活经脉，让血液和气流动顺畅。

艾灸通常可分为明灸和隔物灸两种。前者是将艾炷直接放置于皮肤上，后者将艾条置于身体上方并保持一定距离加热身体特定区域。两者中，隔物灸更为普遍，因为它造成的疼痛感较弱，也可规避灼伤风险。在隔物灸时，针灸医生点燃艾条的一端，并将

indirect type because it comes with a lower risk for pain or burning. In indirect moxibustion, an acupuncture practitioner lights one end of a moxa stick and holds it close to the treatment area for a few minutes until the area turns red. Another form of indirect moxibustion uses both acupuncture needles and moxa.

其靠近治疗区域几分钟，直到区域皮肤变红。有的隔物灸同时使用针灸针和艾条。

4.2 汉译英

（一）四季养生 Seasonal Health Preservation [6-7]

2019 年，习近平主席对中医药工作做出重要指示时，曾指出："中医药学包含着中华民族几千年的健康养生理念及其实践经验，是中华文明的一个瑰宝，凝聚着中国人民和中华民族的博大智慧。"一年之中，春生夏长，秋收冬藏。《黄帝内经》中给出了四季养生的原则。

In 2019, President Xi Jinping, in making important instructions on the work of Traditional Chinese Medicine, pointed out: "Traditional Chinese Medicine accumulates concepts and practical experiences of Chinese nation in staying healthy for thousands of years, which makes it a precious treasure of Chinese civilization, because it condenses the profound wisdom of the Chinese people." Throughout the year, spring is the budding time, summer growth, autumn harvest and winter preservation. The principle of maintaining health according to seasons is manifested in *Yellow Emperor's Canon of Medicine*.

春天是万物生长的季节。人们可着宽松舒适的衣服让形体舒展，将自身与春天欣欣向荣的状态相融。春天

Spring is the season when everything buds. People can wear loose and comfortable clothes to allow the body to

赋予人的生长之气，不要随便损害。若违背了这个道理，就要伤及肝气，那么到夏季就会发生寒性病变。

夏季是万物茂盛的季节。避免发怒，舒展精神，可保持阳气的宣通。如果违背了这个道理，那就要伤及心气，到秋季就容易患疟疾，到冬季还会出现更严重的疾病。

秋季是万物成熟收获的季节。此时天高气爽，秋风劲急。这时人们应早睡早起，起居时间与鸡的活动时间相仿，使精神安定宁静，保持肺气的清肃功能。

stretch, and go into the nature to fully integrate into Spring's thriving state. Spring provides people with the energy of growth, which should not be wasted or disrupted. Violation of such a law of the nature will hurt the energy flow or the flow of Qi in the liver, which in turn will induce cold lesions in summer.

Summer is the season when all things are flourishing. Avoid being angry, and let your spirit be like full blossoms, so that the positive energy or the Qi of Yang will flow freely. Violation of this law will hurt the energy flow in the heart, thus malaria may have a higher incidence in autumn, and more serious diseases will occur in winter.

Autumn is the season of ripening and harvesting. At this time, the sky is clear and the air is refreshing with intermittent gusts of wind. At this time it's better for people to go to bed early and get up early, keeping the bio-clock of the bedtime and rising time with that of a rooster metaphorically speaking, so that the inner calm and serenity is maintained and the clearance function of lungs is preserved as well.

冬季是万物闭藏的季节。这时人们要适应冬季的特点，早睡晚起，待到日光照耀时起床才好，要躲避寒冷，求取温暖。不要使皮肤开泄而令阳气不断地损失。若违背了这个道理，就会损伤肾气，到来年春季就要得痿厥一类的疾病。

Winter is the season when everything stays hidden or shuts down. At this time people have to adapt to the characteristics of winter by going to bed early and getting up late. It is better to stay in bed until the sun is up in the sky to avoid the cold and stay warm. Do not expose the skin to the cold, and the Qi of Yang may escape incrementally. Violation of this law will damage the energy flow in the kidney, then coming together with spring are the higher chances in feeling weak in limbs.

（二）中医预防暴雨洪灾后疾病 TCM Preventing Diseases after Rainstorm and Flooding[8]

暴雨灾害天气会危及人们的生命安全，还可能破坏城乡的自来水系统、下水道系统、污水处理厂、垃圾填埋场、堆肥场等。细菌、病毒、寄生虫等会随洪水扩散，给人民健康带来巨大隐患。水灾后卫生条件差，特别容易出现传染病的暴发流行，应格外注意预防。

Torrential rain (rainstorm) endangers people's lives and safety, and it may also destroy the water supply system, sewerage system, sewage treatment plants, landfills, compost plants, etc. in urban and rural areas. Bacteria, viruses, parasites, etc. will spread with the floods, which poses huge hidden dangers to people's health. Poor sanitation after floods is likely to cause the outbreaks of infectious diseases, therefore special attention and preventative measures are needed.

暴雨让环境发生了巨大的变化，这些变化对蚊蝇、细菌的滋生更加有利。以介水传染病为例，水是它的重要媒介。包括甲肝、血吸虫病、霍乱、痢疾等在内的传染病均可以通过饮用或接触受病原体污染的水而传播。这种传染病的特点之一是，一旦水源受到严重污染，可呈暴发流行，短期内会突然出现大量病人。防大疫，必须做到"一绝不、两防护"。

"一绝不"是指绝不能吃淹死、病死的禽畜和水产品，不吃腐败变质或被污水浸泡过的食物。很多食物在洪水中发生了变化，表面上看不出来，其实微生物在上面繁殖的速度非常快，因此一定不能再食用。

"两防护"：一是防护周边的环

Heavy rains have brought about huge changes in the environment, which are more beneficial to the breeding of mosquitoes, flies and bacteria. In the case of water-borne infectious diseases, water is an important medium. Infectious diseases including hepatitis A, schistosomiasis, cholera, dysentery, etc., can be transmitted through drinking or contact with water contaminated with pathogens. One of the characteristics of these infectious diseases is that once the water source is seriously contaminated, it will have a sudden outbreak of diseases and a large number of patients will be infected in a short time. To prevent the pandemic, we must uphold the principle of "one Never and two Protections".

"One Never" means never eating drowned and sick livestock and aquatic products, or any food that has deteriorated or has been soaked in sewage before. A lot of flood-soaked food has gone bad in the flood. Though we cannot tell from its appearance, microorganisms multiply very fast in the flood-soaked food, therefore it is not edible.

"Two Protections" refers to measures

境，尽快清洁；二是防护皮肤，适当用药。暴雨后容易引发皮肤病，可用龙胆泻肝丸解毒。暴雨后也是急性胃炎高发期，可自行在家准备藿香正气水、黄连素片及葛根芩连片。此外，淋雨后可使用姜汤取暖，同时应注意饮水卫生。

taken to protect the surrounding environment which needs to be cleaned as soon as possible and measures taken to protect the skin, to which some medicine needs to be applied. After heavy rain, people are susceptible to skin diseases. Longdanxiegan pills can be used for detoxification. In the post torrential rain period, acute gastritis also has a high incidence. It can be helpful to have Huoxiangzhengqi liquid, berberine tablets and Gegen Qinlian tablets at home. In addition, ginger soup is a good option for warming the body up after the rain, and attention needs to be paid to the hygiene of drinking water.

（三）中医治疗跌打损伤 TCM Treating External Injuries[9]

体育运动中机械性和物理性因素所造成的伤害，称为运动损伤。在日常生活中，我们有时因为动作幅度过大、动作过快或者用力不当，容易造成脖子、手臂、腰部、臀部和腿部的肌肉拉伤，有时造成脱臼，甚至骨折。

Injuries caused by mechanical and physical factors in sports are called atheletic injuries. In daily life, we are sometimes prone to muscle strains in the neck, arms, waist, hips and legs due to overstretching, sudden and fast initiation of movement, or improper body posture, which sometimes causes joint dislocation or even fractures.

中医认为跌打损伤是由于血淤积在某个部位不散，因此活血化瘀是中医治疗跌打损伤的主要原则。跌打损

Traditional Chinese Medicine believes that the injuries from falls, fractures, contusions and strains are due

伤的治疗可以采取内服或者外用中药的方法，以活血和消痛为主。内服中成药有云南白药、三七片、跌打丸等。外用药有正红花油、活血膏等。

除了使用药物以外，中医还有一些治疗手段也可以用于跌打损伤的治疗，例如针灸、艾灸等。但值得注意的是，传统中医一般不建议对跌打损伤使用冰敷的方式治疗。因为中医讲究气血活通，而冰具有收缩作用。当冰敷患处时，血液和气就会淤堵。冰敷凉爽的感觉可以减轻疼痛是因为皮肤在温度骤降下失去了部分感知能力，但皮肤下的血管收缩是不利的。冰敷阻碍气血流通。

to blood siltation in a certain area, so activating blood circulation and dissolving stasis is the main principle of TCM treatment. The treatment of exterior injuries can be medicine for oral administration or medicine for application on the skin, the purpose of which is mainly to activate the blood and relieve the pain. Yunnan baiyao, sanqi tablets, dieda pills are commonly used internally. Zhenghonghua oil and huoxue ointment are used externally.

In addition to the use of medicine made from herbs, there are some therapies, such as acupuncture, moxibustion and so on. However, it is worth noting that TCM generally does not recommend the use of ice for treating such injuries, because TCM focuses on the circulation of blood and Qi, and ice has a contraction effect. When ice is placed on the surface of the injured parts, the blood and Qi will go into stagnation. The cool feeling may ease the pain, because your skin loses part of the sensation for the drop of the temperature, but the underlying contraction is not good, and it hinders the circulation of blood and Qi.

从中医的角度来看，有其他方法可以冷却受伤部位又不造成气和血液的阻塞。可以在患处敷上有降温作用的草药或者寒性草药，这既减轻了患处肿胀，又让气血能够循环。中医被证明有助于恢复扭伤和拉伤、肌肉肿胀、肩伤、网球肘、高尔夫球肘、膝盖伤、小腿筋膜炎、腹股沟拉伤、跟腱受伤和骨折。

From the perspective of Traditional Chinese Medicine, there are ways to cool down the injured area without creating a blockage of Qi and blood through the application of cooling herbs or herbs that have the nature of coldness, so it helps decrease the swelling, while simultaneously helping circulation. TCM proves effective to help the recovery of sprains and strains, swollen muscles, shoulder injuries, tennis or golf elbow, knee injuries, shin splints, groin pull, Achilles tendon injuries and fractures.

5 口译注释与学习资源

5.1 口译注释

（一）翻译中的概念阐释

中医中有许多概念和疗法都独具特色，属于中华民族特有的，在文化迁移和交流中传入英语世界。对待一种文化中有而另一种文化中没有的概念，宜采取归化和异化相结合的翻译策略，既考虑文化输出又考虑目标读者或者听者的接受度。因此，在中医概念的英译中，**可以采取汉语拼音辅以解释的方式进行翻译。使用汉语拼音是考虑到彰显中国文化的身份属性；辅以解释是为了使目标受众能更好地接受**。例如，"气"是中医中独有的概念，可以译为"Qi, the energy flow"或"Qi, the circulation of energy"。再比如，"阴"和"阳"是中国传统医学中的核心概念，而这一概念对于英语世界来说是全新的，因此可以翻译成"Yin and Yang, the literal meanings of which are negativity and positivity respectively, and the pair constitutes the wholesomeness, thus needs to be maintained at a balanced manner"。解释的程度依据受众、具体语境和口译时间而定。面对对中国文化熟悉的听众可直接使用"Yin and Yang"。

（二）中成药名翻译

中医使用的药物可以是药材本身，也可以是中成药，也就是具有中药成分的制剂，有片剂、胶囊等不同形态。中药的命名大致有以下三个规律特点：（1）直接使用药材名称，如藏红花；（2）药材名称或者药物有效成分＋制剂形态，如麝香牛黄丸；（3）药材本名或药材功能＋修辞手法或文化概念＋制剂形态，如安神补脑液、乌鸡白凤丸。

翻译时对应的方法步骤如下：

（1）直接翻译药材名，如莲子译为"lotus seed"，冬虫夏草译为"Chinese caterpillar fungus"，藏红花译为"（Tibetan）saffron"。

（2）如果药名中有制剂类型，则加上制剂类型相应的英文，如麝香牛黄丸译为"Musk Bezoar Pill"。以下是部分常见制剂类型的英译。

pill 药丸	liquid/syrup 浆/水/糖浆
electuary 冲剂	powder 散/粉
tablet 药片	drop 滴
ointment 软膏	granule 颗粒
capsule 胶囊	patch 贴

（3）如果药名中出现相应的功能描述或者文化修辞手法，则视情况做相应的解释调整，如补充药物成分、介绍药物功能、阐释文化背景。如安神补脑液可译为"anshenbunao liquid which helps neurathenia"。

除此之外，有一些中医药物在海外已经具有一定的知名度，名称已固定下来，比如"虎皮膏药"（也就是"麝香止痛贴"，其包装上有老虎图样）在欧美国家被约定俗成地称为"Tiger Patch"，"乌鸡白凤丸"被约定俗成地称为"Bak Foong Pills"等。翻译这些在海外已经推广并具有较高接受度的中药名称时，可以沿用其约定俗成的英文名称。

有一些药物名称复杂，可采用拼音＋成分或功能解释的方式。如"连花清瘟胶囊"可译为"Lianhua Qingwen Capsule which can relieve symptoms caused by influenza"。上文中的"麝香牛黄丸"也可以译为"Shexiang Niuhuang Pills which are made of musk and bezoar"。具体采取哪种翻译方式，解释多少，根据口译任务性质（如为中医推介会，则需要相应多解释）、听者的接受程度而定。**在普通的看病问诊中，涉及中医的多为汉译英，因此可适当多注重于药物功能的翻译而不是具体药名的字面翻译。**

　　但需要注意的是，药材提取物或者有效成分通常有对应的英文名，如黄连素 berberine、青蒿素 artemisinin、人参皂苷 ginsenoside，不能想当然地使用拼音。

5.2 学习资源

　　登录中国大学 MOOC（慕课），学习"医疗口译"课程中"传统中医"的口译实战示范视频。

参考文献

［1］ The Public Health Advocate（n. d.）. *An introduction to traditional Chinese medicine*. Retrieved November 14, 2021, from https://pha. berkeley. edu/2017/02/01/an-introduction-to-traditional-chinese-medicine/.

［2］ Liew, M.（2017, July 18）. 10 *ancient Chinese herbs that work wonders for different ailments*. Life Advancer. Retrieved November 14, 2021, from https://www. lifeadvancer. com/chinese-herbs/.

［3］ UNESCO.（n. d.）. *Acupuncture and moxibustion of traditional Chinese medicine*. Retrieved November 14, 2021, from https://ich. unesco. org/en/RL/acupuncture-and-moxibustion-of-traditional-chinese-medicine－00425.

［4］ Johns Hopkins Medicine.（n. d.）. *Acupuncture*. Retrieved November 14, 2021, from https://www. hopkinsmedicine. org/health/wellness-and-prevention/acupuncture.

［5］ American Institute of Alternative Medicine.（2020, April 19）. *Moxibustion in acupuncture: What you should know*. Retrieved November 14, 2021, from https://www. aiam. edu/acupuncture/moxibustion/.

［6］《黄帝内经》素问——四气调神大论篇第二（译文）［EB/OL］.［2021－05－19］. http://www. daoisms. org/xuedao/zhujie/info－4385. html.

［7］ 中华中医药学会. 为中华民族伟大复兴打下坚实健康基础——习近平总书记关于健康中国重要论述综述［EB/OL］.［2021－08－09］. http://www. cacm. org. cn/2021/08/09/14634/.

［8］ 中华中医药学会. 暴雨洪灾后常见疾病的中医药预防.［EB/OL］［2021－10－11］. http://www. catcm. org. cn/newsmain. asp?id＝11933.

［9］ Ringsten, S.（2021, August 23）. *Sports injuries & recovery from a Traditional Chinese Medicine Perspective*. Retrieved November 14, 2021, from https://www. sofieringsten. com/blog/sports-injuries-amp-recovery-from-a－traditional-chinese-medicine-perspective.

第二十章

健康中国与健康世界

1 导读

2021 年是中国共产党成立一百周年。一百年风雨兼程，一百年奋斗不息。在中国共产党的坚强领导下，中国发生了翻天覆地的变化。过去一百年的革命和建设经验证明，中国共产党的领导是历史和人民的选择，是实现中华民族伟大复兴的根本保证。

过去三年多，世界各地受到新型冠状病毒感染疫情的影响，面临这场新中国成立以来我国遭遇的传播速度最快、感染范围最广、防控难度最大的突发公共卫生事件，中国共产党始终坚持人民至上、生命至上，最大限度地保护了人民生命安全和身体健康，统筹疫情防控和经济社会发展取得重大积极成果。国家主席习近平于 2021 年 5 月 21 日出席全球健康峰会并发表重要讲话，提出携手推进全球抗疫合作，共建人类卫生健康共同体。

因此，本书在介绍完主要医学科室的基本概念、常见疾病、临床表现、诊断治疗和医学教育之后，加入了第二十章这一特别章节——"健康中国与健康世界"。

本章由口译技巧之口译技术和 6 篇汉译英材料构成。内容选自中华人民共和国主席习近平在全球健康峰会、世界经济论坛"达沃斯议程"对话会，以及第七十五届联合国大会一般性辩论上的讲话。请结合本章口译技巧练习 6 篇口译实战文本，学习如何在重大国际场合讲好中国故事。

2 口译技巧——口译技术

口译是高强度脑力活动，口译技术可以大大降低口译的认知负荷，提升口译员的效率、准确率和职业胜任力。在现代口译活动中，译员应充分发挥口译技术的赋能作用。我们先来了解四个相关的关键概念："机辅口译技术""机器口译技术""口译服务平台""双语平行语料库"。

（1）机辅口译技术。

机辅口译技术是需要口译员现场翻译的辅助技术和解决方案，包括各种现场和远程口译的传输设备及配套软件，以及译前、译中和译后使用的信息检索、电子词典、术语管理、语音识别、自动翻译、翻译记忆等相关技术。

（2）机器口译技术。

机器口译技术是不需要口译员现场翻译的机器口译和解决方案。这种技术基于语音识别、机器翻译、语音合成等自然语言处理和人工智能技术，基于大规模的语音库、语料库和先进的算法库，包括智能口译笔、便携式翻译机、自动口译App 等硬软件。

（3）口译服务平台。

口译服务平台是连接客户和口译员的口译服务传输平台。深受欧美医院、医疗协会及政府机构青睐的远程口译系统如 BEasy 和 LanguageLine 可让用户通过接入 BEasy App 和 InSight Video Interpreting 中的语音或视频获得专业医疗口译人员的即时在线口译服务。疫情暴发以来，ZOOM 等远程会议平台的同声传译功能也被大量使用。需要注意的是，这类共享式口译平台与独享式口译传输设备一样，只负责语言传输，不负责语言转换（翻译）。

（4）双语平行语料库。

双语平行语料库也是重要的口译技术手段，能为口译员的学习和实践提供巨大助力。下面举例说明双语平行语料库的使用。

首先，我们抓取 2020 年全年外交部和国务院新闻办公室官网上的领导人讲话、疫情记者招待会和例行记者招待会的中英文对应语料建库，建成的双语平行语料库规模约为 150 万字。

然后，我们可以通过 Sketch Engine 等语料分析平台来学习和使用这些语料。例如，如果我们想知道 2020 年的高频词语和短语，我们就可以使用 3 - 4 - grams 搜索。虽然是自动分词，但从图 20 - 1 中前 50 个高频词可以看到"新型冠状病毒感染疫情""新冠病毒""人类命运共同体""世界卫生组织""全球公共卫生""国际关系基本准则""中美关系""一个中国原则"等关键话语。

我们可以从中文库和英文库当中分别提取前 10 个关键词，如表 20 - 1 所示。这也能帮助我们看出中国对外话语的一些关键之处。

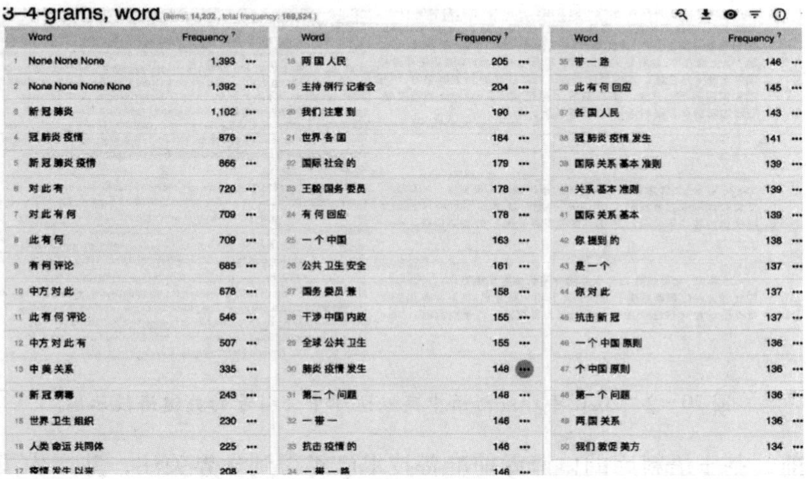

图 20-1　2020 年外宣话语中文库的前 50 个高频 3-4 元词组

表 20-1　2020 年外宣话语中文库和英文库的前 10 个关键词对比

	Target text				Source text		
Rank	Keyword	Keyness	Freq.	Rank	Keyword	Keyness	Freq.
1	疫情	6,847.20	4,587	1	China-US	379.5	350
2	国际	4,182.20	3,423	2	multilateralism	287	317
3	发展	3,772.50	2,597	3	anti-epidemic	279.5	235
4	中国	2,753.80	9,569	4	Pompeo	243.6	460
5	美方	2,753.00	1,895	5	Xinjiang	236	579
6	中方	2,677.30	5,772	6	Wuhan	232	443
7	全球	2,075.20	1,621	7	Jinping	212.6	374
8	问题	1,974.50	2,386	8	CPC	205.7	483
9	维护	1,966.60	1,317	9	ROK	199.6	268
10	抗疫	1,909.90	1,279	10	China-Africa	199.1	177

我们还可以用一些语法标记物来进行搜索，如中文中的引号（""），被引用的词语可能是诗词古话、成语俗语、政策话语等，都是口译工作的关键之处。如图 20-2 所示，通过引号搜索，我们可以学习和参考"一带一路""快捷通道""绿色通道""半边天"等词在不同语境中的译文。

doc#0	<s>三是倡导互利共赢，实现共同发展。</s><s>我们要继续对接发展战略，发挥互补优势，高质量共建"一带一路"。</s><s>当前要有序推进复工复产，建立更多人员往来"快捷通道"和货物出入境"绿色通道"，助力经济社会秩序重启。</s><s>中国正在构建以国内大循环为主体、国内国际双循环相互促进的新发展格局，将推动中国经济更加开放、更有效率、更可持续。</s><s>我们愿同亚洲国家分享发展机遇，实现共同发展。</s>	<s> Third, we need to pursue mutual benefit to achieve common development. </s><s> We should continue to synergize development strategies, leverage our strong complementarities, and advance high-quality Belt and Road cooperation. </s><s> One of the priorities for now is to reopen economies in an orderly way, open more "fast tracks" and "green lanes" to facilitate the flow of people and goods so as to bring business and life back to normal. </s><s> China is shifting t a new development paradigm featuring "dual circulations", with domestic circulation as the mainstay and domestic and international circulations reinforcing each other. </s><s> This aims to make the Chinese economy even more open, efficient and sustainable. </s><s> In this process, we are willing to share development opportunities with fellow Asian countries for common development. </s>
doc#0	<s>25年来，北京世界妇女大会精神不断催生积极变化。</s><s>妇女社会地位显著提高，"半边天"作用日益彰显，性别平等和妇女赋权已成为《联合国2030年可持续发展议程》的重要目标。</s>	<s> Over the past 25 years, the powerful message of the Fourth World Conference on Women held in Beijing has unleashed many positive changes. </s <s> The social status of women is significantly higher. </s><s> Increasingly women are playing an important role of "supporting half of the sky". </s> <s> Indeed, gender equality and women's empowerment are now important goals of the 2030 Agenda for Sustainable Development. </s>
doc#0	<s>25年来，北京世界妇女大会精神不断催生积极变化。</s><s>妇女社会地位显著提高，"半边天"作用日益彰显，性别平等和妇女赋权已成为《联合国2030年可持续发展议程》的重要目标。</s>	<s> Over the past 25 years, the powerful message of the Fourth World Conference on Women held in Beijing has unleashed many positive changes. </s <s> The social status of women is significantly higher. </s><s> Increasingly women are playing an important role of "supporting half of the sky". </s> <s> Indeed, gender equality and women's empowerment are now important goals of the 2030 Agenda for Sustainable Development. </s>

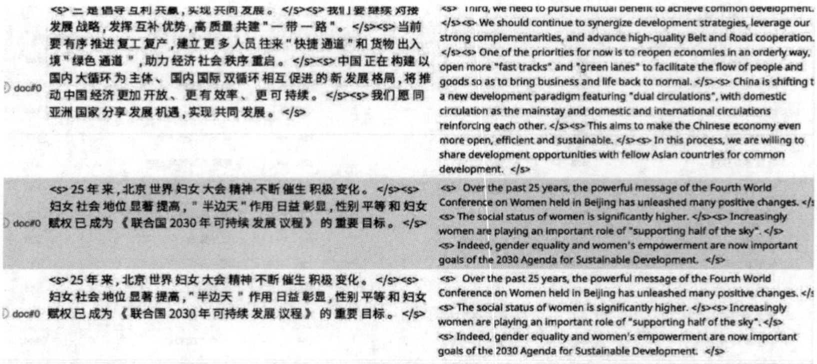

图20-2　2020年外宣话语中英双语库中含引号的关键语段示例

目前，基于语料库的口译译前准备技术已经得到学界关注，并产生了相应成果，感兴趣的同学可以关注徐然等学者的研究[1-2]。在口译技术在口译实践和口译教育中的应用方面，王华树、李智、杨承淑、李德凤等学者[3-6]的研究成果也值得关注。

3　口译词汇与表达

（一）习近平主席在全球健康峰会上的讲话（1）Remarks by President Xi Jinping at the Global Health Summit（1）

人类卫生健康共同体 global community of health for all

德拉吉总理 Prime Minister Mario Draghi

冯德莱恩主席 President Ursula von der Leyen

全球健康峰会 Global Health Summit

应对新冠肺炎特别峰会 Extraordinary Leaders' Summit on COVID-19

利雅得峰会 Riyadh Summit

疫情起伏反复，病毒频繁变异 repeated resurgence and frequent mutations of the coronavirus

正反两方面经验 experience both positive and otherwise

二十国集团成员 G20 members

补短板、堵漏洞、强弱项 remedying deficiencies，closing loopholes and strengthening weak links

坚持科学施策，统筹系统应对 We must follow science-based policies and ensure a coordinated and systemic response.

统筹药物和非药物干预措施 coordinate pharmacological and non-pharmacological interventions

统筹常态化精准防控和应急处置 balance targeted routine COVID-19 protocols and emergency measures

统筹疫情防控和经济社会发展 ensure both epidemic control and socio-economic development

重大突发公共卫生事件 major public health emergencies

缓债 debt suspension

同舟共济 stick together

荣辱与共、命运相连 rise and fall together with a shared future

政治化、标签化、污名化 politicize, label or stigmatize

免疫鸿沟 immunization gap

可及性和可负担性 accessible and affordable

授权生产 authorized production

多边金融机构 multilateral financial institution

新冠肺炎疫苗实施计划 COVID-19 Vaccine Global Access（COVAX）facility

标本兼治 address both the symptoms and root causes

集中检验 extensive test

共商共建共享 extensive consultation, joint contribution and shared benefits

合理诉求 legitimate concern

听取意见 heed the views of

应急物资储备 contingency reserve

（二）习近平主席在全球健康峰会上的讲话（2）Remarks by President Xi Jinping at the Global Health Summit（2）

在这场史无前例的抗疫斗争中 in this unprecedented battle against the pandemic

第七十三届世界卫生大会 the 73rd World Health Assembly

抗疫物资 medical supplies

非洲疾控中心总部大楼 the Africa CDC headquarters

二十国集团"暂缓最贫困国家债务偿付倡议" the G20 Debt Service Suspension Initiative for Poorest Countries

检测试剂盒 testing kits

中非对口医院合作机制 Chinese hospitals to pair up with African hospitals

全球人道主义应急仓库和枢纽 global humanitarian response depot and hub

缓债金额 deferral amount

向发展中国家进行技术转让 transferring technologies to other developing countries

新冠肺炎疫苗知识产权豁免 waiving intellectual property rights on COVID-19 vaccines

利益攸关方 stakeholder

疫苗公平合理分配 fair and equitable distribution of vaccines

古罗马哲人塞涅卡 the ancient Roman philosopher Seneca

（三）习近平主席在世界经济论坛"达沃斯议程"对话会上的特别致辞（节选）Special Address by President Xi Jinping at the World Economic Forum Virtual Event of the Davos Agenda（excerpts）

全球公共卫生面临严重威胁 global public health faced severe threat.

世界经济陷入深度衰退 The world economy was mired in deep recession.

同病魔展开殊死搏斗 battling the deadly coronavirus

疫情还远未结束 The pandemic is far from over.

抗击疫情是国际社会面临的最紧迫任务。Containing the coronavirus is the most pressing task for the international community.

让疫苗真正成为各国人民用得上、用得起的公共产品 to make vaccines public goods that are truly accessible and affordable to people in all countries

医疗专家组 medical expert teams

促进疫苗在发展中国家的可及性和可负担性 to work for greater accessibility and affordability of COVID vaccines in developing countries

（四）习近平主席在第七十五届联合国大会一般性辩论上的讲话（1）Statement by President Xi Jinping at the General Debate of the 75th Session of the United Nations General Assembly（1）

病毒肆虐全球，疫情不断反复 a virus that has ravaged the world and has kept resurging

守望相助 people of different countries have come together

照亮至暗时刻 lit the dark hour

同舟共济 get this through together

反对政治化、污名化 any attempt of politicizing the issue or stigmatization must be rejected

常态化防控措施 long-term control measures

复商复市复工复学 reopen businesses and schools

《联合国 2030 年可持续发展议程》the 2030 Agenda for Sustainable Development

世界百年未有之大变局 profound changes never seen in a century

（五）习近平主席在第七十五届联合国大会一般性辩论上的讲话（2）Statement by President Xi Jinping at the General Debate of the 75th Session of the United Nations General Assembly（2）

互联互通、休戚与共 an interconnected global village with a common stake

以邻为壑、隔岸观火 to pursue a beggar-thy-neighbor policy or just watch from a safe distance when others are in danger

你中有我、我中有你的命运共同体意识 the vision of a community with a shared future in which everyone is bound together

跳出小圈子和零和博弈思维 reject attempts to build blocs to keep others out and oppose a zero-sum approach

像鸵鸟一样把头埋在沙里假装视而不见 burying one's head in the sand like an ostrich in the face of economic globalization

像堂吉诃德一样挥舞长矛加以抵制 trying to fight it with Don Quixote's lance

沿着只讲索取不讲投入、只讲发展不讲保护、只讲利用不讲修复的老路走下去 go down the beaten path of extracting resources without investing in conservation, pursuing development at the expense of protection, and exploiting resources without restoration

国家自主贡献力度 Intended Nationally Determined Contributions

守住道德底线和国际规范 countries should not breach the moral standard and should comply with international norms

（六）习近平主席在第七十五届联合国大会一般性辩论上的讲话（3）Statement by President Xi Jinping at the General Debate of the 75th Session of the United Nations General Assembly（3）

14 亿中国人民不畏艰难、上下同心 the 1.4 billion Chinese, undaunted by the strike of COVID-19

我们永远不称霸，不扩张，不谋求势力范围，无意跟任何国家打冷战热战

We will never seek hegemony, expansion, or sphere of influence. We have no intention to fight either a Cold War or a hot war with any country.

国内国际双循环 domestic and international circulations reinforcing each other

我们不追求一枝独秀，不搞你输我赢 We do not seek to develop only ourselves or engage in a zero-sum game.

联合国全球地理信息知识与创新中心和可持续发展大数据国际研究中心 UN Global Geospatial Knowledge and Innovation Center and an International Research Center of Big Data for Sustainable Development Goals

历史接力棒已经传到我们这一代人手中 the baton of history has been passed to our generation

无愧于人民、无愧于历史的抉择 a choice worthy of the people's trust and of our times.

4 口译实战

（一）习近平主席在全球健康峰会上的讲话（1）Remarks by President Xi Jinping at the Global Health Summit（1）[7-8]

尊敬的德拉吉总理， 尊敬的冯德莱恩主席， 各位同事：	Your Excellency Prime Minister Mario Draghi, Your Excellency President Ursula von der Leyen, Dear Colleagues,
很高兴出席全球健康峰会。去年，二十国集团成功举行了应对新冠肺炎特别峰会和利雅得峰会，就推动全球团结抗疫、助力世界经济恢复达成许多重要共识。	It gives me great pleasure to attend the Global Health Summit. Last year, the G20 successfully held an Extraordinary Leaders' Summit on COVID-19 and the Riyadh Summit. Many important common understandings were reached on promoting global solidarity against the virus and boosting world economic recovery.

一年多来，疫情起伏反复，病毒频繁变异，百年来最严重的传染病大流行仍在肆虐。早日战胜疫情、恢复经济增长，是国际社会的首要任务。二十国集团成员应该在全球抗疫合作中扛起责任，同时要总结正反两方面经验，抓紧补短板、堵漏洞、强弱项，着力提高应对重大突发公共卫生事件能力和水平。下面，我想谈5点意见。

第一，坚持人民至上、生命至上。抗击疫情是为了人民，也必须依靠人民。实践证明，要彻底战胜疫情，必须把人民生命安全和身体健康放在突出位置，以极大的政治担当和勇气，以非常之举应对非常之事，尽最大努力做到不遗漏一个感染者、不放弃一个病患者，切实尊重每个人的生命价值和尊严。同时，要保证人民群众生活少受影响、社会秩序总体正常。

The past year and more have seen repeated resurgence and frequent mutations of the coronavirus. The most serious pandemic in a century is still wreaking havoc. To clinch an early victory against COVID-19 and restore economic growth remains the top priority for the international community. G20 members need to shoulder responsibilities in global cooperation against the virus. In the meantime, we need to draw on experience both positive and otherwise, and lose no time in remedying deficiencies, closing loopholes and strengthening weak links in a bid to enhance preparedness and capacity for coping with major public health emergencies. Here, I want to make five points on what we need to do.

First, we must put people and their lives first. The battle with COVID-19 is one for the people and by the people. What has happened proves that to completely defeat the virus, we must put people's lives and health front and center, demonstrate a great sense of political responsibility and courage, and make extraordinary responses to an extraordinary challenge. No effort must be spared to attend every case, save every patient, and truly respect the value and dignity of every human life. Meanwhile, it is also important to minimize the potential impact on people's life and maintain general order in our society.

第二，坚持科学施策，统筹系统应对。面对这场新型传染性疾病，我们要坚持弘扬科学精神、秉持科学态度、遵循科学规律。抗击疫情是一场总体战，要系统应对，统筹药物和非药物干预措施，统筹常态化精准防控和应急处置，统筹疫情防控和经济社会发展。二十国集团成员要采取负责任的宏观经济政策，加强相互协调，维护全球产业链供应链安全顺畅运转。要继续通过缓债、发展援助等方式支持发展中国家尤其是困难特别大的脆弱国家。

Second, we must follow science-based policies and ensure a coordinated and systemic response. Faced with this new infectious disease, we should advocate the spirit of science, adopt a science-based approach, and follow the law of science. The fight against COVID-19 is an all-out war that calls for a systemic response to coordinate pharmacological and non-pharmacological interventions, balance targeted routine COVID-19 protocols and emergency measures, and ensure both epidemic control and socio-economic development. G20 members need to adopt responsible macro-economic policies and step up coordination to keep the global industrial and supply chains safe and smooth. It is essential to give continued support by such means as debt suspension and development aid to developing countries, especially vulnerable countries facing exceptional difficulties.

第三，坚持同舟共济，倡导团结合作。这场疫情再次昭示我们，人类荣辱与共、命运相连。面对传染病大流行，我们要秉持人类卫生健康共同体理念，团结合作、共克时艰，坚决反对各种政治化、标签化、污名化的企图。搞政治操弄丝毫无助于本国抗疫，只会扰乱国际抗疫合作，给世界各国人民带来更大伤害。

第四，坚持公平合理，弥合"免疫鸿沟"。我在一年前提出，疫苗应该成为全球公共产品。当前，疫苗接种不平衡问题更加突出，我们要摒弃"疫苗民族主义"，解决好疫苗产能和分配问题，增强发展中国家的可及性和可负担性。疫苗研发和生产大国要负起责任，多提供一些疫苗给有急需的发展中国家，支持本国企业同有能力的国家开展联合研究、授权生产。多边金融机构应该为发展中国家采购疫苗提供包容性的融资支持。世界卫生组织要加速推进"新冠肺炎疫苗实施计划"。

Third, we must stick together and promote solidarity and cooperation. The pandemic is yet another reminder that we humanity rise and fall together with a shared future. Confronted by a pandemic like COVID-19, we must champion the vision of building a global community of health for all, tide over this trying time through solidarity and cooperation, and firmly reject any attempt to politicize, label or stigmatize the virus. Political manipulation would not serve COVID-19 response on the domestic front. It would only disrupt international cooperation against the virus and bring greater harm to people around the world.

Fourth, we must uphold fairness and equity as we strive to close the immunization gap. A year ago, I proposed that vaccines should be made a global public good. Today, the problem of uneven vaccination has become more acute. It is imperative for us to reject vaccine nationalism and find solutions to issues concerning the production capacity and distribution of vaccines, in order to make vaccines more accessible and affordable in developing countries. Major vaccine-developing and producing countries need to take up their responsibility to provide more vaccines to developing countries in urgent need, and they also need to support their businesses in joint research and authorized production with other countries having the relevant capacity. Multilateral financial institutions should provide inclusive financing support for vaccine procurement of developing countries. The World Health Organization (WHO) should speed up efforts under the COVID-19 Vaccine Global Access (COVAX) facility.

第五，坚持标本兼治，完善治理体系。这次疫情是对全球卫生治理体系的一次集中检验。我们要加强和发挥联合国和世界卫生组织作用，完善全球疾病预防控制体系，更好预防和应对今后的疫情。要坚持共商共建共享，充分听取发展中国家意见，更好反映发展中国家合理诉求。要提高监测预警和应急反应能力、重大疫情救治能力、应急物资储备和保障能力、打击虚假信息能力、向发展中国家提供支持能力。

Fifth, we must address both the symptoms and root causes as we improve the governance system. The pandemic is an extensive test of the global health governance system. It is important that we strengthen and leverage the role of the UN and the WHO and improve the global disease prevention and control system to better prevent and respond to future pandemics. It is important that we uphold the spirit of extensive consultation, joint contribution and shared benefits, fully heed the views of developing countries, and better reflect their legitimate concerns. It is also important that we enhance our capacity of monitoring, early-warning and emergency response, of treatment of major pandemics, of contingency reserve and logistics, of fighting disinformation, and of providing support to developing countries.

（二）习近平主席在全球健康峰会上的讲话（2）Remarks by President Xi Jinping at the Global Health Summit（2）[7-8]

各位同事！在这场史无前例的抗疫斗争中，中国得到很多国家支持和帮助，中国也开展了大规模的全球人道主义行动。去年5月，我在第七十三届世界卫生大会上宣布中国支持全球抗疫合作的5项举措，正在抓紧落实。在产能有限、自身需求巨大的情况下，中国履行承诺，向80多个有急需的发展中国家提供疫苗援助，向43个国家出口疫苗。

Colleagues, in this unprecedented battle against the pandemic, China has, while receiving support and help from many countries, mounted a massive global humanitarian operation. At the 73rd World Health Assembly held in May last year, I announced five measures that China would take to support global anti-pandemic cooperation. Implementation of those measures is well underway. Notwithstanding the limited production capacity and enormous demand at home, China has honored its commitment by providing free vaccines to more than 80 developing countries in urgent need and exporting vaccines to 43 countries.

中国已为受疫情影响的发展中国家抗疫以及恢复经济社会发展提供了20亿美元援助，向150多个国家和13个国际组织提供了抗疫物资援助，为全球供应了2800多亿只口罩、34亿多件防护服、40多亿份检测试剂盒。中非建立了41个对口医院合作机制，

We have provided 2 billion US dollars in assistance for the COVID-19 response and economic and social recovery in developing countries hit by the pandemic. We have sent medical supplies to more than 150 countries and 13 international organizations, providing

中国援建的非洲疾控中心总部大楼项目已于去年年底正式开工。中国同联合国合作在华设立全球人道主义应急仓库和枢纽也取得了重要进展。中国全面落实二十国集团"暂缓最贫困国家债务偿付倡议",总额超过 13 亿美元,是二十国集团成员中落实缓债金额最大的国家。

为继续支持全球团结抗疫,我宣布:

——中国将在未来 3 年内再提供 30 亿美元国际援助,用于支持发展中国家抗疫和恢复经济社会发展。

——中国已向全球供应 3 亿剂疫苗,将尽己所能对外提供更多疫苗。

more than 280 billion masks, 3. 4 billion protective suits and 4 billion testing kits to the world. A cooperation mechanism has been established for Chinese hospitals to pair up with 41 African hospitals, and construction for the China-assisted project of the Africa CDC headquarters officially started at the end of last year. Important progress has also been made in the China-UN joint project to set up in China a global humanitarian response depot and hub. China is fully implementing the G20 Debt Service Suspension Initiative for Poorest Countries and has so far put off debt repayment exceeding 1. 3 billion US dollars, the highest deferral amount among G20 members.

In continued support for global solidarity against COVID-19, I wish to announce the following:

—China will provide an additional 3 billion US dollars in international aid over the next three years to support COVID-19 response and economic and social recovery in other developing countries.

—Having already supplied 300 million doses of vaccines to the world, China will provide still more vaccines to the best of its ability.

——中国支持本国疫苗企业向发展中国家进行技术转让，开展合作生产。

—China supports its vaccine companies in transferring technologies to other developing countries and carrying out joint production with them.

——中国已宣布支持新冠肺炎疫苗知识产权豁免，也支持世界贸易组织等国际机构早日就此作出决定。

—Having announced support for waiving intellectual property rights on COVID-19 vaccines, China also supports the World Trade Organization and other international institutions in making an early decision on this matter.

——中国倡议设立疫苗合作国际论坛，由疫苗生产研发国家、企业、利益攸关方一道探讨如何推进全球疫苗公平合理分配。

—China proposes setting up an international forum on vaccine cooperation for vaccine-developing and producing countries, companies and other stakeholders to explore ways of promoting fair and equitable distribution of vaccines around the world.

各位同事！古罗马哲人塞涅卡说过，我们是同一片大海的海浪。让我们携手并肩，坚定不移推进抗疫国际合作，共同推动构建人类卫生健康共同体，共同守护人类健康美好未来！

Colleagues, the ancient Roman philosopher Seneca said, "We are all waves of the same sea." Let us join hands and stand shoulder to shoulder with each other to firmly advance international cooperation against COVID-19, build a global community of health for all, and work for a healthier and brighter future for humanity.

（三）习近平主席在世界经济论坛"达沃斯议程"对话会上的特别致辞（节选）Special Address by President Xi Jinping at the World Economic Forum Virtual Event of the Davos Agenda（excerpts）[9-10]

尊敬的施瓦布主席，

女士们，先生们，朋友们：

Professor Klaus Schwab,

Ladies and Gentlemen, Friends,

过去一年，突如其来的新冠肺炎疫情肆虐全球，全球公共卫生面临严重威胁，世界经济陷入深度衰退，人类经历了史上罕见的多重危机。

The past year was marked by the sudden onslaught of the COVID-19 pandemic. Global public health faced severe threat and the world economy was mired in deep recession. Humanity encountered multiple crises rarely seen in human history.

这一年，各国人民以巨大的决心和勇气，同病魔展开殊死搏斗，依靠科学理性的力量，弘扬人道主义精神，全球抗疫取得初步成效。现在，疫情还远未结束，近期又出现反弹，抗疫仍在继续，但我们坚信，寒冬阻挡不了春天的脚步，黑夜遮蔽不住黎明的曙光。人类一定能够战胜疫情，在同灾难的斗争中成长进步、浴火重生。

The past year also bore witness to the enormous resolve and courage of people around the world in battling the deadly coronavirus. Guided by science, reason and a humanitarian spirit, the world has achieved initial progress in fighting COVID-19. That said, the pandemic is far from over. The recent resurgence in COVID cases reminds us that we must carry on the fight. Yet we remain convinced that winter cannot stop the arrival of spring and darkness can never shroud the light of dawn. There is no doubt that humanity will prevail over the virus and emerge even stronger from this disaster.

…… ……

中国将继续积极参与国际抗疫合作。抗击疫情是国际社会面临的最紧迫任务。这既是坚持人民至上、生命至上的基本要求，也是稳定恢复经济的基本前提。我们要深化团结合作，加强信息共享和联防联控，坚决打赢全球疫情阻击战。特别是要加强疫苗研发、生产、分配合作，让疫苗真正成为各国人民用得上、用得起的公共产品。

中国迄今已向 150 多个国家和 13 个国际组织提供抗疫援助，为有需要的国家派出 36 个医疗专家组，积极支持并参与疫苗国际合作。中国将继续同各国分享疫情防控有益经验，向应对疫情能力薄弱的国家和地区提供力所能及的帮助，促进疫苗在发展中国家的可及性和可负担性，助力世界早日彻底战胜疫情。

……

China will continue to take an active part in international cooperation on COVID-19. Containing the coronavirus is the most pressing task for the international community. This is because people and their lives must always be put before anything else. It is also what it takes to stabilize and revive the economy. Closer solidarity and cooperation, more information sharing, and a stronger global response are what we need to defeat COVID-19 across the world. It is especially important to scale up cooperation on the R&D, production and distribution of vaccines and make them public goods that are truly accessible and affordable to people in all countries.

By now, China has provided assistance to over 150 countries and 13 international organizations, sent 36 medical expert teams to countries in need, and stayed strongly supportive and actively engaged in international cooperation on COVID vaccines. China will continue to share its experience with other countries, do its best to assist countries and regions that are less prepared for the pandemic, and work for greater accessibility and affordability of COVID vaccines in developing countries. We hope these efforts will contribute to an early and complete victory over the coronavirus throughout the world.

....

......

（四）习近平主席在第七十五届联合国大会一般性辩论上的讲话（1）

Statement by President Xi Jinping at the General Debate of the 75th Session of the United Nations General Assembly （1）[11-12]

主席先生，
各位同事：

Mr. President,
Colleagues,

今年是世界反法西斯战争胜利 75 周年，也是联合国成立 75 周年。昨天，联合国隆重举行纪念峰会，铭记世界反法西斯战争历史经验和教训，重申对联合国宪章宗旨和原则的坚定承诺，具有重要意义。

This year marks the 75th anniversary of the victory in the World Anti-Fascist War and the founding of the United Nations （UN）. Yesterday, the high-level meeting to commemorate the 75th anniversary of the UN was held. The meeting was a significant one, as it reaffirmed our abiding commitment to the purposes and principles of the UN Charter on the basis of reviewing the historical experience and lessons of the World Anti-Fascist War.

主席先生！人类正在同新冠肺炎疫情进行斗争。病毒肆虐全球，疫情不断反复。我们目睹了各国政府的努力、医务人员的付出、科学工作者的

Mr. President, we humans are battling COVID-19, a virus that has ravaged the world and has kept resurging. In this fight, we have witnessed the efforts of

探索、普通民众的坚守。各国人民守望相助，展现出人类在重大灾难面前的勇气、决心、关爱，照亮了至暗时刻。疫情终将被人类战胜，胜利必将属于世界人民！

——面对疫情，我们要践行人民至上、生命至上理念。要调集一切资源，科学防治，精准施策，不遗漏一个感染者，不放弃一位患者，坚决遏制疫情蔓延。

——面对疫情，我们要加强团结、同舟共济。要秉持科学精神，充分发挥世界卫生组织关键领导作用，推进国际联防联控，坚决打赢全球疫情阻击战，反对政治化、污名化。

——面对疫情，我们要制定全面和常态化防控措施。要有序推进复商复市复工复学，创造就业，拉动经济，恢复经济社会秩序和活力，主要经济

governments, dedication of medical workers, exploration of scientists, and perseverance of the public. People of different countries have come together. With courage, resolve and compassion which lit the dark hour, we have confronted the disaster head on. The virus will be defeated. Humanity will win this battle!

—Facing the virus, we should put people and life first. We should mobilize all resources to make a science-based and targeted response. No case should be missed and no patient should be left untreated. The spread of the virus must be contained.

—Facing the virus, we should enhance solidarity and get this through together. We should follow the guidance of science, give full play to the leading role of the World Health Organization, and launch a joint international response to beat this pandemic. Any attempt of politicizing the issue or stigmatization must be rejected.

—Facing the virus, we should adopt comprehensive and long-term control measures. We should reopen businesses and schools in an orderly way, so as to

体要加强宏观政策协调，不仅要重启本国经济，而且要为世界经济复苏作出贡献。

——面对疫情，我们要关心和照顾发展中国家特别是非洲国家。国际社会要在减缓债务、援助等方面采取及时和强有力举措，确保落实好《联合国 2030 年可持续发展议程》，帮助他们克服困难。

75 年前，中国为赢得世界反法西斯战争胜利作出了历史性贡献，支持建立了联合国。今天，秉持同样的担当精神，中国积极投身国际抗疫合作，为维护全球公共卫生安全贡献中国力量。我们将继续同各国分享抗疫经验和诊疗技术，向有需要的国家提供支持和帮助，确保全球抗疫物资供应链稳定，并积极参与病毒溯源和传播途径全球科学研究。

create jobs, boost the economy, and restore economic and social order and vitality. The major economies need to step up macro policy coordination. We should not only restart our own economies, but also contribute to global recovery.

—Facing the virus, we should show concern for and accommodate the need of developing countries, especially African countries. The international community needs to take timely and robust measures in such fields as debt relief and international assistance, ensure the implementation of the 2030 Agenda for Sustainable Development and help these countries overcome their difficulties.

Seventy-five years ago, China made historic contributions to winning the World Anti-Fascist War and supported the founding of the United Nations. Today, with the same sense of responsibility, China is actively involved in the international fight against COVID-19, contributing its share to upholding global public health security. Going forward, we will continue to share our epidemic control practices as well as diagnostics and therapeutics with other countries, provide support and assistance to countries in need, ensure stable global anti-epidemic supply chains, and actively participate in the global research on tracing the source and transmission routes of the virus.

中国已有多支疫苗进入Ⅲ期临床试验，研发完成并投入使用后将作为全球公共产品，优先向发展中国家提供。中国将落实好两年提供 20 亿美元国际援助的承诺，深化农业、减贫、教育、妇女儿童、气候变化等领域国际合作，助力各国经济社会恢复发展。

At the moment, several COVID-19 vaccines developed by China are in Phase Ⅲ clinical trials. When their development is completed and they are available for use, these vaccines will be made a global public good, and they will be provided to other developing countries on a priority basis. China will honor its commitment of providing US $2 billion of international assistance over two years, further international cooperation in such fields as agriculture, poverty reduction, education, women and children, and climate change, and support other countries in restoring economic and social development.

主席先生！人类社会发展史，就是一部不断战胜各种挑战和困难的历史。新冠肺炎疫情全球大流行和世界百年未有之大变局相互影响，但和平与发展的时代主题没有变，各国人民和平发展合作共赢的期待更加强烈。新冠肺炎疫情不会是人类面临的最后一次危机，我们必须做好携手迎接更多全球性挑战的准备。

Mr. President, the history of development of human society is a history of our struggles against all challenges and difficulties and our victories over them. At present, the world is battling the COVID-19 pandemic as it goes through profound changes never seen in a century. Yet, peace and development remain the underlying trend of the times, and people everywhere crave even more strongly for peace, development and win-

win cooperation. COVID-19 will not be the last crisis to confront humanity, so we must join hands and be prepared to meet even more global challenges.

（五）习近平主席在第七十五届联合国大会一般性辩论上的讲话（2）
Statement by President Xi Jinping at the General Debate of the 75th Session of the United Nations General Assembly（2）[9]

第一，这场疫情启示我们，我们生活在一个互联互通、休戚与共的地球村里。各国紧密相连，人类命运与共。任何国家都不能从别国的困难中谋取利益，从他国的动荡中收获稳定。如果以邻为壑、隔岸观火，别国的威胁迟早会变成自己的挑战。

First, COVID-19 reminds us that we are living in an interconnected global village with a common stake. All countries are closely connected and we share a common future. No country can gain from others' difficulties or maintain stability by taking advantage of others' troubles. To pursue a beggar-thy-neighbor policy or just watch from a safe distance when others are in danger will eventually land one in the same trouble faced by others.

我们要树立你中有我、我中有你的命运共同体意识，跳出小圈子和零和博弈思维，树立大家庭和合作共赢理念，摒弃意识形态争论，跨越文明冲突陷阱，相互尊重各国自主选择的发展道路和模式，让世界多样性成为人类社会进步的不竭动力、人类文明多姿多彩的天然形态。

This is why we should embrace the vision of a community with a shared future in which everyone is bound together. We should reject attempts to build blocs to keep others out and oppose a zero-sum approach. We should see each other as members of the same big family, pursue win-win cooperation, and rise above ideological disputes and do not fall into the trap of "clash of civilizations". More importantly, we should respect a country's independent choice of development path and model. The world is diverse in nature, and we should turn this diversity into a constant source of inspiration driving human advancement. This will ensure that human civilizations remain colorful and diversified.

　　第二，这场疫情启示我们，经济全球化是客观现实和历史潮流。面对经济全球化大势，像鸵鸟一样把头埋在沙里假装视而不见，或像堂吉诃德一样挥舞长矛加以抵制，都违背了历史规律。世界退不回彼此封闭孤立的状态，更不可能被人为割裂。我们不能回避经济全球化带来的挑战，必须直面贫富差距、发展鸿沟等重大问题。

Second, COVID-19 reminds us that economic globalization is an indisputable reality and a historical trend. Burying one's head in the sand like an ostrich in the face of economic globalization or trying to fight it with Don Quixote's lance goes against the trend of history. Let this be clear: The world will never return to isolation, and no one can sever the ties between countries. We should not dodge the challenges of economic globalization. Instead, we must face up to major issues such as the wealth gap and the development divide.

　　我们要处理好政府和市场、公平和效率、增长和分配、技术和就业的关系，使发展既平衡又充分，发展成果公平惠及不同国家不同阶层不同人群。我们要秉持开放包容理念，坚定不移构建开放型世界经济，维护以世

We should strike a proper balance between the government and the market, fairness and efficiency, growth and income distribution, and technology and employment so as to ensure full and balanced development that delivers

界贸易组织为基石的多边贸易体制，旗帜鲜明反对单边主义、保护主义，维护全球产业链供应链稳定畅通。

第三，这场疫情启示我们，人类需要一场自我革命，加快形成绿色发展方式和生活方式，建设生态文明和美丽地球。人类不能再忽视大自然一次又一次的警告，沿着只讲索取不讲投入、只讲发展不讲保护、只讲利用不讲修复的老路走下去。应对气候变化《巴黎协定》代表了全球绿色低碳转型的大方向，是保护地球家园需要采取的最低限度行动，各国必须迈出决定性步伐。

benefit to people from all countries, sectors and backgrounds in an equitable way. We should pursue open and inclusive development, remain committed to building an open world economy, and uphold the multilateral trading regime with the World Trade Organization as the cornerstone. We should say no to unilateralism and protectionism, and work to ensure the stable and smooth functioning of global industrial and supply chains.

Third, COVID-19 reminds us that humankind should launch a green revolution and move faster to create a green way of development and life, preserve the environment and make Mother Earth a better place for all. Humankind can no longer afford to ignore the repeated warnings of Mother Nature and go down the beaten path of extracting resources without investing in conservation, pursuing development at the expense of protection, and exploiting resources without restoration. The Paris Agreement on climate change charts the course for the world to transition to green and low-carbon development. It outlines the minimum steps to be taken to protect the Earth, our shared homeland, and all

中国将提高国家自主贡献力度，采取更加有力的政策和措施，二氧化碳排放力争于2030年前达到峰值，努力争取2060年前实现碳中和。各国要树立创新、协调、绿色、开放、共享的新发展理念，抓住新一轮科技革命和产业变革的历史性机遇，推动疫情后世界经济"绿色复苏"，汇聚起可持续发展的强大合力。

第四，这场疫情启示我们，全球治理体系亟待改革和完善。疫情不仅是对各国执政能力的大考，也是对全球治理体系的检验。我们要坚持走多边主义道路，维护以联合国为核心的国际体系。全球治理应该秉持共商共建共享原则，推动各国权利平等、机会平等、规则平等，使全球治理体系符合变化了的世界政治经济，满足应对全球性挑战的现实需要，顺应和平发展合作共赢的历史趋势。

countries must take decisive steps to honor this Agreement.

China will scale up its Intended Nationally Determined Contributions by adopting more vigorous policies and measures. We aim to have CO_2 emissions peak before 2030 and achieve carbon neutrality before 2060. We call on all countries to pursue innovative, coordinated, green and open development for all, seize the historic opportunities presented by the new round of scientific and technological revolution and industrial transformation, achieve a green recovery of the world economy in the post-COVID era and thus create a powerful force driving sustainable development.

Fourth, COVID-19 reminds us that the global governance system calls for reform and improvement. COVID-19 is a major test of the governance capacity of countries; it is also a test of the global governance system. We should stay true to multilateralism and safeguard the international system with the UN at its core. Global governance should be based on the principle of extensive consultation, joint contribution and shared benefits so as to ensure that all countries enjoy equal rights and opportunities and follow the same rules. The global governance system should adapt itself to evolving global political and economic dynamics, meet global challenges and embrace the underlying trend of peace, development and win-win cooperation.

国家之间有分歧是正常的，应该通过对话协商妥善化解。国家之间可以有竞争，但必须是积极和良性的，要守住道德底线和国际规范。大国更应该有大的样子，要提供更多全球公共产品，承担大国责任，展现大国担当。

It is natural for countries to have differences. What's important is to address them through dialogue and consultation. Countries may engage in competition, but such competition should be positive and healthy in nature. When in competition, countries should not breach the moral standard and should comply with international norms. In particular, major countries should act like major countries. They should provide more global public goods, take up their due responsibilities and live up to people's expectations.

（六）习近平主席在第七十五届联合国大会一般性辩论上的讲话（3）
Statement by President Xi Jinping at the General Debate of the 75th Session of the United Nations General Assembly （3）[9]

主席先生！今年以来，14 亿中国人民不畏艰难、上下同心，全力克服疫情影响，加快恢复生产生活秩序。我们有信心如期全面建成小康社会，如期实现现行标准下农村贫困人口全

Mr. President, since the start of this year, we, the 1.4 billion Chinese, undaunted by the strike of COVID-19, and with the government and the people united as one, have made all-out efforts

部脱贫，提前 10 年实现《联合国2030 年可持续发展议程》减贫目标。

中国是世界上最大的发展中国家，走的是和平发展、开放发展、合作发展、共同发展的道路。我们永远不称霸，不扩张，不谋求势力范围，无意跟任何国家打冷战热战，坚持以对话弥合分歧，以谈判化解争端。我们不追求一枝独秀，不搞你输我赢，也不会关起门来封闭运行，将逐步形成以国内大循环为主体、国内国际双循环相互促进的新发展格局，为中国经济发展开辟空间，为世界经济复苏和增长增添动力。

to control the virus and speedily restore life and economy to normalcy. We have every confidence to achieve our goals within the set time frame, that is, to finish the building of a moderately prosperous society in all respects, lift out of poverty all rural residents living below the current poverty line, and meet ten years ahead of schedule the poverty eradication target set out in the 2030 Agenda for Sustainable Development.

China is the largest developing country in the world, a country that is committed to peaceful, open, cooperative and common development. We will never seek hegemony, expansion, or sphere of influence. We have no intention to fight either a Cold War or a hot war with any country. We will continue to narrow differences and resolve disputes with others through dialogue and negotiation. We do not seek to develop only ourselves or engage in a zero-sum game. We will not pursue development behind closed doors. Rather, we aim to foster, over time, a new development paradigm with domestic circulation as the mainstay and domestic and international circulations reinforcing each other. This will create more space for China's economic development and add impetus to global economic recovery and growth.

中国将继续做世界和平的建设者、全球发展的贡献者、国际秩序的维护者。为支持联合国在国际事务中发挥核心作用，我宣布：

China will continue to work as a builder of global peace, a contributor to global development and a defender of international order. To support the UN in playing its central role in international affairs, I hereby announce the following steps to be taken by China:

——中国将向联合国新冠肺炎疫情全球人道主义应对计划再提供 5000 万美元支持；

—China will provide another US $50 million to the UN COVID-19 Global Humanitarian Response Plan.

——中国将设立规模 5000 万美元的第三期中国－联合国粮农组织南南合作信托基金；

—China will provide US $50 million to the China-FAO South-South Cooperation Trust Fund (Phase III).

——中国－联合国和平与发展基金将在 2025 年到期后延期 5 年；

—China will extend the Peace and Development Trust Fund between the UN and China by five years after it expires in 2025.

——中国将设立联合国全球地理信息知识与创新中心和可持续发展大数据国际研究中心，为落实《联合国 2030 年可持续发展议程》提供新助力。

—China will set up a UN Global Geospatial Knowledge and Innovation Center and an International Research Center of Big Data for Sustainable Development Goals to facilitate the implementation of the 2030 Agenda for Sustainable Development.

主席先生、各位同事！历史接力棒已经传到我们这一代人手中，我们必须作出无愧于人民、无愧于历史的抉择。让我们团结起来，坚守和平、发展、公平、正义、民主、自由的全人类共同价值，推动构建新型国际关系，推动构建人类命运共同体，共同创造世界更加美好的未来！

Mr. President, Colleagues, the baton of history has been passed to our generation, and we must make the right choice, a choice worthy of the people's trust and of our times. Let us join hands to uphold the values of peace, development, equity, justice, democracy and freedom shared by all of us and build a new type of international relations and a community with a shared future for mankind. Together, we can make the world a better place for everyone.

5 口译注释与学习资源

5.1 口译注释

成员与成员国（members vs member countries or states）

国际组织分为政府间国际组织（International Governmental Organization）和非政府间国际组织（International Non-governmental Organizations），前者包括联合国、欧盟、非盟、东盟、世界贸易组织等，后者有国际足联、国际奥委会、国际红十字会等。口译员切记不可"嘴瓢"，将"成员"误译为"成员国"，犯下"大是大非"的错误。其中，口译员特别需要关注亚太经合组织（APEC），因为该组织的构成是成员（members）或成员经济体（member economies），而非成员国（member countries or states）。

5.2 学习资源

登录中国大学 MOOC（慕课），学习"医疗口译"课程汉译外的口译实战示范视频。关注和学习中国外交部、"两会"、政府工作报告、政府白皮书等汉译外双语资源。

参考文献

[1] Xu, R. (2018). Corpus-based terminological preparation for simultaneous interpreting. *Interpreting*, 20 (1), 29–58.

[2] 徐然. 基于语料库技术的口译译前准备模式建构 [J]. 中国翻译, 2018 (03): 53–59.

[3] 王华树. 人工智能时代口译技术应用研究 [M]. 北京: 知识产权出版社, 2020.

[4] 王华树, 李智. 口译技术研究现状、问题与展望 (1988—2019)——一项基于相关文献的计量分析 [J]. 上海翻译, 2020 (03): 50–55+95–96.

[5] 王华树, 杨承淑. 人工智能时代的口译技术发展: 概念、影响与趋势 [J]. 中国翻译, 2019 (06): 69–79+191–192.

[6] 李智, 李德凤. 人工智能时代口译员信息技术素养研究 [J]. 中国翻译, 2019 (06): 80–87.

[7] 习近平. 携手共建人类卫生健康共同体——在全球健康峰会上的讲话 [EB/OL]. [2021.05.21]. https://www.fmprc.gov.cn/web/ziliao_674904/zyjh_674906/t1877663.shtml.

[8] Xi, J. (2021, May 21). *Working together to build a global community of health for all.* Ministry of Foreign Affairs of the People's Republic of China. Retrieved November 15, 2021, from https://www.fmprc.gov.cn/mfa_eng/wjdt_665385/zyjh_665391/t1877666.shtml.

[9] 习近平. 让多边主义的火炬照亮人类前行之路——在世界经济论坛"达沃斯议程"对话会上的特别致辞 [EB/OL]. [2021-01-25]. https://www.fmprc.gov.cn/web/zyxw/t1848322.shtml.

[10] Xi, J. (2021, January 25). *Let the torch of multilateralism light up Humanity's Way Forward.* Ministry of Foreign Affairs of the People's Republic of China. Retrieved November 15, 2021, from https://www.fmprc.gov.cn/mfa_eng/wjdt_665385/zyjh_665391/t1848323.shtml.

[11] 习近平. 习近平在第七十五届联合国大会一般性辩论上的讲话 [EB/OL]. [2020-09-22]. https://www.fmprc.gov.cn/web/zyxw/t1817092.shtml.

[12] Xi, J. (2020, September 22). *Statement by H. E. Xi Jinping president of the People's Republic of China at the general debate of the 75th session of the United Nations General Assembly.* Ministry of Foreign Affairs of the People's Republic of China. Retrieved November 15, 2021, from https://www.fmprc.gov.cn/mfa_eng/wjdt_665385/zyjh_665391/t1817098.shtml.